# CHILDREN AND YOUTH
## Social Problems and Social Policy

# CHILDREN AND YOUTH
Social Problems and Social Policy

# CHILDREN'S BUREAU STUDIES

Introduction by

William M. Schmidt

ARNO PRESS
A New York Times Company
New York — 1974

Reprint Edition 1974 by Arno Press Inc.

Infant Mortality and Habit Clinics For Child Guidance were reprinted from copies in The University of Illinois Library

CHILDREN AND YOUTH
Social Problems and Social Policy
ISBN for complete set: 0-405-05940-X
See last pages of this volume for titles.

Manufactured in the United States of America

**Library of Congress Cataloging in Publication Data**

Main entry under title:

Children's Bureau studies.

(Children and youth: social problems and social policy)

Reprint of Infant mortality, by E. Duke, first published in 1915; of Maternal mortality from all conditions connected with childbirth in the United States and certain other countries, by G. L. Meigs, first published in 1917; of The nutrition and care of children in a mountain county of Kentucky, by L. Roberts, first published in 1922; of Maternal deaths; a brief report of a study made in 15 states, issued by the United States Children's Bureau, first published in 1933; and of Habit clinics for child guidance, by D. A. Thom, first published in 1939.

1. Infants (Newborn)--Mortality--Statistics. 2. United States--Statistics, Medical. 3. Mothers--Mortality--Statistics. I. United States. Children's Bureau. II. Title. III. Series. [DNLM: W1 UN6181 WS100 U575]

RJ59.C54 1974 618.9'2 74-1676
ISBN 0-405-05955-8

## CONTENTS

## Introduction

The Children's Bureau was established by an Act of Congress in 1912. It was charged to "investigate and report . . . upon all matters pertaining to the welfare of children and child life among all classes of our people . . ." First on the list of specific subjects which follow the general mandate in the Act of 1912, and which serve to make its intent plain, is the problem of the excessively high infant mortality rate. Less than five months after actual operations of the Children's Bureau began, field work was started on a series of studies of factors related to deaths of infants in their first year of life.

Infant mortality rates were not then available for the United States as a whole. Accurate registration of births is needed in order to calculate infant death rates, and only a few states and cities had relatively complete registration of births in 1912. Indeed, "the birth rate" was another in the list of subjects the Children's Bureau was charged to study. The Bureau joined with governmental and non-governmental organizations — notably the General Federation of Women's Clubs — to campaign for complete birth registration. It required twenty years before all states had attained sufficiently complete birth registration for admission to the national birth registration area.

However, in 1912 there was an immediate need for data on social, economic, and health factors affecting the chance of survival of infants, as a basis for action. Six cities which already had fairly complete birth registration were selected for study which was planned to be illustrative of the national problem. The first of these was Johnstown, Pennsylvania. The report of the Johnstown study is the first document of this volume.

In contrast to studies based solely upon the deaths of infants, the Johnstown study takes as its point of departure *all births* occurring within the city during an entire year. Each newborn baby was followed to determine whether it survived its first year of life, or, if not, to ascertain the factors related to its death from examination of the death certificate, and especially from detailed inquiry into the environmental and social circumstances of the infant and his family.

No other study in the United States until that time had so thoroughly and fully established the correlation of income level, housing, physical environment, and nutrition with the risk of death in infancy.

Important as these factors were found to be, still another claimed close attention: the prenatal care of the mother, and the qualifications of the attendant at birth. It was found that the protection of the lives and health of mothers during pregnancy, labor and delivery, and the post-partum period were so closely bound up with the reduction of the high infant mortality rate that the two could not be separated. Studies of maternity care, and of maternal mortality were needed.

"Maternal Mortality from all Conditions Connected with Childbirth", the second document of this volume, is a statistical study, drawing together data from states and cities insofar as it was then available. It shows the trend — not a very encouraging one — in the risk of death from conditions associated with pregnancy and childbirth from 1890 to 1913. It offers comparisons of rates in rural and urban areas, and of states and cities with each other and with foreign countries. Crude as the basic data were, it was shown that the rate for the reporting area of the United States was "considerably higher" than for any foreign country in the group studied: England, Scotland, a number of European countries, New Zealand, and Japan. The next step was to secure exact information about the circumstances of each maternal death — its causes and preventability.

This was done, and reported in "Maternal Mortality in Fifteen States" (1934) Document #3 in this volume. The "Fifteen State Study" (as it came to be referred to) had decisive influence on practices in maternity care, and led to the dramatic, progressive drop in maternal mortality which began just a few years later.

Many of the procedures adopted for the Fifteen State Study became standard in subsequent state studies. For example, certificates of death were matched with corresponding birth certificates; visits by physicians were made to interview the attending physician in the case, or others who signed the death certificate, as attendant at birth. Clinical case records were also carefully reviewed for additional information.

The wealth of detailed information thus obtained established the relative frequency of complications causing death, and provided clinical data on which an advisory committee of obstetric specialists based their recommendations to the medical profession and to the general public. One recommendation, to the profession, was: "Medical societies and departments of health should investigate each maternal death within a few weeks of the death." This recommendation has been widely carried out, and, in one state after another, has contributed to better maternity care and reduced maternal mortality, as well as reduced risks for the fetus and the newborn infant.

To the general public, one of the recommendations was that "There should be widespread education of the general public as to the following: . . . That the community has a definite responsibility to provide adequate medical and nursing facilities for the care of women during pregnancy, labor and the post-partum period." Despite remarkable improvement in the quality of maternity care, this recommendation still awaits its total fulfillment. Too many women still do not secure early and adequate prenatal care, and when adverse factors create a situation of high risk for the maternity patient, not all patients are provided with equal access to the specialized facilities and staff needed for intensive care of complex problems. Such expert care is not yet readily available in all areas, and to patients of all social classes.

In these and other studies some attention had been given to questions of nutrition, but by 1922 it was decided that since malnutrition was one of the "diseases of children" in the list of problems assigned to the Children's Bureau, a major survey study focussed directly on the nutrition of children should be undertaken. A rural county in Kentucky was the site chosen, and *every home* within the study area in which there was a child aged 2 to 11 years, was visited. Accurate data was secured on foods consumed, living conditions, and hygienic practices. Medical examinations of the children completed this first nutrition survey on a population sample by the Children's Bureau. The report, the fourth of this volume, presents a picture of poverty, isolation, a meagre life in many respects, and evidence of inadequate diets and poor nutritional status of the children. The findings lead to proposals for improving the situation. But improvement came slowly, malnutrition has not been eliminated, and its continued existence is not because of lack of knowledge, but because public policy does not provide means for the problem to be squarely met, and fully dealt with.

The last of the reports of this volume, "Habit Clinics for Child Guidance" (1939) is a revision and enlargement of a publication of 1923. It is a recognition of the importance of the preschool years to child development. A number of concepts are developed which have become generally accepted, although far from fully implemented. Thus, the family unit is shown to be an essential concern in the care and treatment of young children. Visits to the family at home are suggested, and the role of the public health nurse in the clinic program is delineated. Social work in the assessment of children's problems, and in providing services to families is given a prominent role. The report is based chiefly on experience gained in a specialized clinic, but a proposal is made that "mental health" services could appropriately be placed in general health clinics.

These five reports show how the Children's Bureau carried out its task to "investigate and report". It could do no more at that time because, during the first ten years of the Bureau's existence there was no national program to give material help to states and localities to develop services for mothers and children. Studies, recommendations, advice, consultation, were all good, but not enough. Material help too was needed. Its very first publication (1912) describing the Children's Bureau to the public concluded with the sentences "It will endeavor to secure pertinent facts and to present them clearly for use and popular distribution. Its effectiveness must depend upon the use made of these facts by the people of the United States".

Such reports as these did indeed inform a concerned public, and laid the groundwork for support for the first Maternity and Infancy Act (Sheppard-Towner) which provided grants-in-aid to states to develop health services for mothers and infants. Despite attacks on the bill from some members of Congress, elements of the medical profession, and other conservative groups, it was enacted in 1921. It remained in effect, enabling states to develop their programs, until 1929 when it lapsed during a period of setbacks for social programs. Six years later, however, in a period of renewed social progress, even more extensive provisions for maternal and child health and welfare came into being as Title V of the Social Security Act (1935).

Under the leadership of Julia Lathrop, Grace Abbott, Katharine Lenroot and Martha Eliot the Children's Bureau was the federal agency which, more than any other, was concerned with promoting the health and welfare of children and young persons. These reports are their work as well as the work of men and women who came to be associated with them in the Children's Bureau in the first fifty-five years of its history.

William M. Schmidt, M.D.
April 22, 1974
Brookline, Massachusetts

U. S. DEPARTMENT OF LABOR
CHILDREN'S BUREAU
JULIA C. LATHROP, Chief

# INFANT MORTALITY

## RESULTS OF A FIELD STUDY IN JOHNSTOWN, PA., BASED ON BIRTHS IN ONE CALENDAR YEAR

BY

EMMA DUKE

INFANT MORTALITY SERIES No. 3
Bureau Publication No. 9

WASHINGTON
GOVERNMENT PRINTING OFFICE
1915

# CONTENTS.



## GENERAL TABLES.

## APPENDIXES.



## ILLUSTRATIONS.

# LETTER OF TRANSMITTAL.

U. S. DEPARTMENT OF LABOR,
CHILDREN'S BUREAU,
*Washington, August 24, 1914.*

SIR: I transmit herewith a statement of the first study in the field inquiry contemplated by the Children's Bureau into the subject of infant mortality in the United States. This study was made in Johnstown, Pa., during the first year of the bureau's existence, and is submitted as the first item in a proposed series of studies into infant mortality to be made in a number of typical communities throughout the country.

The city of Johnstown was selected because of its interest as a type of town in which there are no large factories employing women and because its size and its good birth registration permitted a study by the staff which the bureau could at first assign to this work.

The subject of infant mortality was chosen, first, because of its obvious importance as recognized by the fact that it is the first subject mentioned in the law creating the bureau; second, because of its fundamental value to further work of the bureau; and third, because it was practicable to make a single study, complete in itself, which would yet form part of an integral whole as it became possible to extend the field inquiry.

The restricted and tentative character of this first study is recognized. Its results will be constantly compared and collated with those of following similar studies in other communities. Doubtless the method of the general field inquiry may be modified from time to time, but the essential basal material of the schedules will be comparable throughout.

Infant mortality is a subject of profound social importance. The modern view has ceased to be fatalistic; infant mortality is now regarded as a preventable waste, injurious to survivors as well as destructive to infants, and cruelly increasing the burden of rearing a family. Sir Arthur Newsholme, the great English authority, has said, "Infant mortality is the most sensitive index we possess of social welfare and of sanitary administration, especially under urban conditions." Nationally, the United States has as yet no means of measuring the extent and significance of its infant mortality. If it were practicable, it would be illuminating to visit each one of the

2,500,000 children who, it is estimated, are born in this country yearly, and to take note of the varying social and economic conditions under which some 300,000 of them die and the others survive. As this is manifestly impossible, the nearest approach is to consider certain communities typical of the whole, and it is believed that in the course of a few years' study such data can be presented as will give the United States a fairly adequate measure of the conditions under which American-born infants survive or perish, and of the possibilities of modifying those conditions by local action.

Brilliant work for infant welfare has been done in many localities, notably by the public-health authorities and volunteer organizations of the larger cities, and incidental thereto much information regarding infant mortality has been gathered; but in the greater part of the country, especially in the smaller cities and rural communities, it is as yet hardly recognized that the problems which confront the crowded quarters of the great cities may also exist in less congested areas.

In accordance with the plans for a general inquiry into infant mortality, Mr. Ethelbert Stewart, the first statistical expert of the Children's Bureau, directed the preparation of the schedule and the field work at Johnstown.

This study considers all the babies born in Johnstown within a single calendar year. Since the work was begun in January, 1913, it was necessary to select the year 1911 as the latest in which all babies born could have attained a full year of life.

Mr. Stewart preceded the agents by a visit to Johnstown in which he explained the purposes of the inquiry, and the courtesy with which the agents were received by the general public—the press, the clergy, civic and volunteer organizations, and especially by the mothers themselves—was a valuable factor in making the inquiry successful.

Above all, the bureau wishes to express its obligation to the mothers of Johnstown, without whose generous understanding and help the inquiry could not have been conducted. Their good will is evidenced by the fact that, out of 1,553 mothers visited, only two refused information. The readiness with which the information was given undoubtedly depended upon the appeal to the mothers to cooperate with the Government in the effort to learn how to save babies' lives and to the fact that the agents could show that the information given was not to be used in any personal way.

The schedules were taken by Miss Emma Duke, Miss Sophia Vogt, and Miss Emily Miladofsky, special agents of the bureau, while the preliminary work of transferring to the schedules the information contained on the State records of birth was done by Mr. A. V. Parsons, special agent of the bureau, who also took the photographs reproduced.

Just as the work of filling out the schedules was being completed in Johnstown, Mr. Stewart was transferred to the Bureau of Labor Statistics, and his loss, together with other bureau exigencies, delayed the completion of the report. Miss Emma Duke has written the text and she has had the assistance of Miss Sophia Vogt and Miss Ella A. Merritt in making the tabulations. Mr. Lewis Meriam, Assistant Chief of the Children's Bureau, was interested in the inquiry from the start, and on Mr. Stewart's transfer was placed in charge of the statistics. The bureau wishes to acknowledge its indebtedness to all those who have aided in the preparation of this study by preliminary advice and by criticism of the schedule or manuscript.

The method of the inquiry is in one respect unique, so far as we are aware. Instead of taking as its point of departure the death records of children who have not survived their first year, the birth records are first secured for all children born within a certain calendar year, and each child is then traced through the first 12 months of life, or as much of that period as he survives, in order to obtain information as to the conditions which surround all the children of the town born during the given year. It is evident that this inquiry can be carried on effectively only in communities which have birth registration, and its extension to include typical units throughout the country must depend largely upon the further extension of birth registration.

The law creating the bureau provided for no medical officer upon the staff, and the inquiry was necessarily restricted to a consideration of family, social, industrial, and civic factors. The original material of the schedule was secured through personal interviews between individual mothers and the women agents. As the text shows, certain facts regarding the civic surroundings of the families were secured in addition to the interviews, but the chief value of the inquiry lies in the information afforded by the mothers. It is plain, however, that a study thus limited must omit certain important considerations. It is not fair nor practicable to enter a home and ask questions regarding conditions which, if they exist, are considered personally humiliating. Hence it was necessary to omit questions bearing on matters of personal character or behavior, and therefore to omit all consideration of two recognized factors in infant mortality—alcoholism and venereal disease. It is anticipated that the bureau will be in a position later to consider these and other factors, notably those connected with the employment of mothers and with industrial diseases, by methods independent of family inquiry.

The emphasis of the inquiry, as shown throughout the text, was upon certain of the more obvious economic, social, and civic factors which have surrounded the lives of the children of Johnstown born within the given year. Civic action can remedy defective sewerage and scavenger systems and dirty unpaved streets which are instrumental in creating conditions that endanger the lives of infants. The extension of city water to all houses; improved methods for sewage disposal, garbage collections, and general scavenging; the paving of streets and inhabited alleys; the widening of alleys; the improved grading of streets and alleys; the relief of house and lot congestion; the abolition of wells and yard privies; sewer connection for all houses; the abatement of the smoke nuisance—all of these are needed improvements for the infant health and the general health of Johnstown.

But the public's responsibility does not end merely in remedying such conditions as those just noted. There is a growing tendency on the part of municipalities to accept responsibility for furnishing information and instruction to its citizens. Some cities have reduced their infant mortality rate by having expectant mothers instructed in prenatal care; others by sending instructive visiting nurses, immediately after the birth of a child, into homes that need them. Other means which have been found effective in reducing excessive infant mortality rates are baby welfare stations, consultation stations for expectant and nursing mothers, and the distribution of sound literature on prenatal care, the care and feeding of infants, the care of milk, and other hygienic matters.

The importance of a pure milk supply in reducing infant mortality has been repeatedly demonstrated. The direct effects of impure milk on the health of Johnstown babies could not be ascertained in this investigation, but the careless handling of milk was obvious, and at the request of the Johnstown Board of Health and the local health officer the Children's Bureau secured the cooperation of the Bureau of Animal Industry of the Department of Agriculture in making a comprehensive investigation of the milk supply in Johnstown. The findings of the experts, L. B. Cook, C. E. Clement, and B. J. Davis, printed in full on pages 89 to 93 of this report (Appendix III), justify the citizens' campaign for clean milk now under way in Johnstown.

In many directions public spirit is active in Johnstown. The city is awakening to its needs and to its responsibilities as well. It supports a strong civic club and other associations which are studying ways and means to proceed. Its newspapers are virile and progressive and plans are being made to remedy insanitary conditions. Through private effort a visiting nurse has been secured to instruct mothers in the care of their homes and their children.

The Johnstown report shows a coincidence of underpaid fathers, overworked and ignorant mothers, and those hazards to the life of the offspring which individual parents can not avoid or control because they must be remedied by community action. All this points toward the imperative need of ascertaining a standard of life for the American family, a standard which must rest upon such betterment of conditions of work and pay as will permit parents to safeguard infants within the household. Toward the slow working out of the essentials of such a standard it is hoped that the bureau's continued studies into infant mortality may contribute.

While the bureau has not yet determined upon all the units of the inquiry, it is the purpose at present to study localities outside those great urban areas whose spectacular needs have secured costly and effective work by municipal and volunteer organizations. Such work should be equally valuable and, on the whole, equally applicable in smaller towns and even in rural communities. That similar problems and needs exist also in our less congested areas is proved by the 1913 report of the New York State Health Commission, which has made plain the unfavorable health showing of the State as a whole as compared with that of the city of New York. This report and the studies upon which it is based have furnished the impetus for new legislation which extends throughout the State certain measures for improving the health of children which have already proved effective in the largest city of the State. In various parts of the world the history of intelligent efforts to surround babies with healthful conditions shows a progressively lessening infant mortality rate and leads to the belief that the problems of infant mortality can be solved.

Sir Arthur Newsholme, who has already been quoted above, says in the Forty-Second Annual Report of the Local Government Board (1912–13), "It is obvious that the complex problems involved (excessive infant and child mortality) can not be effectively stated in a single report, and that investigation is called for in nearly every center of excessive mortality."

It is therefore desired to pursue this inquiry in various typical communities throughout the country so that the facts may secure popular attention. Clearly the law creating the Children's Bureau, framed by experts in child welfare, embodies the conviction that if the Government can "investigate and report" upon infant mortality, the conscience and power of local communities can be depended upon for necessary action.

Respectfully submitted.

JULIA C. LATHROP, *Chief.*

Hon. WILLIAM B. WILSON,
*Secretary of Labor.*

# INFANT MORTALITY: JOHNSTOWN, PA.

## INTRODUCTION.

The term infant mortality, used technically, applies to deaths of babies under 1 year of age. An infant mortality rate is a statement of the number of deaths of such infants in a given year per 1,000 births in the same year. Some countries include stillbirths in making the computations, but this method is not generally followed in this country nor has it been followed in this report.

Ordinary procedure is to compare the live births in a single calendar year with the deaths of babies under 12 months of age occurring in that same year, even though those who died may not have been born within the calendar year of their death. The infant mortality rates in this report, however, have not been computed on the usual basis, but for the purpose of securing greater accuracy in measuring the incidence of death this bureau has considered, in making the computation, only so many of the babies born in the year 1911 as could be located by its agents, and has compared with this number the number of deaths within this group of babies who died within one year of birth, even though some of these deaths may have occurred during the calendar year 1912.[1]

Infant mortality can be accurately measured in no other way than by means of a system of completely registering all births as well as all deaths. In 1911 the United States Bureau of the Census regarded the registration of deaths as being "fairly complete (at least 90 per cent of the total)" in 23 States, but the same degree of completeness in the registration of births was found only in the New England States, Pennsylvania, and Michigan, and in New York City and Washington, D. C. An exact infant mortality rate for the United States as a whole can not be computed owing to this generally incomplete registration. In the 1911 census report on mortality statistics,[2] however, the infant mortality rate is estimated at 124 per 1,000 live births. How this estimated rate compared with the computed rates for other countries is shown in the following summary:

---

[1] For more detailed description of method see Appendix II, pp. 86 to 88.

[2] Bulletin 112, Bureau of the Census, p. 23.

DEATHS OF CHILDREN UNDER 1 YEAR OF AGE PER 1,000 LIVE BIRTHS, BY QUINQUENNIAL PERIODS FROM 1901 TO 1910, AND ALSO FOR THE SINGLE CALENDAR YEARS 1909 AND 1910.[1]

| COUNTRY. | 1901 to 1905 | 1906 to 1910 | 1909 | 1910 |
|---|---|---|---|---|
| Chile | 306 | 315 | 315 | 313 |
| Russia (European) | (2) | ...... | ...... | ...... |
| Austria | 215 | ...... | ...... | ...... |
| Hungary | 212 | 204 | 212 | 194 |
| Prussia | 190 | 168 | 164 | 157 |
| Jamaica | 174 | 191 | 174 | 188 |
| Spain | 173 | ...... | ...... | ...... |
| Ceylon | 171 | 189 | 202 | 176 |
| Italy | 168 | ...... | 155 | ...... |
| Japan | 154 | ...... | 166 | ...... |
| Servia | 149 | ...... | ...... | ...... |
| Belgium | 148 | ...... | 137 | ...... |
| Bulgaria | 148 | ...... | ...... | ...... |
| France | 139 | ...... | 120 | ...... |
| England and Wales | 138 | 117 | 109 | 105 |
| The Netherlands | 136 | 114 | 99 | 108 |
| Switzerland | 134 | ...... | 115 | ...... |
| Finland | 131 | 117 | 111 | 118 |
| Scotland | 120 | ...... | 108 | ...... |
| Denmark | 119 | ...... | 98 | ...... |
| Province of Ontario | 114 | 127 | 131 | 123 |
| Ireland | 98 | 94 | 92 | 95 |
| Australian Commonwealth | 97 | 78 | 72 | 75 |
| Sweden | 91 | ...... | 72 | ...... |
| Norway | 81 | ...... | 72 | ...... |
| New Zealand | 75 | 70 | 62 | 68 |

1 From the Seventy-third Annual Report of the Registrar General of Births, Deaths, and Marriages in England and Wales (1910). London, 1912.
2 Available only for the period from 1896 to 1900, when it was 261.

When it had been decided by the Children's Bureau to make infant mortality the subject of its first field study and to include all babies born in a given calendar year, regardless of whether they lived or died during their first year, advice and cooperation were enlisted of mothers, physicians, nurses, and others experienced in the care of children, and also of trained investigators and statisticians, in the preparation of a schedule which was submitted to them for criticism.

With its limited force and funds it was not possible for the Children's Bureau to extend its inquiries throughout the entire United States. It was therefore decided to make intensive studies of babies born in a single calendar year in each of a number of typical areas throughout the country that offered contrasts in climate and in economic and social conditions, the results to be eventually combined and correlated. It was necessary to restrict the choice of the first area to a place of such size as could be covered thoroughly within a reasonable time by the few agents available for the work.

Johnstown, Pa., was the first place selected. It is in a State where birth registration prevails, and hence a record of practically all babies could be secured; it is of such size that the work could be done by a small force within a reasonable period, and it seemed to present conditions that could with interest be contrasted with conditions typical of other communities. Moreover, the State commissioner of health and the State registrar of vital statistics were both working zealously to enforce birth-registration laws; both were actively interested in reducing infant mortality, and they welcomed a study of the subject in their State. In Johnstown the mayor, the president of the board of health, the health officer, and other local officials all showed the same spirit of hearty cooperation and interest.

Inasmuch as the study was confined to babies born in a single calendar year and work was begun in January, 1913, the latest year in which the babies could have been born and still have attained at least one full year of life was 1911.

Work was begun on January 15, 1913, with the transcription from the original records at Harrisburg of the names and other essential facts entered on the birth certificates of babies born in 1911, and, if the baby had died during its first year of life, items on the death certificate were also copied.

In the meantime the people of Johnstown through the press, and through the clergy in the foreign sections, had been informed of the purpose and plan of the investigation. Without the friendly spirit thus aroused and the interest manifested by the Civic Club and other organizations the work could not have been brought to a successful issue. The investigation was absolutely democratic; every mother of a baby born in 1911, rich or poor, native or foreign, was sought, and it is interesting to note refusals were met with in but two cases.

The original plan was to limit the investigation to those babies born in the calendar year selected whose births had been registered, the purpose being to secure facts concerning a definite group and not to measure the completeness of birth registration. Shortly after beginning the work, however, agents of this bureau were told that the Servian women in Johnstown seldom had either a midwife or a physician at childbirth; that they called in a neighbor or depended upon their husbands for help at such times, or that they managed alone for themselves, and that therefore their babies usually escaped registration. The omission of these babies meant the exclusion of a number of mothers in a group that was too important racially to be omitted from an investigation embracing all races and classes. Accordingly a list of babies christened in the Servian Church and born in the year 1911 was secured and an attempt made to locate them. In addition an agent called at each house in the principal Servian quarter to inquire concerning births in 1911. A number of unregistered babies of Servian mothers were thus found and included in the investigation.

The agents were sometimes approached by mothers of babies born in 1911 who resented being omitted from the investigation simply for the reason that their babies' births had not been registered. The agents were therefore instructed to interview mothers thus accidentally encountered and to include their babies in the investigation. But no additional baptismal records were copied nor was a house-to-house canvass made of the city; in fact, no further means were resorted to to locate unregistered babies for the purpose of including them in the investigation.

There were 1,763 certificates copied at Harrisburg, and 1,383 of the babies named in them were reached by the agents. In addition, 168 babies for whom there were no birth certificates, but who were located in the ways just noted, were included, making a total of 1,551 completed schedules secured.

Of the 380 not included in the investigation there were 149 who could not be located at all; 220 others had moved out of reach—that is, into another city or State; 6 of the mothers had died; 3 could not be found at home after several calls, and 2 refused to be interviewed.

From the following summary of data recorded on the certificates of the 380 unlocated babies just referred to it appears that the infant mortality rate (134.3) among them is almost the same as that (134) shown in Table 1 for babies included in the investigation. In reality, however, it is perhaps a little higher, as some of these babies no doubt died outside of Johnstown and their deaths were recorded elsewhere.

| NATIONALITY OF MOTHER. | Total births. | Live births. | Still-births. | SEX OF BABY. | | ATTENDANT AT BIRTH. | | | Certificate showing deaths during first year. |
|---|---|---|---|---|---|---|---|---|---|
| | | | | Male. | Female. | Physician. | Midwife. | Unknown. | |
| Total | 380 | 350 | 30 | 227 | 153 | 158 | 189 | 33 | 47 |
| Native | 134 | 118 | 16 | 76 | 58 | 122 | 5 | 7 | 12 |
| Foreign | 246 | 232 | 14 | 151 | 95 | 36 | 184 | 26 | 35 |
| Slovak, Polish, etc | 43 | 41 | 2 | 27 | 16 | 4 | 37 | 2 | 3 |
| Croatian and Servian | 13 | 11 | 2 | 10 | 3 | | 7 | 6 | 5 |
| Magyar | 1 | 1 | | 1 | | | 1 | | |
| German | 8 | 8 | | 6 | 2 | 2 | 5 | 1 | 2 |
| Italian | 41 | 39 | 2 | 26 | 15 | 3 | 36 | 2 | 4 |
| Syrian and Greek | 7 | 6 | 1 | 3 | 4 | 3 | 4 | | 1 |
| British | 7 | 7 | | 3 | 4 | 5 | 2 | | |
| Austrian (not otherwise specified) | 123 | 116 | 7 | 73 | 50 | 19 | 89 | 15 | 20 |
| Not reported | 3 | 3 | | 2 | 1 | | 3 | | |

## RELATION OF INFANT MORTALITY TO ENVIRONMENT.

### NEIGHBORHOOD INCIDENCE.

The rate of infant mortality is regarded as a most reliable test of the sanitary condition of a district. (Sir Arthur Newsholme, Elements of Vital Statistics, p. 120. London, 1899.)

Johnstown is a hilly, somewhat Y-shaped area of about 5 square miles which spreads itself out into long, narrow, irregularly shaped strips, detached by rivers and runs and steep hills. In some places it is not over a quarter of a mile wide, but its extreme length is about 4 miles. The city is composed of 21 wards and is an aggregation of what were formerly separate unrelated boroughs or towns. The names of these different sections, together with the numerical designations of the wards included in or comprising them, are shown in the following table. This table gives for each section not only the total population according to the Federal census of 1910, but also the number of live-born babies included in the investigation and the number and proportion of deaths among such babies during their first year.

TABLE 1.—DISTRIBUTION OF POPULATION, LIVE BIRTHS, AND DEATHS DURING FIRST YEAR, AND INFANT MORTALITY RATE ACCORDING TO SECTION OF JOHNSTOWN, FOR ALL CHILDREN INCLUDED IN THIS INVESTIGATION.

| SECTION OF CITY AND WARD. | Population, 1910.[1] | Total live-born babies. | Deaths during first year of babies born in 1911. | Infant mortality rate. |
|---|---|---|---|---|
| The whole city | 55,482 | 1,463 | 196 | 134.0 |
| Down-town section (wards 1, 2, 3, 4) | 5,944 | 80 | 4 | 50.0 |
| Kernville (wards 5, 6) | 6,070 | 104 | 6 | 57.7 |
| Hornerstown (ward 7) | 4,476 | 109 | 17 | 156.0 |
| Roxbury (ward 8) | 2,862 | 85 | 10 | 117.6 |
| Conemaugh Borough (wards 9, 10) | 5,282 | 136 | 16 | 117.6 |
| Woodvale (ward 11) | 3,945 | 107 | 29 | 271.0 |
| Prospect (ward 12) | 1,893 | 55 | 11 | 200.0 |
| Peelorville (ward 13) | 1,443 | 18 | 1 | (2) |
| Minersville (ward 14) | 2,403 | 72 | 9 | 125.0 |
| Cambria City (wards 15, 16) | 8,706 | 310 | 55 | 177.4 |
| Moxham (ward 17) | 5,735 | 157 | 14 | 89.2 |
| Morrellville (wards 18, 19, 20) | 5,757 | 194 | 16 | 82.5 |
| Coopersdale (ward 21) | 966 | 36 | 8 | (2) |

[1] Federal census of 1910.
[2] Total live births less than 50; base therefore considered too small to use in computing an infant mortality rate.

To learn where the babies die is perhaps the first step in solving the infant mortality problem. The modern health officer recognizes this and generally has in his office a wall map upon which are indicated sections, wards, city blocks, and sometimes even houses. As infant deaths are reported, pins are stuck in the map in the proper places, a density of pins on any part of the map indicating, of course, where deaths are most numerous, although the percentage of infant deaths may not be the highest. The next table shows the comparative frequency of infant deaths in each of the several sections of Johnstown as well as the rate of infant mortality, total population, proportion of foreign population, proportion of foreign mothers, and total births in the year 1911 in each.

TABLE 2.—RELATIVE RANK OF SECTIONS OF JOHNSTOWN, ACCORDING TO INFANT MORTALITY RATE FOR ALL CHILDERN INCLUDED IN THIS INVESTIGATION, TOTAL POPULATION, TOTAL FOREIGN BORN, PERCENTAGE OF FOREIGN BORN IN TOTAL POPULATION, NUMBER OF BABIES BORN ALIVE IN 1911, PROPORTION OF FOREIGN-BORN MOTHERS, AND NUMBER OF INFANT DEATHS.

| Section of city and ward. | Rank of the several sections of the city according to— | | | | | | |
|---|---|---|---|---|---|---|---|
| | Infant mortality rate. | Total population.[1] | Total foreign-born population.[1] | Per cent of foreign-born population.[1] | Babies included in investigation. | | |
| | | | | | Number live born. | Proportion of foreign mothers. | Number of infant deaths. |
| Woodvale (ward 11) | 1 | 8 | 2 | 1 | 6 | 2 | 2 |
| Prospect (ward 12) | 2 | 11 | 8 | 5 | 11 | 5 | 7 |
| Cambria City (wards 15, 16) | 3 | 1 | 1 | 2 | 1 | 1 | 1 |
| Hornerstown (ward 7) | 4 | 7 | 10 | 11 | 5 | 11 | 3 |
| Minersville (ward 14) | 5 | 10 | 4 | 3 | 10 | 3 | 9 |
| Conemaugh borough (wards 9, 10) | 6 | 6 | 3 | 4 | 4 | 4 | 4 |
| Roxbury (ward 8) | 7 | 9 | 12 | 13 | 8 | 12 | 8 |
| Moxham (ward 17) | 8 | 5 | 6 | 8 | 3 | 7 | 6 |
| Morrellville (wards 18, 19, 20) | 9 | 4 | 7 | 9 | 2 | 6 | 5 |
| Kernville (wards 5, 6) | 10 | 2 | 9 | 12 | 7 | 13 | 11 |
| Down town (wards 1, 2, 3, 4) | 11 | 3 | 5 | 7 | 9 | 9 | 12 |
| Peelorville (ward 13) | (2) | 12 | 11 | 6 | 13 | 10 | 13 |
| Coopersdale (ward 21) | (2) | 13 | 13 | 10 | 12 | 8 | 10 |

[1] According to Federal census of 1910.
[2] Total live births less than 50; base therefore considered too small to use in computing an infant mortality rate.

The highest infant mortality rate, 271, is found in the eleventh ward, known as Woodvale, although this is neither the most populous ward nor the one having the largest number of births. The infant mortality rate here, however, is double the rate for the city as a whole and more than five times as great as it is for the most favorable ward.

This is where the poorest, most lowly persons of the community live—families of men employed to do the unskilled work in the steel mills and the mines. They are for the most part foreigners, 78 per cent of the mothers interviewed in this ward being foreign born.

Through Woodvale runs the main line of the Pennsylvania Railroad. To the north of the tracks rises a steep hill, toward the top of which is Woodvale Avenue, the principal street north of the railroad. (See plate A.) Sewer connection is possible for the houses along this avenue, as a sewer main has recently been installed, but the people have not in all cases gone to the expense of having the connection made, and in other cases where they have done so sometimes only the sinks are connected with the sewer and the yard privy is retained.

On the streets above Woodvale Avenue dwellings are more scattered and the appearance is more rural. A few of the families still have to depend upon more or less distant springs for their water, although city water is quite generally available throughout Woodvale.

The streets near the bottom of the hill, as Plum Street, for example, are so much below the level of the sewer mains that they cannot be properly drained into the sewer. Private drain pipes from houses are buried a few feet below the surface and protrude from the sides of the hills, dripping with house drainage which flows slowly into ditches and forms slimy pools. (See Plates B and C.)

None of the streets on the north side of the railroad track are paved; sidewalks and gutters are lacking. In cold weather the streets are icy and slippery and even dangerous on account of the grade. In warm weather they are frequently slippery and slimy with mud.

Maple Avenue is the principal street of that part of Woodvale lying to the south of the railroad tracks, and it is the only properly paved and graded street in Woodvale. The streets on this side of the tracks, however, are not in as bad a condition as those to the north, nor are the drainage and general sewerage conditions as offensive as north of the tracks, but many of the streets are nevertheless muddy and filthy. (See Plate D.)

Prospect ranks next to Woodvale in infant mortality, having a rate of 200. This section, lying along a steep hill and above one of the big plants of the steel company, has not a single properly graded, drained, and paved street. The sewers are of the open-ditch type, and the natural slope of the land toward the river is depended upon for carrying off the surface water that does not seep into the soil. The closets are generally in the yard and are either dry privies or they are situated over cesspools. Some of the people who live on the lower part of the slope have wells sunk directly in the course of the drainage from above. (See Plate E.)

Cambria City, which is composed of the two most populous wards of Johnstown, has the third highest infant mortality rate, 177.4. It has a large foreign element, as is evidenced by the fact that 90.6 per cent of the mothers interviewed were foreign born. It is situated along the river, between the hills of Minersville and Morrellville, and somewhat to the north of Prospect. The sewage from other residential sections and from the steel mills above them empties into the river at this point. In warm, dry seasons the river is low, flows slowly, and forms foul-smelling pools.

Sewer connection is possible for most of the houses in Cambria City, although all are not connected. Some, on the streets bordering the river, have private drain pipes that empty out into the stream. Others have their kitchen sinks connected with the sewer but still retain yard privies, which, of course, are not sewer connected.

There is considerable crowding of houses on lots, rear houses being commonly built on lots intended for but one house. Density of population and house congestion are greater here than elsewhere in the city.

The streets of Cambria City are somewhat better graded and more generally paved than those of Woodvale, but muddy streets and unpaved sidewalks nevertheless exist here. Broad Street, however, which is the business thoroughfare and runs through the center of the section, is the widest and best constructed street in Johnstown. Bradley Alley, on the other hand, running the length of Cambria City and parallel to Broad Street, is the most conspicuous example in the city of a narrow lane or alley used as a residence street. A number of small dwellings, generally housing more than one family, have their frontage on this alley, which is 19 feet 10 inches in width and without sidewalks. It is unpaved and in bad condition, generally being either muddy or dusty and littered with bottles, cans, and other trash. (See Plates F and G.)

Hornerstown has an infant mortality rate of 156, ranking fourth among the several sections of Johnstown in this respect. It has a fairly prosperous and somewhat suburban appearance, but its comparatively high infant mortality rate can perhaps be partly accounted for by the bad street conditions and the fact that refuse of all sorts is dumped into the shallow river at this point.

Minersville is a district where a high rate would be expected from prevailing conditions. The rate is 125, or less than the average for the city but more than double that for the most favorable sections. This ward is built on a hill and so located that the rising clouds of grit-laden smoke from the steel mills envelop it much of the time. Only one street in this section is well paved, and this is seldom clean. Houses on some of the streets near the top of the hill are not sewer connected; and streams of waste water trickle down the hill and give rise to unpleasant odors. (See Plates H and I.)

Conemaugh Borough, with an infant mortality rate of 117.6, ranks sixth in this respect among the sections into which Johnstown has been divided. It comprises wards 9 and 10 and begins at the edge of the downtown section and spreads upward over the hills to the southwest. Some of the houses on streets near the top of the hill are not sewer connected, and streams of water constantly trickle down the numerous alleys and streets that descend the hill. (See Plate J.) This section makes a very unfavorable first impression because of the open drainage and of the many dirty, badly paved streets. (See Plate K.) Unlike some of the other wards, it has a rather evenly distributed population and is without the vast uninhabited areas and acutely congested spots found in some other sections. On the whole there is little crowding on the lots and there are many good-sized yards. One-third of the population is foreign born. Of these the Italians are the most numerous. Despite certain ugly spots this section has not the unwholesome atmosphere that characterizes Woodvale and to a lesser extent Prospect, Cambria City, and Minersville.

The infant mortality rate of 117.6 per thousand in Roxbury is the same as that of Conemaugh Borough. For reasons not plainly apparent the rate here is higher than in Moxham, Morrellville, Kernville, or the down-town section, although it appears to be as favorably conditioned as these sections are from a social, economic, and sanitary standpoint. Here, as in all these sections, however, are many conditions not conducive to health. For example, parts of Franklin Street are in bad repair. The roadway is full of ruts and holes; the street, which is seldom sprinkled, is dusty in dry weather and muddy in wet weather, and in front of good houses along one section of this street runs an open ditch that receives house drainage.

Moxham has the eighth highest infant mortality rate, it being 89.2. Conditions here are generally rather favorable, although there is some complaint that at "high water" the sewage received by one of the runs in this section backs into some of the houses and then the sinks and water-closets overflow. Some of the homes here, near the city limits, are not supplied with city water but are still dependent upon wells and springs.

One of the three wards constituting Morrellville (ward 18) has a rural appearance; there is little house crowding on lots, big yards are common, and the streets are not paved. It is, however, marred by an offensive open-ditch sewer. Ward 19 of Morrellville has a more finished, less rural appearance. One of its objectionable features is that house drainage and the bloody waste of slaughterhouses are emptied into a shallow stream that flows through it. Ward 20 adjoins ward 19, and although it spreads out into a suburb it appears for the most part to be a comfortable and busy little village. Strayer's Run winds about here and receives sewage. The fact that it is without a guardrail in some places and that the railing is inadequate in others makes it a source of danger, and according to common report such accidents as children falling into the stream have occurred. The infant mortality rate for Morrellville is 82.5.

Kernville, a section with a considerable proportion of prosperous people, has a very favorable infant mortality rate, it being 57.7. Parts of this section, however, are on a hill stretching upward from Stony Creek, which is both unsightly and offensive in warm weather and when the water is low.

The down-town section, i. e., wards 1, 2, 3, and 4, where are to be found many of the best conditioned houses, the homes of many of the well-to-do people, has the lowest infant mortality rate in the city, it being but 50.

No infant mortality rate is presented in the tables for Coopersdale or for Peelorville. In the first-named section only 36 live-born infants were considered, and 8 of them died in their first year. But this high rate need not be considered as especially significant, as the base number is small for such a computation. Coopersdale, however, is a suburban-appearing community in which one would expect the infant mortality rate to be low.

Peelorville is that part of the thirteenth ward which adjoins Prospect. A number of company houses are located here in which sanitary conditions are fairly good. The ward seems to have good drainage and no sewage nuisances. It is a community of wage earners and not of prosperous homes. Only 18 babies are included in the report for this district, one of whom died. With such a small base the infant mortality rate is not significant. (See Plate L.)

### SANITARY CONDITIONS—SEWERAGE, PAVEMENTS, GARBAGE COLLECTIONS.

The general inadequacy of the sewerage system which has been indicated for the city as a whole is due in part to the fact that the city is largely an aggregation of sections, formerly independent of Johnstown itself, which have been annexed at different periods. Some of these boroughs had sewer systems more or less developed when they were taken into Johnstown; others had none. Not only the sewage of Johnstown but that of outlying boroughs pollutes the two shallow rivers, the Conemaugh and the Stony Creek, that flow through Johnstown. These are burdened with more waste than they can properly carry away, and the deposits which are left on the rocks in various sections of both rivers create nuisances that are the subject of much complaint, especially during the warm summer months. (See Plates M, N, O, and P.) At various times agitation has been started to improve the rivers which, as they flow through Johnstown, are, at the low-water stage, little better than swamps of reeking slime from the waste matter emptied into them from the hundreds of sewers along their banks. The pipes through which waste matter is emptied into the streams go only to the river edge, leaving their mouths uncovered and making the river beds at times pools of slowly flowing filth. These unsightly, malodorous conditions could be remedied if pipes were extended out into the middle of the streams, where the water is deeper.

With the exception of sprinkling a few wagon loads of lime along the banks of the streams each year, the city has done nothing to abate the nuisances arising from the use of these rivers as sewers or to restrain the coal and steel companies from allowing the drainage from mines and mills to enter the streams.

The engineer's records show that Johnstown had in 1911 a total of 41.1 miles of sewers and 36 sewer outlets, and 82 miles of streets, 52.7 miles being paved. The alleys in Johnstown are generally inhabited. They are narrow and without sidewalks. Their length is 52.88 miles and 47.35 miles are unpaved. The combined length of streets and alleys is 134.88 miles. A comparison of this combined length of streets and alleys with the 41.1 miles of sewers having 36 outlets shows the inadequacy of the sewer system.

Not only is there an absence of paving, but the roadways are in very bad condition. A protest by "A Citizen" in the Democrat of June 26, 1913, says that there are nine months in the year when it would be impossible for the proposed fire-department automobile engines to attend a fire in the seventh, eighth, eleventh, seventeenth, eighteenth, nineteenth, twentieth, and twenty-first wards owing to the condition of the streets.

The scavenger system is also very defective. Citizens are required to pay for the removal of their ashes, trash, and garbage. Garbage collections are not made by the municipality, but by private contractors, and any sort of receptacle, covered or uncovered, can or box, is pressed into service by householders. It is by no means uncommon to find streets and alleys littered with ashes, garbage, bottles, tin cans, beer cases, and small kegs. Dirty streets are by no means exceptional in Johnstown, even though the State of Pennsylvania has a law (act of Apr. 20, 1905) which provides for the punishment of any person who litters paved streets. It reads, in part, as follows (sec. 7 of Pamphlet Laws, 227):

> From and after the passage of this act, it shall be unlawful, and is hereby forbidden, for any person or persons to throw waste paper, sweepings, ashes, household waste, nails, or rubbish of any kind into any street in any city, borough, or township in this Commonwealth, or to interfere with, scatter, or disturb the contents of any receptacle or receptacles containing ashes, garbage, household waste, or rubbish which shall be placed upon any of said paved streets or sidewalks for the collection of the contents thereof.
>
> Any person or persons who shall violate any of the provisions of this act shall, upon conviction thereof before any magistrate, be sentenced to pay the cost of prosecution and to forfeit and pay a fine not exceeding $10 for each offense, and in default of the payment thereof shall be committed and imprisoned in the county jail of the proper county for a period not exceeding ten days.

In a report on infant mortality to the registrar general of Ontario, 1910, Dr. Helen MacMurchy says: "Improve the water supply, the sewerage system, and the system of disposing of refuse; introduce better pavements, such as asphalt, and at once there is a decline in infantile mortality." All these are sanitary features in need of great improvement in Johnstown, and unquestionably a lowered infant mortality rate would reward any efforts for their betterment.

## HOUSING.

In Johnstown the so-called "double" house predominates, usually frame. The double house is in reality two semidetached houses built upon a single lot. Rows of three or more houses of two, three, or four rooms each are common, and they are known locally as three-family, or six-family houses, as the case may be. Sometimes these are "rear houses," that is, they are built behind other houses that face the street, on the same lots and in fact are approached by way of a narrow alley running alongside the house that has its frontage directly on the street. For this type of house water-closets or privies are often in rows in the yard or court that is used in common by all families. (See Plates Q and R.) In some places they are too few in number to permit each family to have the exclusive use of one.

Johnstown has three or four comparatively high-grade apartment houses, and in several office buildings rooms are rented to families for housekeeping. These are generally taken by native families.

In one of these office buildings the two lower floors are used for business purposes and the two upper floors are given over entirely to tenement purposes. From 40 to 50 families live here, many of whom have but one room. To serve the 20 or 25 families on each floor there is one bath and toilet room for men and another for women. Adjoining the toilet rooms is a small room containing garbage cans and trash receptacles for the use of the tenants.

The sanitary conditions in some of the best tenements or apartments, however, are not up to the standards of other cities, and in those occupied by the poorer people conditions are much worse than are usually permitted to exist in cities having large tenement houses in great numbers, where a tenement-house problem is recognized as such and active efforts are made by the municipality to improve conditions.

An absolute measure of the importance of each single housing defect in a high mortality rate can not be secured from this study. But it is not without interest to note that in homes where water is piped into the house the infant mortality rate was 117.6 per thousand, as compared with a rate of 197.9 in homes where the water had to be carried in from outdoors. Or that in the homes of 496 live-born babies where bathtubs were found the infant mortality rate was 72.6, while it was more than double, or 164.8, where there were no bathtubs. Desirable as a bathtub and bodily cleanliness may be, this does not prove that the lives of the babies were saved by the presence of the tub or the assumed cleanliness of the persons having them. In a city of Johnstown's low housing standards, the tub is an index of a good home, a suitable house from a sanitary standpoint, a fairly comfortable income, and all the favorable conditions that go with such an income.

The same trend of a high infant mortality rate in connection with other housing defects is noted in the next table.

TABLE 3.—DISTRIBUTION OF LIVE BIRTHS AND OF DEATHS DURING FIRST YEAR, AND INFANT MORTALITY RATE, ACCORDING TO HOUSING CONDITIONS.

| HOUSING CONDITIONS. | Live births. | DEATHS DURING FIRST YEAR. | |
|---|---|---|---|
| | | Number. | Infant mortality rate. |
| Total | 1,463 | 196 | 134.0 |
| Dry homes | 808 | 99 | 122.5 |
| Moderately dry homes | 336 | 47 | 139.9 |
| Damp homes | 319 | 50 | 156.7 |
| Bath | 496 | 36 | 72.6 |
| No bath | 965 | 159 | 164.8 |
| Not reported | 2 | 1 | (1) |
| Water supply in house | 1,173 | 138 | 117.6 |
| Water supply outside | 288 | 57 | 197.9 |
| Not reported | 2 | 1 | (1) |
| City water available | 1,333 | 176 | 132.0 |
| City water not available | 128 | 19 | 148.4 |
| Not reported | 2 | 1 | (1) |
| Yard clean | 801 | 80 | 99.9 |
| Yard not clean | 632 | 107 | 169.3 |
| No yard | 28 | 8 | (1) |
| Not reported | 2 | 1 | (1) |
| Water-closet | 739 | 80 | 108.3 |
| Yard privy | 722 | 115 | 159.3 |
| Not reported | 2 | 1 | (1) |

1 Total live births less than 50; base therefore considered too small to use in computing an infant mortality rate.

The following summary may be of interest in indicating some relation between infant mortality and cleanliness or uncleanliness combined with dryness or dampness of homes:

TABLE 4.—DISTRIBUTION OF LIVE BIRTHS AND OF DEATHS DURING FIRST YEAR, AND INFANT MORTALITY RATE, ACCORDING TO CLEANLINESS AND DRYNESS OF HOME.

| TYPE OF HOME. | Live births. | DEATHS DURING FIRST YEAR. | |
|---|---|---|---|
| | | Number. | Infant mortality rate. |
| All types | 1,463 | 196 | 134.0 |
| Clean | 943 | 107 | 113.5 |
| Moderately clean | 354 | 58 | 163.8 |
| Dirty | 166 | 31 | 186.7 |
| Dry | 807 | 99 | 122.7 |
| Damp | 656 | 97 | 147.9 |
| Clean: | | | |
| Dry | 581 | 61 | 105.0 |
| Damp | 362 | 46 | 127.1 |
| Moderately clean: | | | |
| Dry | 158 | 27 | 170.9 |
| Damp | 196 | 31 | 158.2 |
| Dirty: | | | |
| Dry | 68 | 11 | 161.8 |
| Damp | 98 | 20 | 204.1 |

Dirt is doubtless unhealthful, but the amount of ill health or the number of infant deaths caused by a home being dirty can hardly be measured, when, as is usually the case, the dirt is accompanied by so many other bad conditions arising from poverty. For example, a home in close proximity to railroad tracks or mills whose stacks send forth clouds of soot, smoke, and ashes is generally the poorly built home of those who have neither time nor means to secure and retain cleanliness under such difficulties.

Overcrowding in homes is another factor the relative importance of which can not be exactly determined, because of its close connection with other ills. But the degree of overcrowding is greatest in the small cheaper houses, those of one, two, three, or four rooms. The average number of persons per room in the homes of all live-born babies for whom the data were secured was found to be 1.38. Homes of four rooms were more numerous than those of any other size and they housed an average of 1.58 persons per room. The number of babies in homes of various sizes with the number of persons per room for homes of each size was as follows:

TABLE 5.—NUMBER OF BABIES LIVING IN HOMES OF EACH SPECIFIED SIZE, AND AVERAGE NUMBER OF PERSONS PER ROOM IN HOMES OF EACH SIZE.

| SIZE OF HOME. | Live-born babies. | Persons per room. | SIZE OF HOME. | Live-born babies. | Persons per room. |
|---|---|---|---|---|---|
| All homes | 1,463 | | 8 rooms | 43 | 0.83 |
| | | | 9 rooms | 22 | .93 |
| 1 room | 33 | 4.42 | 10 rooms | 4 | .88 |
| 2 rooms | 165 | 2.27 | 11 rooms | 4 | .64 |
| 3 rooms | 147 | 1.83 | 12 rooms | 1 | .75 |
| 4 rooms | 526 | 1.58 | 13 rooms | 1 | .69 |
| 5 rooms | 222 | 1.22 | 14 rooms | 2 | .43 |
| 6 rooms | 233 | 1.07 | Not reported | 22 | |
| 7 rooms | 38 | .96 | | | |

In homes of one, two, three, or four rooms or where the number of occupants ranged from 4.42 to 1.58 persons per room the infant mortality rate was 155, as compared with a rate of but 101.8 in larger homes, where the number ranged from 1.22 to 0.43 persons per room.

The 1910 census returns show that the greatest overcrowding was in ward 15, where the average number of persons per dwelling was 9.9. Wards 16, 11, and 14 came next with rates of 8.3, 7.7, and 7.2, respectively. The infant mortality rate for these four wards is 190.2, which is over one-third more than the rate for the whole city.

The mortality rate among infants who slept in a room with no other person than their parents was much lower than among those who slept in a room with more than two persons. The babies that slept in separate beds also had a much lower infant mortality rate than those who did not sleep alone, as shown in the next table.

TABLE 6.—DISTRIBUTION OF BIRTHS AND OF DEATHS DURING FIRST YEAR AMONG BABIES SURVIVING AT LEAST 1 MONTH, AND INFANT MORTALITY RATE, ACCORDING TO CERTAIN CONDITIONS IN BABY'S SLEEPING ROOM

| CONDITIONS IN BABY'S SLEEPING ROOM. | BABIES WHO LIVED AT LEAST 1 MONTH. | | |
|---|---|---|---|
| | Total. | Deaths during first year. | |
| | | Number. | Rate per 1,000 of those who lived 1 month. |
| Total | 1,389 | 122 | 87.8 |
| Number of others sleeping in same room with baby: | | | |
| 2 or less | 600 | 40 | 66.7 |
| 3 to 5 | 725 | 71 | 97.9 |
| Over 5 | 57 | 7 | 122.8 |
| Not reported | 7 | 4 | (1) |
| Baby sleeping alone in separate bed: | | | |
| Yes | 575 | 32 | 55.7 |
| No | 810 | 88 | 108.6 |
| Not reported | 4 | 2 | (1) |

[1] Total number of babies less than 50; base therefore considered too small to use in computing rate.

In presenting statistics on sleeping and ventilation, only the babies who lived at least one month have been considered, for the reason that so many deaths during the first month of life were due to prenatal causes.

The incidence shown in the foregoing table is significant, even though it can by no means be deduced therefrom that the health of a large proportion of babies was so impaired by sleeping with older and more or less unhealthy persons that death resulted. But irregular night feeding and overfeeding are undoubtedly harmful, and the mother is tempted to subject the baby to this when it sleeps with her and disturbs her rest.

Of the 1,389 babies who lived at least one month, 600, or 43.2 per cent, lived in homes where the baby slept in a room with not more than two other persons. The fact that the baby slept in a room with no more persons than its parents generally argues that the family's means permitted them to have one or more additional rooms for other members of the family, but in other cases, of course, merely that there were no other persons in the family.

Almost every home visited had means for good ventilation of the baby's room at night, yet but 604, or 43.5 per cent, of the 1,389 babies who lived at least a month slept at night in well-ventilated rooms—that is, in rooms where, according to the mother's statement, a window was open all night. Some mothers opened windows when the weather was neither cold nor damp; or opened them in a hall or room adjoining that where the baby slept; others emphatically stated that at night the windows were "always shut tight." The babies subjected to differences of ventilation show corresponding variations in infant mortality rates.

TABLE 7.—DISTRIBUTION OF BIRTHS AND OF DEATHS DURING FIRST YEAR, AND INFANT MORTALITY RATE AMONG BABIES SURVIVING AT LEAST 1 MONTH, ACCORDING TO VENTILATION OF BABY'S ROOM.

| VENTILATION OF BABY'S ROOM. | BABIES WHO LIVED AT LEAST 1 MONTH. | | |
|---|---|---|---|
| | Total. | Died during first year. | |
| | | Number. | Rate per 1,000 of those who lived 1 month. |
| Total | 1,389 | 122 | 87.8 |
| Good | 604 | 17 | 28.1 |
| Fair | 392 | 36 | 91.8 |
| Poor | 390 | 66 | 169.2 |
| Not reported | 3 | 3 | (1) |

1 Total number of babies less than 50; base therefore considered too small to use in computing rate.

A high death rate in badly ventilated homes can not be charged wholly to bad air. The mother who did not, or could not, provide proper ventilation was generally the mother without the means or the knowledge necessary to enable her to care for her baby properly in other respects, and yet the marked differences suggest that ventilation is itself a very important ally of the baby in its first year of struggle for existence.

In many rooms that were poorly ventilated, windows were not opened for the reason that the room was not properly heated and the houses themselves were flimsy and drafty. The problem in such houses is to keep warm. If the windows were frequently or constantly opened, the houses would be too cold to live in. In some localities the outside air is so laden with soot, ashes, dirt. and smoke that every effort is made to keep it out of the house.

The foreigners, who generally have the most miserable homes, are not dirty people who select bad living conditions through innate poor judgment, low standards, and lack of taste. The squalid homes which housed the natives and later the Germans and the Irish until the present type of immigrants came to do the more poorly paid work were the only homes available within the purchasing power of their low wages. The new immigrants demanded practically nothing and the owners did practically nothing in the matter of improving these homes, which naturally became more and more squalid as time went on. An excessive infant mortality rate and insanitary homes in unhealthful sections were found to be coexistent.

## NATIONALITY.

### GENERAL NATIVITY.

The investigation embraced 860 babies of native mothers (of whom 6 were negroes) and 691 babies of foreign mothers, making a total of 1,551. The infant mortality rate for the entire group was 134 per 1,000 live births; for the babies of native mothers 104.3, and for those of foreign mothers 171.3. The stillbirth rate for native mothers having children in 1911 was less than that for foreign mothers, being 52.3, as compared with 62.2 per 1,000 total births.

The line between the natives and foreigners is very sharply drawn in Johnstown. The native population as a rule knows scarcely anything about the foreigners, except what appears in the newspapers about misdemeanors committed in foreign sections. The report of the Immigration Commission[1] comments "on the attitude of the police department toward foreigners * * * with regard to Sunday desecration," and states that "the Croatians are accustomed to spend Sunday in singing, drinking, and noisy demonstrations. The police have been instructed to show no leniency on account of ignorance of the municipal regulations, and, without any attempt at explaining the laws; they arrest the offenders in large numbers." Again, it states: "They are arrested more often for crimes that make them a nuisance to the native population than for mere infractions of the law * * *. Few arrests are made for immorality among foreigners." "Sabbath desecration" is the crime foreigners are most frequently charged with.

Foreigners are employed largely in the less skilled occupations of the steel mills, which operate 24 hours a day, seven days a week. At the time the investigation was made some of the men in the steel mills worked for a period of two weeks on a night shift of 14 hours, then two weeks on a day shift of 10 hours, and back again to the night shift of 14 hours for another two weeks, and so on. When shifts were changed, one group of men was required to work throughout a period of 24 hours instead of for the usual 10 or 14 hour period and another group had 24 hours off duty. Some departments of the steel mills, however, shut down on Sundays, and in some departments for certain occupations an eight-hour day prevails, but these more favorable conditions do not prevail among the majority of the unskilled foreign workers whose homes were visited.

The foreigners who work on a 24-hour shift in a mill on one Sunday frequently "desecrate" their alternate free Sabbath by "singing, drinking, and noisy demonstrations," in spite of the known danger

1 United States Immigration Commission Reports, Volume VIII, "Immigrants in Industries: Part 2, Iron and Steel Manufacturing in the East," p. 387. Reference is to Johnstown and is a very true picture of various immigrant institutions and of the comparative progress and assimilation of different races there. Although the immigration report was made five years before our investigation, conditions remain practically the same.

of arrest for "crimes that make them a nuisance to the native population" or for "Sabbath desecration," laws concerning which are strictly enforced in Johnstown; for example, children are not permitted to play in public playgrounds on Sunday and mercantile establishments are required to be closed on that day. Also, it is "unlawful for any person or persons to deliver ice cream, or to sell or deliver milk from wagon or by person carrying same, within the city on the Sabbath day, commonly called Sunday, after 12 o'clock m." The ordinance from which the foregoing sentence was quoted became a law on January 25, 1914.

## SERBO-CROATIAN.

The foreign group having the highest infant mortality rate is the Serbo-Croatian[1] where, as shown in the next table, infant deaths numbered 263.9 per 1,000 live births.

TABLE 8.—DISTRIBUTION OF BIRTHS, LIVE BIRTHS, AND DEATHS DURING FIRST YEAR, AND INFANT MORTALITY RATE, ACCORDING TO NATIONALITY OF MOTHER.

| NATIONALITY OF MOTHER. | Total births. | Total live births. | DEATHS DURING FIRST YEAR. | |
|---|---|---|---|---|
| | | | Number. | Infant mortality rate. |
| All nationalities | 1,551 | 1,463 | 196 | 134.0 |
| Native | 860 | 815 | 85 | 104.3 |
| Foreign | 691 | 648 | 111 | 171.3 |
| Slovak, Polish, etc | 394 | 367 | 65 | 177.1 |
| Serbo-Croatian | 76 | 72 | 19 | 263.9 |
| Italian | 75 | 71 | 13 | 183.1 |
| German | 53 | 47 | 6 | (1) |
| Magyar | 38 | 38 | 4 | (1) |
| British | 33 | 31 | 4 | (1) |
| Syrian and Greek | 12 | 12 | | |
| Hebrew | 10 | 10 | | |

[1] Total live births less than 50; base therefore considered too small to use in computing an infant mortality rate.

The men of the Serbo-Croatian group are fine looking and powerful and are employed in the heavy unskilled work of the steel mills and the mines. They greatly outnumber the women of their race in Johnstown, and a man with a wife frequently becomes a "boarding boss"; that is, he fills his rooms with beds and rents out sleeping space to his fellow countrymen at from $2.50 to $3 a month each.

[1] A distinct and homogenous race, from a linguistic point of view, among Slavic peoples. They are divided into the groups "Croatian" and "Servian," on political and religious grounds, the former being Roman Catholics and the latter Greek Orthodox. Their spoken language is the same but they can not read each other's publications, for the Croatians use the Roman alphabet, or sometimes the strange old Slavic letters, while the Servians use the Russian characters fostered by the Greek Church.

Three Krainers have also, for convenience, been included in this group. Krainers are Slovenians from the Austro-Hungarian Province of Carniola and are designated "close cousins of the Croatians but with a different though nearly related language" by Emily Greene Balch in her book entitled "Our Slavic Fellow Citizens."

The same bed and bedding is sometimes in service both night and day to accommodate men on the night and the day shifts of the steel mills.

The wife, without extra charge, makes up the beds, does the washing and ironing, and buys and prepares the food for all the lodgers. Usually she gets everything on credit and the lodgers pay their respective shares biweekly. These conditions exist to some extent among other foreigners, but are not as prevalent among other nationalities in Johnstown as among the Serbo-Croatians.

In a workingman's family, it is sometimes said, the woman's workday is two hours longer than the man's. But if this statement is correct in general, the augmentation stated is insufficient in these abnormal homes where the women are required to have many meals and dinner buckets ready at irregular hours to accommodate men working on different shifts.

The Serbo-Croatian women who, more than any of the others, do all this work are big, handsome, and graceful, proud and reckless of their strength. During the progress of the investigation, in the winter months, they were frequently seen walking about the yards and courts, in bare feet, on the snow and ice-covered ground, hanging up clothes or carrying water into the house from a yard hydrant.

Whether it harmed them to expend their force and vigor as they did could not be determined in individual cases, but their babies are the ones who died off with the greatest rapidity, their infant mortality rate being 263.9, as compared with the rates of 171.3 for all the foreign; 104.3 for the natives; and 134 for the entire group as shown in Table 8. Excluding babies of Serbo-Croatian mothers, the infant mortality rate for babies of foreign mothers is but 159.7.

### ITALIAN.

The Italian mothers visited in Johnstown bore 75 children in 1911, 4 being stillborn. The infant mortality rate among the live born was 183.1, the highest of any racial group excepting the Serbo-Croatian, where it was 263.9.

The Italians have been in Johnstown somewhat longer than the Serbo-Croatians and they seem to have a little firmer grip on the community life there. Their homes are a shade better, a trifle cleaner, and somewhat less crowded than those of the Serbo-Croatians, although their hygienic standards seem little if any higher and they rank no better in literacy. The women do not perform the arduous duties that are the lot of so many of the Serbo-Croatian women; they have not the robust physique of the latter and the men are not found in those branches of the steel industry which require the extraordinary strength possessed by the Serbo-Croatians. The occupations of the Italian fathers were found to be more diversified than those of the Serbo-Croatians, some being fruit, grocery, or cheese merchants;

steamship agents; bricklayers, carpenters, or workers at other skilled and semiskilled trades.

### SLOVAK, POLISH, ETC.

The infant mortality rate in the group designated "Slovak, Polish, etc.," is 177.1. In this group are included all the Slavic races represented in the investigation excepting the Serbo-Croatian. The babies of Slovak[1] mothers were found to be most numerous, there being 276 of them. There were 108 babies of Polish,[2] 2 of Bohemian,[3] and 7 of Ruthenian[4] mothers. In addition, one baby of a Scandinavian (Danish) mother was included, not because Scandinavians bear the least racial resemblance to the Slavic races, but because the few Scandinavians in Johnstown happened to be on about the same economic footing as the "Slovak, Polish, etc."

The rate for this group is lower than that for either the Serbo-Croatians or the Italians, but it is nevertheless very high and one exceeded by only a few European countries, as shown by the table on page 12.

Some of the "Slovaks, Poles, etc.," live in the same squalid sections as the Serbo-Croatians, and in the same type of inferior houses, but on the whole they have been in Johnstown longer, are more prosperous, and are therefore beginning to move from Cambria City and Woodvale, where formerly practically all lived, into more desirable sections. Those who have been in this country longest and intend to stay here are buying homes with large yards in the less crowded sections and are raising vegetables and flowers. Others, however, still remain in poor neighborhoods and sometimes buy houses there for from $300 to $600 each, built close together on rented ground.

Lodgers are by no means uncommon among the people in this group, but usually their homes are cleaner, less crowded, and possessed of more comforts than those of the Serbo-Croatians and Italians.

### OTHER NATIONALITIES.

The British[5] infant mortality rate in Johnstown is 129 and the German 127.7. The British and Germans in Johnstown are more prosperous than the Slavic, Magyar, Jewish, Italian, Syrian, and Greek peoples, and regard the others as "foreigners." It was strange

[1] Slovaks occupy practically all except the Ruthenian territory of northern Hungary; also found in great numbers in southeast Moravia. They are the Moravians conquered by Hungary. In physical type no dividing line can be drawn between Slovaks and Moravians. It is often claimed that Slovak is a Bohemian dialect.

[2] The west Slavic race native to the former Kingdom of Poland. For the most part they adhere to the Roman rather than the Greek Orthodox Catholic Church.

[3] The westernmost division or dialect of the Czech and the principal people or language of Bohemia. Czech is the westernmost race or linguistic division of the Slavic (except Wendish, in Germany), the race or people residing mainly in Bohemia and Moravia.

[4] Also known as Little Russians; live principally in southern Russia; also share Galicia with the Poles but greatly surpassed by Poles in number. In language and physical type resemble Slovaks. Generally Greek Orthodox, but a few are Greek Catholics of the Roman Catholic Church, whose priests marry, and are separated from other Roman Catholics by marked religious differences.

[5] English, Irish, Scotch, and Welsh included in the term British.

to hear a man, one who could hardly speak English, say, "We are not foreigners; we are Germans." The British and Germans occupy the same relative position economically that they occupy in the infant mortality scale with relation to other races.

In the Magyar[1] group, of 38 babies born alive 4 died in their first year, making an infant mortality rate of 105.3, which is almost as low as that for babies of native mothers. The Magyars are little if any better off than the other "foreigners" among whom they live, but they possess somewhat higher standards of living. They live in poor neighborhoods and have inferior houses, but their homes are cleaner and they themselves somewhat more alert, personally cleaner, and less illiterate than the other foreigners.

There were but 10 babies of Hebrew mothers and 12 of Syrian and Greek mothers; among these there were no deaths. These groups are too small numerically to be significant in a comparative race study of infant mortality.

## STILLBIRTHS.

In all there were but 88 stillbirths included in the investigation. They were more numerous proportionately among the Germans than among the mothers of any of the other nationalities. No single nationality group, however, has a very large representation, and hence a comparison of the rate for one with that for another nationality is not as significant as the difference in rate between native and foreign mothers. Although a special study of the causes of stillbirths was not made in connection with a study of deaths of infants during their first year of life, nevertheless the incidence of these births among the different nationality groups is believed to be of some interest, and therefore shown in the next table.

TABLE 9.—DISTRIBUTION OF BIRTHS AND OF STILLBIRTHS, AND RATE OF STILLBIRTHS PER 1,000 BIRTHS, ACCORDING TO NATIONALITY OF MOTHER.

| NATIONALITY OF MOTHER. | Total births. | STILLBIRTHS. | |
|---|---|---|---|
| | | Number. | Rate per 1,000 births. |
| All nationalities | 1,551 | 88 | 56.7 |
| Native | 860 | 45 | 52.3 |
| Foreign | 691 | 43 | 62.2 |
| Slovak, Polish, etc | 394 | 27 | 68.5 |
| Serbo-Croatian | 76 | 4 | 52.6 |
| Italian | 75 | 4 | 53.3 |
| German | 53 | 6 | 113.2 |
| Magyar | 38 | | |
| British | 33 | 2 | 60.6 |
| Syrian and Greek | 12 | | |
| Hebrew | 10 | | |

[1] The race of Finno-Tatar origin that invaded Hungary about the ninth century and is now dominant there; commonly called Hungarians.

## ATTENDANT AT BIRTH.

The native mother usually had a physician at childbirth; the foreign-born, a midwife. The more prosperous of the foreign mothers, however, departed from their traditions or customs and had physicians, while the American-born mothers, when very poor, resorted to midwives. The midwives usually charged $5, and sometimes only $3; they waited for payment or accepted it in installments, and they performed many little household services that no physician would think of rendering.

TABLE 10.—NUMBER AND PER CENT OF BIRTHS ACCORDING TO ATTENDANT AT BIRTH AND NATIVITY OF MOTHER.

| NATIVITY OF MOTHER. | ALL BIRTHS. | | MOTHER ATTENDED BY— | | | | | | | |
|---|---|---|---|---|---|---|---|---|---|---|
| | | | Physician. | | Midwife. | | Neighbor, relative, or friend. | | No one. | |
| | Number. | Per cent. | Number. | Per cent. | Number. | Per cent. | Number. | Per cent. | Number. | Per cent. |
| All | 1.551 | 100.0 | 928 | 59.8 | 588 | 37.9 | 14 | 0.9 | 21 | 1.4 |
| Native mothers | 860 | 100.0 | 774 | 90.0 | 84 | 9.8 | 2 | 0.2 | | |
| Foreign mothers | 691 | 100.0 | 154 | 22.3 | 504 | 72.9 | 12 | 1.7 | 21 | 3.6 |

Two-thirds of those having no attendant were Serbo-Croatians It was a Polish woman, however, who gave the following accoun of the birth of her last child:

> At 5 o'clock Monday evening went to sister's to return washboard, having jus finished day's washing. Baby born while there; sister too young to assist in an way; woman not accustomed to midwife anyway, so she cut cord herself; washe baby at sister's house; walked home, cooked supper for boarders, and was in bed b 8 o'clock. Got up and ironed next day and day following; it tired her, so she the stayed in bed two days. She milked cows and sold milk day after baby's birth but being tired hired some one to do it later in week.
>
> This woman keeps cows, chickens, and lodgers; also earns money doing laundr and char work. Husband deserts her at times; he makes $1.70 a day. A 15-year-ol son makes $1.10 a day in coal mine. Mother thin and wiry; looks tired and worn Frequent fights in home.

The infant mortality rate was lower for babies delivered by phy sicians than for those delivered by midwives or for those at whos birth no properly qualified attendant was present. This is not neces sarily an indication of the quality of the care at birth, although i some cases the inefficiency of the midwife may have directly or ind rectly caused deaths, just as in some instances a physician's ineff ciency may have caused them. The midwife, however, is resorte to by the poor, and in their homes are found other conditions th create a high infant mortality rate.

TABLE 11.—DISTRIBUTION OF BIRTHS AND OF DEATHS DURING FIRST YEAR, AND INFANT MORTALITY RATE, ACCORDING TO ATTENDANT AT BIRTH AND NATIVITY OF MOTHER.

| ATTENDANT AT BIRTH AND NATIVITY OF MOTHER. | Total live births. | DEATHS DURING FIRST YEAR. | |
|---|---|---|---|
| | | Number. | Infant mortality rate. |
| All births | 1,463 | 196 | 134.0 |
| Physician in attendance | 866 | 87 | 100.5 |
| Native mothers | 730 | 68 | 93.2 |
| Foreign mothers | 136 | 19 | 139.7 |
| Midwife in attendance | 562 | 101 | 179.7 |
| Native mothers | 83 | 15 | 180.7 |
| Foreign mothers | 479 | 86 | 179.5 |
| Other person or no attendant | 35 | 8 | (1) |
| Native mothers | 2 | 2 | (1) |
| Foreign mothers | 33 | 6 | (1) |

1 Total live births less than 50; base therefore considered too small to use in computing an infant mortality rate.

Frequently the Serbo-Croatian women dispense altogether with any assistance at childbirth; sometimes not even the husband or a neighbor assists. Over 30 per cent of the births among the women of this race took place without a qualified attendant. More than one-half of those delivered by midwives, less than one-fifteenth of those delivered by physicians, and about one-fifth of those delivered without a qualified attendant had babies who died in their first year of life, as shown in the next tabulation:

TABLE 12.—DISTRIBUTION OF BIRTHS AND OF DEATHS DURING FIRST YEAR, ACCORDING TO ATTENDANT AT BIRTH, FOR BABIES OF SERBO-CROATIAN MOTHERS.

| ATTENDANT AT BIRTH. | ALL BIRTHS TO SERBO-CROATIAN MOTHERS. | | Live births. | Deaths during first year. |
|---|---|---|---|---|
| | Number. | Per cent. | | |
| Total | 76 | 100.0 | 72 | 19 |
| Physician | 31 | 40.8 | 28 | 2 |
| Midwife | 22 | 28.9 | 21 | 12 |
| Other person | 9 | 11.8 | 9 | 2 |
| No one | 14 | 18.4 | 14 | 3 |

Fifteen of the 19 Serbo-Croatian women whose babies died under 1 year of age kept lodgers.

In Johnstown the midwife is resorted to principally by the poor. Recent laws that the State is now trying to enforce require that the standard for the practice of midwifery be raised. If this can be done midwives might become definitely helpful persons in the community. One or two of the intelligent graduate midwives in Johnstown have been an educational force among the foreign mothers for some years past. On the other hand there were others who were so dirty and so ignorant that they were a menace to the public health.

## MOTHERS.

### LITERACY.[1]

There are differences in the infant mortality rate between the babies of literate and the babies of illiterate mothers; between those with mothers who can speak English and those with mothers who can not; and between babies of the mothers who have been in this country for a considerable period and those of the newer arrivals. Comparisons of this nature are confined to the foreign mothers, as only three cases of illiteracy were found among native mothers, and the other comparisons would not, of course, be applicable in any case to native mothers.

The next table shows that the infant mortality rate among the children of illiterate foreign mothers was 214, or 66 per thousand greater than the rate among literate foreign mothers.

TABLE 13.—DISTRIBUTION OF BIRTHS AND OF DEATHS DURING FIRST YEAR, INFANT MORTALITY RATE, AND NUMBER AND PER CENT OF STILLBIRTHS, ACCORDING TO LITERACY OF FOREIGN MOTHERS.

| LITERACY OF FOREIGN MOTHERS. | Total births. | Live births. | STILLBIRTHS. | | DEATHS DURING FIRST YEAR. | |
|---|---|---|---|---|---|---|
| | | | Number. | Per cent. | Number. | Infant mortality rate. |
| Foreign mothers | 691 | 648 | 43 | 6.2 | 111 | 171.3 |
| Literate | 445 | 419 | 26 | 5.8 | 62 | 148.0 |
| Illiterate | 246 | 229 | 17 | 6.9 | 49 | 214.0 |

### ABILITY TO SPEAK ENGLISH.

The next table shows that babies whose mothers can not speak English were characterized by a more unfavorable infant mortality rate than other babies.

TABLE 14.—DISTRIBUTION OF BIRTHS AND OF DEATHS DURING FIRST YEAR, INFANT MORTALITY RATE, AND NUMBER AND PER CENT OF STILLBIRTHS, ACCORDING TO ABILITY OF FOREIGN MOTHER TO SPEAK ENGLISH.

| ABILITY TO SPEAK ENGLISH. | Total births. | Live births. | STILLBIRTHS. | | DEATHS DURING FIRST YEAR. | |
|---|---|---|---|---|---|---|
| | | | Number. | Per cent. | Number. | Infant mortality rate. |
| Foreign mothers | 691 | 648 | 43 | 6.2 | 111 | 171.3 |
| Speak English | 263 | 247 | 16 | 6.1 | 36 | 145.7 |
| Can not speak English | 428 | 401 | 27 | 6.3 | 75 | 187.0 |

[1] By literacy is meant ability to read and write in any language and not simply in English.

## YEARS IN THE UNITED STATES.

In addition to a consideration of the babies according to their mothers' ability to speak English, it is of interest to note the infant mortality rates among babies whose mothers have been in this country for different periods of time.

TABLE 15.—DISTRIBUTION OF BIRTHS AND OF DEATHS DURING FIRST YEAR, AND INFANT MORTALITY RATE, ACCORDING TO LENGTH OF RESIDENCE OF FOREIGN MOTHER IN THE UNITED STATES.

| YEARS IN THE UNITED STATES. | Total live births. | DEATHS DURING FIRST YEAR. | |
|---|---|---|---|
| | | Number. | Infant mortality rate. |
| Foreign mothers | 648 | 111 | 171.3 |
| 5 years or less | 168 | 36 | 214.3 |
| Over 5 years | 480 | 75 | 156.3 |

The high infant mortality rate for the children of newer immigrants, illiterates, and those who can not speak English is perhaps affected by the fact that they are at the same time generally of the poorest families and are housed in the most insanitary and unhealthful part of the city.

## AGE.

The age of the mother is frequently believed to be a factor in the health of the child. The highest infant mortality rate was found to be that for the group of babies with mothers over 40 years of age, and the lowest for babies of mothers from 20 to 24 years of age.

TABLE 16.—DISTRIBUTION OF BIRTHS AND OF DEATHS DURING FIRST YEAR, INFANT MORTALITY RATE, AND NUMBER AND PER CENT OF STILLBIRTHS, ACCORDING TO AGE OF MOTHER.

| AGE OF MOTHER. | Total births. | Live births. | STILLBIRTHS. | | DEATHS. | |
|---|---|---|---|---|---|---|
| | | | Number. | Per cent of total. | Number. | Infant mortality rate. |
| All mothers | 1,551 | 1,463 | 88 | 5.7 | 196 | 134.0 |
| Under 20 | 105 | 95 | 10 | 9.5 | 13 | 136.8 |
| 20 to 24 | 476 | 454 | 22 | 4.6 | 55 | 121.1 |
| 25 to 29 | 410 | 391 | 19 | 4.6 | 56 | 143.2 |
| 30 to 39 | 480 | 449 | 31 | 6.5 | 61 | 135.9 |
| 40 and over | 80 | 74 | 6 | 7.5 | 11 | 148.6 |

The youngest mothers have a higher stillbirth rate than other mothers, and the oldest group of mothers has the next highest rate. In this connection not only the foregoing table is of interest, but also Table XII on page 70, based upon the entire reproductive histories of the mothers included in this study. As all the children borne by these mothers are included, the base numbers in the latter table are larger and the figures therefore somewhat more significant.

## BABY'S AGE AT DEATH AND CAUSE (DISEASE) OF DEATH.

A baby who comes into the world has less chance to live one week than an old man of 90, and less chance to live a year than one of 80.—*Bergeron.*

The most dangerous time of life is early infancy; even old age seldom has greater risk. Death strikes most often in infancy. The Johnstown babies died during their first year of life at the rate of 134 per 1,000 born alive, and they paid their heaviest toll in their very earliest days. If the total of 196 deaths had been distributed evenly throughout the 12 months, 8.3 per cent of the babies would have died each month and 25 per cent during each quarter. But instead of that 37.8 per cent died in the first month; 9.2 per cent in the second, and 8.2 per cent in the third, or over 55 per cent in the first quarter.

TABLE 17 —NUMBER AND PER CENT DISTRIBUTION OF DEATHS OF BABIES, BY AGE AT DEATH.

| AGE AT DEATH. | DEATHS OF BABIES OF ALL MOTHERS. Number. | Per cent distribution. |
|---|---|---|
| Total deaths in first year | 196 | 100.0 |
| First quarter | 108 | 55.1 |
| First month | 74 | 37.8 |
| First week | 45 | 23.0 |
| Less than 1 day and 1 day | 30 | 15.3 |
| 2 days | 4 | 2.0 |
| 3 to 6 days | 11 | 5.6 |
| Second week | 14 | 7.1 |
| Third week | 7 | 3.6 |
| Fourth week | 8 | 4.1 |
| Second month | 18 | 9.2 |
| Third month | 16 | 8.2 |
| Second quarter | 42 | 21.4 |
| Third quarter | 31 | 15.8 |
| Fourth quarter | 15 | 7.7 |

The large number of deaths in the first few hours or days of life indicates that many babies are born with some handicap and that in many instances the mother has been subjected to some condition which resulted in the birth of a child incapable of withstanding the ordinary strain of life. Of the 45 babies who died in Johnstown less than a week after birth, 38 died of prematurity, congenital debility or malformations, or injuries received at birth. In one other case the cause of death was given as "bowel trouble" and in six other cases it was not clearly defined. In addition to the 45 babies just referred to as having died in their first week, 12 died later either from prematurity or from congenital defects.

Of the deaths from causes arising after birth, 52 were attributed by the attending physicians to diarrhea and enteritis, 50 to respiratory diseases, and 44 to some other or to some ill-defined cause.

TABLE 18.—DISTRIBUTION OF DEATHS DURING FIRST YEAR AND INFANT MORTALITY RATE, ACCORDING TO CAUSE OF DEATH AND NATIVITY OF MOTHER.

| CAUSE OF DEATH. | DEATHS DURING FIRST YEAR OF BABIES OF— All mothers. | | Native mothers. | | Foreign mothers. | |
|---|---|---|---|---|---|---|
| | Number. | Infant mortality rate. | Number. | Infant mortality rate. | Number. | Infant mortality rate. |
| All causes | 196 | 134.0 | 85 | 104.3 | 111 | 171.3 |
| Diarrhea and enteritis | 52 | 35.5 | 17 | 20.9 | 35 | 54.0 |
| Respiratory diseases | 50 | 34.2 | 19 | 23.3 | 31 | 47.8 |
| Premature births | 24 | 16.4 | 11 | 13.5 | 13 | 20.1 |
| Congenital debility or malformation | 19 | 12.9 | 5 | 6.1 | 14 | 21.6 |
| Injuries at birth | 7 | 4.8 | 6 | 7.4 | 1 | 1.5 |
| Other causes or not reported | 44 | 30.1 | 27 | 33.1 | 17 | 26.2 |

The latest census report on mortality statistics characterizes diarrhea and enteritis as the "most important preventable cause of infant mortality" in the United States, and numerically at least it proves to be the most important cause of infant death in Johnstown.

Holt [1] says that one of the most striking facts about diarrheal diseases in infants is their prevalence during the summer season. In Johnstown the infant diarrheal deaths were least prevalent in the first quarter of the year, next in the second, next prevalent in the fourth, and most prevalent in the third or summer quarter.

TABLE 19.—DISTRIBUTION OF DEATHS, ACCORDING TO CAUSE OF DEATH AND QUARTER OF CALENDAR YEAR IN WHICH DEATH OCCURRED.

| CAUSE OF DEATH. | All deaths. | QUARTER OF CALENDAR YEAR IN WHICH DEATH OCCURRED. First. | Second. | Third. | Fourth. |
|---|---|---|---|---|---|
| All causes | 196 | 54 | 29 | 74 | 39 |
| Diarrhea and enteritis | 52 | 3 | 5 | 32 | 12 |
| Respiratory diseases | 50 | 24 | 8 | 7 | 11 |
| Premature births | 24 | 7 | 5 | 9 | 3 |
| Congenital debility or malformation | 19 | 5 | 2 | 8 | 4 |
| Injuries at birth | 7 | 5 | 1 | ........ | 1 |
| Other causes or not reported | 44 | 10 | 8 | 18 | 8 |

[1] The Diseases of Infancy and Childhood, by L. Emmett Holt. p. 345. New York, 1912.

Our figures are too small to admit of broad generalizations or a very full discussion of infant deaths according to the period of the year.

This excess of infant deaths from diarrhea in the summer months has been established by statistics in many countries, and the cause of such an excess has been the subject of much discussion, but as yet there is no general agreement. Liefmann and Lindemann[1] conclude, however, that in this field of controversy there are certain facts which are at present well established, these being the dependence of the high summer mortality on methods of feeding, on hot weather, and on the living and social condition of the parents. The last factor mentioned by these authors, including as it does housing conditions, economic status, and degree of intelligence, is becoming more and more the subject of study and investigation. It has been shown that the distinctly harmful effect of hot weather on the infant is increased when the housing conditions are bad; in overcrowded homes with bad ventilation the indoor temperature may be many degrees higher than the outdoor temperature. The ignorance and carelessness of mothers has also been shown to increase the bad effect of hot weather. With hygienic care, including cool baths, much fresh air, and careful feeding, many infants are able to pass through extremely hot weather without diarrheal disturbances.

Respiratory diseases were reported as a cause of death with almost as great frequency as diarrheal diseases. As shown by Table 19, these deaths occurred principally in the colder months of the first and fourth quarters of the calendar year.

## FEEDING.

Food is recognized as of such importance in relation to infant mortality that studies of this subject frequently resolve themselves into studies of feeding only. Invariably these demonstrate the truth of the statement of Dr. G. F. McCleary[2] that "in human milk we have a unique and wonderful food for which the ingenuity of man may toil in vain to find a satisfactory substitute." Many mothers, however, still fail to appreciate the risk their young babies face in being given any except the natural infant food, and consequently babies are in large numbers wholly or partly weaned from the breast in the earliest months of their lives.

---

[1] Liefmann, H., and Lindemann, H., Die Lokalization der Säuglingsterblichkeit und ihre Beziehungen zur Wohnungsfrage. Med. Klinik 1912, pp. 8, 1074.

[2] Infantile Mortality and Infants' Milk Depots. London.

Breast feeding is far more general, comparatively, among the poorer mothers than among the well to do, as shown by the following summary which gives the number and per cent of babies of mothers with husbands earning varying incomes, who had been completely weaned from the breast when they were 3, 6, or 9 months of age, respectively. For each of the periods indicated the percentage completely weaned from the breast is much greater in the groups where earnings are highest.

TABLE 20.—DISTRIBUTION OF BABIES ALIVE AT 3, 6, AND 9 MONTHS OF AGE BY TYPE OF FEEDING AT EACH OF SAID AGES, ACCORDING TO ANNUAL EARNINGS OF FATHER AND NATIVITY OF MOTHER.

| ANNUAL EARNINGS OF FATHER AND NATIVITY OF MOTHER. | BABIES LIVING AT AGE OF— | | | | | | | | |
|---|---|---|---|---|---|---|---|---|---|
| | 3 months. | | | 6 months. | | | 9 months. | | |
| | Total. | Completely weaned from breast. | | Total. | Completely weaned from breast. | | Total. | Completely weaned from breast. | |
| | | Number. | Per cent. | | Number. | Per cent. | | Number. | Per cent. |
| Total | 1,355 | 193 | 14.2 | 1,313 | 250 | 19.0 | 1,282 | 353 | 27.5 |
| Under $624 | 341 | 22 | 6.5 | 322 | 32 | 9.9 | 309 | 57 | 18.4 |
| $625 to $899 | 358 | 48 | 13.4 | 351 | 63 | 17.9 | 342 | 85 | 24.9 |
| $900 and over [1] | 629 | 114 | 18.1 | 616 | 146 | 23.7 | 608 | 201 | 33.1 |
| Not reported [2] | 27 | 9 | 33.3 | 24 | 9 | 37.5 | 23 | 10 | 43.3 |
| Mother native | 765 | 155 | 20.3 | 747 | 195 | 26.1 | 735 | 251 | 34.1 |
| Under $624 | 69 | 10 | 14.5 | 66 | 13 | 19.7 | 65 | 18 | 27.7 |
| $625 to $899 | 180 | 36 | 20.0 | 177 | 46 | 26.0 | 173 | 55 | 31.8 |
| $900 and over [1] | 491 | 100 | 20.4 | 482 | 127 | 26.3 | 476 | 168 | 35.3 |
| Not reported [2] | 25 | 9 | 36.0 | 22 | 9 | 40.9 | 21 | 10 | 47.6 |
| Mother foreign | 590 | 38 | 6.4 | 566 | 55 | 9.7 | 547 | 102 | 18.6 |
| Under $624 | 272 | 12 | 4.4 | 256 | 19 | 7.4 | 244 | 39 | 16.0 |
| $625 to $899 | 178 | 12 | 6.7 | 174 | 17 | 9.8 | 169 | 30 | 17.8 |
| $900 and over [1] | 138 | 14 | 10.1 | 134 | 19 | 14.2 | 132 | 33 | 25.0 |
| Not reported [2] | 2 | | | 2 | | | 2 | | |

[1] Includes those reported as earning "ample." "Ample," as used in this report has a somewhat technical meaning; when information concerning the father's earnings was not available and the family showed no evidences of poverty, the word "ample" was used. When, however, the family was clearly in a state of abject poverty, it was included in the group "Under $521."

[2] Unmarried mothers' babies also included.

Breast feeding, wholly or in part, is continued for a longer period by foreign than by native mothers, as indicated in the preceding table, showing that 20.3, 26.1, and 34.1 per cent of the native mothers' babies as compared with 6.4, 9.7, and 18.6 per cent of the foreign mothers' babies had been weaned from the breast at the age of 3, 6, and 9 months, respectively.

Some additional details concerning the type of feeding of babies of native and foreign mothers are given in the next table.

TABLE 21.—NUMBER AND PER CENT OF BABIES AGED 3, 6, AND 9 MONTHS WHO RECEIVED SPECIFIED TYPE OF FEEDING, ACCORDING TO NATIVITY OF MOTHER.

| TYPE OF FEEDING AND NATIVITY OF MOTHER. | AGE OF BABY. | | | | | |
|---|---|---|---|---|---|---|
| | 3 months. | | 6 months. | | 9 months. | |
| | Number. | Per cent. | Number. | Per cent. | Number. | Per cent. |
| All babies | 1,355 | 100.0 | 1,313 | 100.0 | 1,282 | 100.0 |
| Exclusively breast fed | 987 | 72.8 | 616 | 46.9 | 220 | 17.2 |
| Partly breast fed | 175 | 12.9 | 447 | 34.0 | 709 | 55.3 |
| Exclusively artificially fed | 193 | 14.2 | 250 | 19.0 | 353 | 27.5 |
| Native mothers' babies | 765 | 100.0 | 747 | 100.0 | 735 | 100.0 |
| Exclusively breast fed | 512 | 66.9 | 307 | 41.1 | 87 | 11.8 |
| Partly breast fed | 98 | 12.8 | 245 | 32.8 | 397 | 54.0 |
| Exclusively artificially fed | 155 | 20.3 | 195 | 26.1 | 251 | 34.1 |
| Foreign mothers' babies | 590 | 100.0 | 566 | 100.0 | 547 | 100.0 |
| Exclusively breast fed | 475 | 80.5 | 309 | 54.6 | 133 | 24.3 |
| Partly breast fed | 77 | 13.1 | 202 | 35.7 | 312 | 57.0 |
| Exclusively artificially fed | 38 | 6.4 | 55 | 9.7 | 102 | 18.6 |

The following table shows that artificially fed babies die at a much more rapid rate than breast-fed babies. In the very earliest months exclusive breast feeding seems to be the only safe method. After four months the danger of giving some other food in addition to the breast milk does not seem to be so great.

TABLE 22.—DISTRIBUTION OF BABIES ALIVE AT END OF EACH MONTH, FROM SECOND TO TENTH, INCLUSIVE, ACCORDING TO TYPE OF FEEDING DURING EACH MONTH SPECIFIED, NUMBER OF DEATHS DURING FIRST YEAR, AND RATE PER 1,000 ALIVE IN EACH GROUP.

| TYPE OF FEEDING AT TIME SPECIFIED. | LIVE-BORN BABIES. | | |
|---|---|---|---|
| | Number alive at specified time. | Deaths during first year. | |
| | | Number. | Rate per 1,000 alive at specified time. |
| Second month | 1,389 | 122 | 87.8 |
| Breast exclusively | 1,181 | 85 | 72.0 |
| Mixed (i. e., breast and other) | 77 | 6 | 77.9 |
| Artificial (i. e., no breast milk) | 131 | 31 | 236.6 |
| Third month | 1,371 | 104 | 75.9 |
| Breast exclusively | 1,112 | 60 | 54.0 |
| Mixed | 98 | 9 | 91.8 |
| Artificial | 161 | 35 | 217.4 |
| Fourth month | 1,355 | 88 | 64.9 |
| Breast exclusively | 987 | 46 | 46.6 |
| Mixed | 175 | 10 | 57.1 |
| Artificial | 193 | 32 | 165.8 |
| Fifth month | 1,337 | 70 | 52.4 |
| Breast exclusively | 871 | 33 | 37.9 |
| Mixed | 253 | 10 | 39.5 |
| Artificial | 213 | 27 | 126.8 |

TABLE 22.—DISTRIBUTION OF BABIES ALIVE AT END OF EACH MONTH, FROM SECOND TO TENTH, INCLUSIVE, ETC.—Continued.

| TYPE OF FEEDING AT TIME SPECIFIED. | LIVE BORN BABIES. | | |
|---|---|---|---|
| | Number alive at specified time. | Deaths during first year. | |
| | | Number. | Rate per 1,000 alive at specified time. |
| Sixth month | 1,318 | 51 | 38.7 |
| Breast exclusively | 780 | 20 | 25.6 |
| Mixed | 310 | 10 | 32.3 |
| Artificial | 228 | 21 | 92.1 |
| Seventh month | 1,313 | 46 | 35.0 |
| Breast exclusively | 616 | 18 | 29.2 |
| Mixed | 447 | 10 | 22.4 |
| Artificial | 250 | 18 | 72.0 |
| Eighth month | 1,305 | 38 | 29.1 |
| Breast exclusively | 502 | 13 | 25.9 |
| Mixed | 541 | 11 | 20.3 |
| Artificial | 262 | 14 | 53.4 |
| Ninth month | 1,291 | 24 | 18.6 |
| Breast exclusively | 395 | 7 | 17.7 |
| Mixed | 611 | 10 | 16.4 |
| Artificial | 285 | 7 | 24.6 |
| Tenth month | 1,282 | 15 | 11.7 |
| Breast exclusively | 220 | 3 | 13.6 |
| Mixed | 709 | 8 | 11.3 |
| Artificial | 353 | 4 | 11.3 |

The next table differentiates between babies of native and foreign mothers, giving the statistics by three-month periods instead of by single months.

TABLE 23.—DISTRIBUTION OF BABIES ALIVE AT THE END OF 3, 6, AND 9 MONTHS, RESPECTIVELY, ACCORDING TO TYPE OF FEEDING, NUMBER OF DEATHS DURING FIRST YEAR, AND RATE PER 1,000 ALIVE IN EACH GROUP, BY NATIVITY OF MOTHER.

| AGE OF BABY AND NATIVITY OF MOTHER. | Babies alive at age indicated. | BREAST FED EXCLUSIVELY. | | | MIXED FOOD: BREAST AND OTHER. | | | ARTIFICIAL FOOD: NO BREAST MILK. | | |
|---|---|---|---|---|---|---|---|---|---|---|
| | | Total. | Deaths in first year. | | Total. | Deaths in first year. | | Total. | Deaths in first year. | |
| | | | Number. | Rate per 1,000 alive at specified age. | | Number. | Rate per 1,000 alive at specified age. | | Number. | Rate per 1,000 alive at specified age. |
| ALL | | | | | | | | | | |
| 3 months | 1,355 | 987 | 46 | 46.6 | 175 | 10 | 57.1 | 193 | 32 | 165.8 |
| 6 months | 1,313 | 616 | 18 | 29.2 | 447 | 10 | 22.4 | 250 | 18 | 72.0 |
| 9 months | 1,282 | 220 | 3 | 13.6 | 709 | 8 | 11.3 | 353 | 4 | 11.3 |
| NATIVE. | | | | | | | | | | |
| 3 months | 765 | 512 | 12 | 23.4 | 98 | 2 | 20.4 | 155 | 21 | 135.5 |
| 6 months | 747 | 307 | 2 | 6.5 | 245 | 1 | 4.1 | 195 | 14 | 71.8 |
| 9 months | 735 | 87 | 1 | 11.5 | 397 | 1 | 2.5 | 251 | 3 | 12.0 |
| FOREIGN. | | | | | | | | | | |
| 3 months | 590 | 475 | 34 | 71.6 | 77 | 8 | 103.9 | 38 | 11 | 289.5 |
| 6 months | 566 | 309 | 16 | 51.8 | 202 | 9 | 44.6 | 55 | 4 | 72.7 |
| 9 months | 547 | 133 | 2 | 15.0 | 312 | 7 | 22.4 | 102 | 1 | 9.8 |

These statistics show that the manner of feeding is one of the most important considerations in the life and health of a baby. But a comparison of the number of deaths among babies whose fathers earn specified sums (Table 31) shows that the influence of poverty reaches even the breast-fed baby. When the fathers' earnings are small a larger proportion of babies die despite breast feeding.

## SEX.

The Johnstown investigation comprehended 1,551 births in the year 1911, male births numbering 813 and female 738, the proportion being as 1,101.6 male to 1,000 female births; or, stated inversely, 907.7 female to 1,000 male births. Newsholme[1] says that "male infants always suffer from a higher infant mortality rate than female infants," and in Johnstown we find this true for the group as a whole, the rates being as shown in the next table:

TABLE 24.—DISTRIBUTION OF LIVE BIRTHS AND STILLBIRTHS AND OF DEATHS DURING FIRST YEAR, AND INFANT MORTALITY RATE, ACCORDING TO SEX OF BABY.

| SEX OF BABY. | All births. | Live births. | STILLBIRTHS. | | DEATHS IN FIRST YEAR. | |
|---|---|---|---|---|---|---|
| | | | Total. | Rate per 1,000 births. | Total. | Infant mortality rate. |
| Total babies | 1,551 | 1,463 | 88 | 56.7 | 196 | 134.0 |
| Male | 813 | 761 | 52 | 64.0 | 105 | 138.0 |
| Female | 738 | 702 | 36 | 48.8 | 91 | 129.6 |

Among foreign mothers male births were considerably in excess of female births; among native mothers the reverse was true. The more favorable mortality rate for female infants does not prevail among the children of foreign mothers, as can be seen in the next table, which shows an infant mortality rate of 177.5 for girls as compared with one of 166.2 for boys.

[1] Thirty-ninth Annual Report of the Local Government Board. London, 1910.

TABLE 25.—DISTRIBUTION OF ALL BIRTHS, LIVE BIRTHS, AND STILLBIRTHS AND OF DEATHS DURING FIRST YEAR, AND INFANT MORTALITY RATE, ACCORDING TO SEX OF BABY AND NATIVITY OF MOTHER.

| SEX OF BABY AND NATIVITY OF MOTHER. | All births. | Live births. | Stillbirths. | | Deaths during first year. | |
|---|---|---|---|---|---|---|
| | | | Total. | Rate per 1,000 births. | Total. | Infant mortality rate. |
| BABIES OF NATIVE MOTHERS. | | | | | | |
| Total number | 860 | 815 | 45 | 52.3 | 85 | 104.3 |
| Male: | | | | | | |
| Number | 433 | 406 | 27 | 62.4 | 46 | 113.3 |
| Per cent | 50.3 | 49.8 | 60.0 | .......... | 54.1 | .......... |
| Female: | | | | | | |
| Number | 427 | 409 | 18 | 42.2 | 39 | 95.4 |
| Per cent | 49.7 | 50.2 | 40.0 | .......... | 45.9 | .......... |
| BABIES OF FOREIGN MOTHERS. | | | | | | |
| Total number | 691 | 648 | 43 | 62.2 | 111 | 171.3 |
| Male: | | | | | | |
| Number | 380 | 355 | 25 | 65.8 | 59 | 166.2 |
| Per cent | 55.0 | 54.8 | 58.1 | .......... | 53.2 | .......... |
| Female: | | | | | | |
| Number | 311 | 293 | 18 | 57.9 | 52 | 177.5 |
| Per cent | 45.0 | 45.2 | 41.9 | .......... | 46.8 | .......... |

## MOTHER'S HOUSEHOLD DUTIES, CESSATION AND RESUMPTION OF.

The extent to which the native and foreign mothers in Johnstown relinquished a part of their household duties as the time for their confinement approached is shown below:

TABLE 26.—DISTRIBUTION OF BIRTHS ACCORDING TO TIME OF THE MOTHER'S RELINQUISHMENT OF PART OF HOUSEHOLD DUTIES BEFORE CONFINEMENT, BY NATIVITY OF MOTHER.

| TIME OF RELINQUISHMENT OF PART OF HOUSEHOLD DUTIES BEFORE CONFINEMENT. | All births. | To native mothers. | To foreign mothers. |
|---|---|---|---|
| All mothers | 1,551 | 860 | 691 |
| No household duties relinquished to day of confinement | 1,350 | 695 | 655 |
| Part of duties relinquished: | | | |
| Less than 7 days before confinement | 3 | 1 | 2 |
| 7 to 13 days before confinement | 7 | 5 | 2 |
| 2 weeks to 1 month before confinement | 16 | 12 | 4 |
| 1 month or more before confinement | 174 | 146 | 28 |
| Had no household duties | 1 | 1 | .......... |

Among the 174 babies of mothers who relinquished part of their household duties a month before confinement, the infant mortality rate was 112.5, as compared with 136.7 for those of other mothers.

TABLE 27.—DISTRIBUTION OF BIRTHS AND OF DEATHS DURING FIRST YEAR, AND INFANT MORTALITY RATE, ACCORDING TO TIME OF RELINQUISHMENT OF PART OF HOUSEHOLD DUTIES OF MOTHER BEFORE CONFINEMENT.

| TIME OF RELINQUISHMENT OF PART OF HOUSEHOLD DUTIES BEFORE CONFINEMENT. | All births. | Live births. | Deaths during first year. | Infant mortality rate. |
|---|---|---|---|---|
| All mothers | 1,551 | 1,463 | 196 | 134.0 |
| No cessation or less than 1 month | 1,376 | 1,302 | 178 | 136.7 |
| 1 month or more | 174 | 160 | 18 | 112.5 |
| No housework | 1 | 1 | .......... | .......... |

To what extent the relinquishment of household duties at a given time directly affected the health of the child can not be definitely shown. A relation may exist, but on the other hand the difference in the mortality rate may be due to the fact that the mothers could afford to give consideration to their condition and escape some of their heaviest tasks as their pregnancy approached its end, and were members of families who were thoughtful of them and relieved them of these tasks or employed extra household assistance at such times.

Another indication of intelligence and of comfortable surroundings is the care given a mother in the early days of her baby's life, particularly if she is a nursing mother. The duration of her rest period before the resumption of part of her household duties is one measure of this. The foreign mothers, with less education, more numerous and arduous tasks, less opportunity for leisure, and smaller incomes, begin to resume their housework sooner than the native mothers with young babies

TABLE 28.—DISTRIBUTION OF LIVE BIRTHS AND OF DEATHS DURING FIRST YEAR, AND INFANT MORTALITY RATE, ACCORDING TO TIME OF MOTHER RESUMING PART OF HOUSEHOLD DUTIES AFTER CONFINEMENT, BY NATIVITY OF MOTHER.

| TIME OF RESUMING PART OF HOUSEHOLD DUTIES AFTER CONFINEMENT. | LIVE BIRTHS TO— | | | DEATHS DURING FIRST YEAR. | |
|---|---|---|---|---|---|
| | All mothers. | Native mothers. | Foreign mothers. | Total. | Infant mortality rate. |
| Total | 1,463 | 815 | 648 | 196 | 134.0 |
| 8 days or less | 467 | 44 | 423 | 79 | 169.2 |
| 9 to 13 days | 560 | 446 | 114 | 70 | 125.0 |
| 14 days or more | 427 | 318 | 109 | 41 | 96.0 |
| Mother died or not reported | 9 | 7 | 2 | 6 | (1) |

[1] Total number of live births less than 50; base therefore considered too small to use in computing an infant mortality rate.

The fact that a mother takes up her housework in the early days of her baby's life does not necessarily increase the danger of its death. In some cases, however, mothers stated that the quantity of their breast milk was noticeably impaired when they got up and resumed their work too soon. Naturally this would affect the baby's nutrition. In other cases a mother's cares and duties may be so absorbing that she can not give the baby full attention. Whatever the exact explanation, attention should be called to the greater frequency of infant deaths when the mother resumed household duties very soon after childbirth.

A statement of the time of the mother's resumption of household duties in full, like that giving the time of resumption in part, shows that the native mothers have the longer period of rest.

TABLE 29.—DISTRIBUTION OF LIVE BIRTHS AND OF DEATHS DURING FIRST YEAR, AND INFANT MORTALITY RATE, ACCORDING TO TIME OF MOTHER RESUMING ALL HOUSEHOLD DUTIES AFTER CONFINEMENT, BY NATIVITY OF MOTHER.

| TIME OF RESUMING ALL HOUSEHOLD DUTIES AFTER CONFINEMENT. | LIVE BIRTHS TO— | | | DEATHS DURING FIRST YEAR. | |
|---|---|---|---|---|---|
| | All mothers. | Native mothers. | Foreign mothers. | Total. | Infant mortality rate. |
| Total | 1,463 | 815 | 648 | 196 | 134.0 |
| 8 days or less | 219 | 13 | 206 | 37 | 168.9 |
| 9 to 13 days | 182 | 132 | 50 | 30 | 164.8 |
| 14 days or more | 1,053 | 663 | 390 | 123 | 116.8 |
| Mother died or not reported | 9 | 7 | 2 | 6 | (1) |

1 Total live births less than 50; base therefore considered too small to use in computing an infant mortality rate.

The infant mortality rates for all mothers in the group just referred to, according to the time of resuming housework in full after childbirth, show fewer infant deaths proportionately when the mother has had a longer rest; that is, a rest of two weeks or more.

## ECONOMIC FACTORS.

### EARNINGS OF FATHER.

A grouping of babies according to the income of the father shows the greatest incidence of infant deaths where wages are lowest, and the smallest incidence where they are highest, indicating clearly the relation between low wages and ill health and infant deaths.

For all live babies born in wedlock the infant mortality rate is 130.7. It rises to 255.7 when the father earns less than $521 a year or less than $10 a week, and falls to 84 when he earns $1,200 or more or if his earnings are "ample."[1] The variation in the infant mortality rate from one earnings group to another is not perfectly regular and consistent, but if any two or more consecutive groups are combined an invariable lowering of the infant mortality rate from one such combined group to that next higher results.

1 "Ample" as used in this report has a somewhat arbitrary meaning. When information concerning the father's earnings was not available and the family showed no evidences of actual poverty, the word "ample" was used. If no information concerning earnings was available when, on the other hand, the family was clearly in a state of abject poverty, then the income was tabulated as "Under $521."

TABLE 30.—DISTRIBUTION OF LIVE BIRTHS AND OF DEATHS DURING FIRST YEAR, AND INFANT MORTALITY RATE, ACCORDING TO ANNUAL EARNINGS OF FATHER AND NATIVITY OF MOTHER, FOR LEGITIMATE LIVE-BORN BABIES.

| ANNUAL EARNINGS OF FATHER ACCORDING TO NATIVITY OF WIFE. | Total live births. | Deaths during first year. | Infant mortality rate. |
|---|---|---|---|
| Total | 1,431 | 187 | 130.7 |
| Under $625 | 384 | 82 | 213.5 |
| Under $521 | 219 | 56 | 255.7 |
| $521 to $624 | 165 | 26 | 157.6 |
| $625 to $899 | 385 | 47 | 122.1 |
| $625 to $779 | 224 | 24 | 107.1 |
| $780 to $899 | 161 | 23 | 142.9 |
| $900 or more | 186 | 18 | 96.8 |
| $900 to $1,199 | 138 | 14 | 101.4 |
| $1,200 or more | 48 | 4 | 83.3 |
| Ample [1] | 476 | 40 | 84.0 |
| Husbands with native wives | 785 | 76 | 96.8 |
| Under $625 | 80 | 16 | 200.0 |
| Under $521 | 32 | 9 | (2) |
| $521 to $624 | 48 | 7 | 145.8 |
| $625 to $899 | 193 | 20 | 103.6 |
| $625 to $779 | 86 | 6 | 69.8 |
| $780 to $899 | 107 | 14 | 130.8 |
| $900 or more | 129 | 10 | 77.5 |
| $900 to $1,199 | 92 | 7 | 76.1 |
| $1,200 or more | 37 | 3 | (2) |
| Ample [1] | 383 | 30 | 78.3 |
| Husbands with foreign wives | 646 | 111 | 171.8 |
| Under $625 | 304 | 66 | 217.1 |
| Under $521 | 187 | 47 | 251.3 |
| $521 to $624 | 117 | 19 | 162.4 |
| $625 to $899 | 192 | 27 | 140.6 |
| $625 to $779 | 138 | 18 | 130.4 |
| $780 to $899 | 54 | 9 | 166.7 |
| $900 or more | 57 | 8 | 140.6 |
| $900 to $1,199 | 46 | 7 | 152.2 |
| $1,200 or more | 11 | 1 | (2) |
| Ample | 93 | 10 | 107.5 |

[1] See note on page 45.
[2] Total live births less than 50; base therefore considered too small to use in computing an infant mortality rate.

In considering the babies of native and of foreign mothers separately in the foregoing table, similar variations in mortality rates according to earnings of father are found, although the foreign infant death rate is higher in each group. The foreign are less numerous both actually and relatively in the higher wage groups.

The foreigners of a given wage group almost always live in a poorer neighborhood than the natives earning the same amount. The foreigners go where they find their own countrymen, most of whom are poor, and hence even those who earn a fair wage find themselves, until they become Americanized, surrounded by poor conditions and an ignorant class of people.

It is of interest to note what per cent of the native and what per cent of the foreign are in the several earnings groups. The next table shows this for all married mothers and not simply for those of live-born babies as in the foregoing table.

TABLE 31.—NUMBER AND PER CENT OF MOTHERS BY NATIVITY, ACCORDING TO THE ANNUAL EARNINGS OF HUSBAND.

| ANNUAL EARNING OF HUSBAND. | ALL MOTHERS. | | NATIVE MOTHERS. | | FOREIGN MOTHERS. | |
|---|---|---|---|---|---|---|
| | Number. | Per cent. | Number. | Per cent. | Number. | Per cent. |
| Total | 1,491 | 100.0 | 816 | 100.0 | 675 | 100.0 |
| Under $521 | 233 | 15.6 | 36 | 4.4 | 197 | 29.2 |
| $521 to $624 | 174 | 11.7 | 50 | 6.1 | 124 | 18.4 |
| $625 to $779 | 229 | 15.4 | 86 | 10.5 | 143 | 21.2 |
| $780 to $899 | 166 | 11.1 | 108 | 13.2 | 58 | 8.6 |
| $900 to $1,199 | 146 | 9.8 | 98 | 12.0 | 48 | 7.1 |
| $1,200 and over | 50 | 3.4 | 39 | 4.8 | 11 | 1.6 |
| Ample[1] | 493 | 33.1 | 399 | 48.9 | 94 | 13.9 |

[1] See note on page 45.

The 1,491 married mothers included in the foregoing table bore 1,517 babies in 1911, the excess being due to plural births. The 33 unmarried mothers and their 34 babies (one mother had twins), although included in some of the general tables, are not included in those relative to the earnings of the husband.

## GAINFUL WORK OF MOTHER.

In localities where large numbers of women are engaged in industrial work, comparisons are frequently made of the death rates among their babies with those of the babies of mothers not so engaged. In Johnstown, however, industrial occupations are not open to women, and but 3.1 per cent of the mothers visited went outside their homes to earn money. All mothers who gained money by keeping lodgers or in any other way are, for convenience, designated "wage-earning" mothers, even though their earnings were not in the form of a definite wage at stated periods.

Although not industrially engaged, nearly one-fifth of the mothers did resort to some means of supplementing the earnings of their husbands. Usually they kept lodgers. This was done by the foreign mothers principally, exactly one-third of whom had lodgers, as compared with less than 1 per cent of the native women. Usually work done outside the home consisted either of char work or of assisting husbands in their stores. Generally these stores were in the same building with the home.

When a mother of a young baby does not give her full time to her duties within the home but resorts to means of earning money, it generally indicates poverty. This is true to a greater degree in Johnstown than in places which have many inducements for women to work. In Johnstown, with its excess of males, especially in the foreign population, the woman's services are particularly needed to make the home.

In the group where the husband earns $10 a week or less—that is, under $521 a year—many of the women are wage earners. In each group showing better earnings for the husband the number and percentage of wage-earning wives decline. Such a tabulation as the following almost automatically fixes the minimum wage on which a man, wife, and a child or two can live with any degree of comfort in Johnstown at about $780 a year. When the husband's wage is less than $780 a year, it is shown that the wives, in considerable number, must be wage earners. As shown in the next table, in nearly half of the families where the husband earns $10 a week or less (less than $521 a year), the wife resorted to some means of earning money; when he earned as much as $900 a year, only 8.9 per cent of the wives worked, and in the small group where the man earns as much as $1,200 a year, only 1 in 50.

TABLE 32.—NUMBER AND PER CENT OF HUSBANDS WITH WAGE-EARNING WIVES, BY NATIVITY OF WIFE AND ANNUAL EARNINGS OF HUSBAND.

| ANNUAL EARNINGS OF HUSBAND. | TOTAL HUSBANDS. | | | HUSBANDS HAVING NATIVE WIVES. | | | HUSBANDS HAVING FOREIGN WIVES. | | |
|---|---|---|---|---|---|---|---|---|---|
| | Number. | Husbands with wage-earning wives. | | Number. | Husbands with wage-earning wives. | | Number. | Husbands with wage-earning wives. | |
| | | Number. | Per cent. | | Number. | Per cent. | | Number. | Per cent. |
| Total | 1,491 | 278 | 18.6 | 816 | 26 | 3.2 | 675 | 252 | 37.3 |
| Under $521 | 233 | 111 | 47.6 | 36 | 9 | 25.0 | 197 | 102 | 51.8 |
| $521 to $624 | 174 | 57 | 32.8 | 50 | 3 | 6.0 | 124 | 54 | 43.5 |
| $625 to $779 | 229 | 51 | 22.3 | 86 | 4 | 4.7 | 143 | 47 | 32.9 |
| $780 to $899 | 166 | 25 | 15.1 | 108 | 6 | 5.6 | 58 | 19 | 32.8 |
| $900 to $1,199 | 146 | 13 | 8.9 | 98 | 1 | 1.0 | 48 | 12 | 25.0 |
| $1,200 and over | 50 | 1 | 2.0 | 39 | ........ | ........ | 11 | 1 | 9.1 |
| "Ample"[1] | 493 | 20 | 4.1 | 399 | 3 | .8 | 94 | 17 | 18.1 |

[1] See note on page 45.

It is impossible to judge from statistics alone whether or not the work done by an individual woman, either her own housework or work for money, is so excessive as to affect her during pregnancy or while nursing to the extent of reacting on the health of the baby; but the fact is that the infant mortality rate is higher among the babies of wage-earning mothers than among others, being 188 as compared with a rate of 117.6 among the babies of nonwage-earning mothers. Wage-earning mothers and low-wage fathers are in practically the same groups, and it is difficult to secure an exact measurement of the comparative weight of the two factors in the production of a high infant mortality rate.

TABLE 33.—DISTRIBUTION OF LIVE BIRTHS AND OF DEATHS DURING FIRST YEAR, AND INFANT MORTALITY RATE FOR BABIES OF WAGE-EARNING AND NONWAGE-EARNING MOTHERS, ACCORDING TO ANNUAL EARNINGS OF FATHER.

| ANNUAL EARNINGS OF FATHER. | MOTHER A WAGE EARNER. | | MOTHER NOT A WAGE EARNER. | | INFANT MORTALITY RATE. | |
|---|---|---|---|---|---|---|
| | Live births. | Number of deaths in first year. | Live births. | Number of deaths in first year. | Mother a wage earner. | Mother not a wage earner. |
| Total | 266 | 50 | 1,165 | 137 | 188.0 | 117.6 |
| Under $521 | 105 | 26 | 114 | 30 | 247.6 | 263.2 |
| $521 to $624 | 53 | 8 | 112 | 18 | 150.9 | 160.7 |
| $625 to $779 | 48 | 6 | 176 | 18 | 127.1 | 102.3 |
| $780 or over, or "ample"[1] | 60 | 10 | 763 | 71 | 166.7 | 93.1 |

[1] See note on page 45.

## ILLEGITIMACY.

Of the 1,551 births included in this investigation 34, or 2.2 per cent, occurred out of wedlock. Nine of the 32 illegitimate babies who were born alive died during their first year. It is recognized that these figures are a very small base from which to draw conclusions concerning the effect of illegitimacy on the infant mortality rate. It is of interest, nevertheless, to note that the findings for this small group are similar to those of countries which compute an infant mortality rate for legitimate and illegitimate children separately, that is, a rate for illegitimates more than twice as high as for children born in wedlock.

TABLE 34.—DISTRIBUTION OF BIRTHS AND OF DEATHS DURING FIRST YEAR, AND INFANT MORTALITY RATE, ACCORDING TO LEGITIMACY.

| LEGITIMACY. | Total births. | Live births. | DEATHS DURING FIRST YEAR. | |
|---|---|---|---|---|
| | | | Number. | Infant mortality rates. |
| Illegitimate | 34 | 32 | 9 | 281.3 |
| Legitimate | 1,517 | 1,431 | 187 | 130.7 |

Thirty-two, or 3.7 per cent, of the 860 native mothers, as compared with 2, or 0.3 per cent, of the 691 foreign mothers visited, had illegitimate children in 1911.

61112°—15——4

## REPRODUCTIVE HISTORIES.

In addition to the data relating exclusively to babies born in 1911, a statement was secured from each mother as to the number and duration of each of her pregnancies and the result thereof; that is, the number of children she had borne, alive or dead, the number of miscarriages she had had, and the age at death of each live-born child who had died. Although this information was secured for all mothers, tabulations are presented of the data furnished by married mothers only. Comparatively few single mothers reported more than one child, and information from them on this point is not believed to be as reliable as that from married mothers.

The 1,491 married mothers of babies born in 1911 had had an aggregate of 5,554 pregnancies, resulting in 5,617 births, the excess of 63 births over pregnancies being due to plural births. Eight hundred and four of these children died under 1 year of age, making an infant mortality rate of 149.9 for all their babies, as compared with the rate of 134 for those born in 1911. The stillbirths of these women numbered 194, or 4.5 per cent of the total number of births; miscarriages reported numbered 191, but these were not added to the total reportable[1] pregnancies.

Details as to the infant mortality rates for all babies born to native and foreign mothers included in this study, not only in the year 1911 but at any other time, are presented in the next table, which classifies the babies according to the total number of reportable pregnancies that their mothers had had, to and including the pregnancy resulting in the 1911 birth.

TABLE 35.—DISTRIBUTION OF MOTHERS, OF LIVE BIRTHS, AND OF DEATHS DURING FIRST YEAR, AND INFANT MORTALITY RATE FOR BABIES OF NATIVE AND FOREIGN MARRIED MOTHERS, ACCORDING TO THE NUMBER OF REPORTABLE PREGNANCIES.

| REPORTABLE PREGNANCIES FOR MARRIED MOTHERS. | Number of married mothers. | NUMBER OF BABIES. | | INFANT MORTALITY RATE AMONG BABIES OF— | | |
|---|---|---|---|---|---|---|
| | | Born alive. | Died in first year. | All mothers. | Native mothers. | Foreign mothers. |
| Total | 1,491 | 5,363 | 804 | 149.9 | 113.1 | 184.6 |
| 1 | 339 | 322 | 35 | 108.7 | 75.9 | 183.7 |
| 2 | 283 | 544 | 59 | 108.5 | 76.5 | 156.7 |
| 3 | 214 | 626 | 92 | 147.0 | 118.0 | 177.6 |
| 4 | 186 | 723 | 78 | 107.9 | 99.4 | 116.3 |
| 5 | 147 | 704 | 103 | 146.3 | 86.1 | 191.5 |
| 6 | 94 | 546 | 88 | 161.2 | 157.4 | 163.6 |
| 7 | 83 | 555 | 78 | 140.5 | 100.0 | 173.8 |
| 8 | 54 | 426 | 95 | 223.0 | 157.6 | 272.7 |
| 9 | 33 | 283 | 41 | 144.9 | 128.4 | 155.2 |
| 10 or more | 58 | 634 | 135 | 212.9 | 164.5 | 257.6 |

The statistics, based upon the results of all her reportable pregnancies, show a generally higher infant mortality rate where the mother has had many pregnancies, but there is not always an increase from

[1] "Reportable" pregnancies are those terminating either in the birth of a live child or of a dead child when the period of gestation exceeds 28 weeks; that is, when its registration or report is required by law.

one pregnancy to the next. This is more clearly shown when the pregnancies are grouped as in the next table.

TABLE 36.—INFANT MORTALITY RATE FOR ALL CHILDREN BORNE BY MARRIED MOTHERS, ACCORDING TO SPECIFIED NUMBER OF REPORTABLE PREGNANCIES.

| REPORTABLE PREGNANCIES FOR MARRIED MOTHERS. | Infant mortality rate. |
|---|---|
| Total | 149.9 |
| 1 and 2 | 108.5 |
| 3 and 4 | 126.0 |
| 5 and 6 | 152.8 |
| 7 and 8 | 176.4 |
| 9 or more | 191.9 |

This tendency is shown in still another form of summary: Combinations of four or less pregnancies are, for convenience, considered as group 1, while the combinations of over four are designated group 2. The differences in rates in the two groups are notable. The infant mortality rate is much lower for the first than for the second group.

TABLE 37.—INFANT MORTALITY RATE FOR ALL CHILDREN BORNE BY MARRIED MOTHERS, ACCORDING TO SPECIFIED NUMBER OF REPORTABLE PREGNANCIES, BY GROUPS.

| REPORTABLE PREGNANCIES FOR MARRIED MOTHERS. | Infant mortality rate. | REPORTABLE PREGNANCIES FOR MARRIED MOTHERS. | Infant mortality rate. |
|---|---|---|---|
| GROUP 1. | | GROUP 2. | |
| 2 or less | 108.5 | Over 4 | 171.5 |
| 3 or less | 124.7 | Over 5 | 178.8 |
| 4 or less | 119.2 | Over 6 | 183.9 |

This influence of the size of the family upon the infant mortality rate is shown in the computations giving the relative infant mortality rate for the different children borne by married mothers. The rate is most favorable for the second-born child, being 131.2. Among first born it is 143.6; for tenth or later born children 252.3.

TABLE 38.—INFANT MORTALITY RATE FOR ALL CHILDREN BORNE BY MARRIED MOTHERS, ACCORDING TO THE ORDER IN WHICH THE CHILD WAS BORN.

| ORDER OF BIRTH. | Infant mortality rate. | ORDER OF BIRTH. | Infant mortality rate. |
|---|---|---|---|
| First-born child | 143.6 | Seventh-born child | 192.1 |
| Second-born child | 131.2 | Eighth-born child | 165.4 |
| First and second born children | 138.3 | Seventh and eighth born children | 181.5 |
| Third-born child | 144.2 | Ninth-born child | 128.2 |
| Fourth-born child | 142.0 | Tenth or later born child | 252.3 |
| Third and fourth born children | 143.2 | Ninth and later born children | 201.1 |
| Fifth-born child | 178.1 | | |
| Sixth-born child | 175.5 | | |
| Fifth and sixth born children | 177.0 | | |

The next table gives a further elaboration of the same data; that is, it shows the infant mortality rate where such rates are lowest and highest, respectively, according to the age of the mother at the child's birth and the order in which the child was born. Attention is again directed to the fact that the statistics presented in this section on "Reproductive histories" are based upon the total number of reportable pregnancies; that is, in addition to the pregnancies resulting in births in 1911, all prior pregnancies of the women considered in the investigation have been included.

TABLE 39.—LOWEST AND HIGHEST INFANT MORTALITY RATES, ACCORDING TO AGE OF MOTHER AT BIRTH OF CHILD AND THE ORDER IN WHICH CHILD WAS BORN.

| ORDER OF BIRTH. | INFANT MORTALITY RATES, ACCORDING TO MOTHER'S AGE. | | | |
|---|---|---|---|---|
| | Lowest mortality. | | Highest mortality. | |
| | Mother's age. | Mortality rate. | Mother's age. | Mortality rate. |
| All children | 20–24 | 140.0 | Under 17 | 367.3 |
| First child | 25–29 | 92.1 | 17–19 | 190.4 |
| Second child | 25–29 | 100.3 | 17–19 | 178.6 |
| Third child | 30–39 | 106.4 | 25–29 | 160.8 |
| Fourth child | 30–39 | 122.4 | 20–24 | 155.0 |
| Fifth child | 30–39 | 105.8 | 25–29 | 236.6 |
| Sixth child | 30–39 | 164.8 | 25–29 | 171.4 |

The differences in size of family for native and foreign mothers of different ages are indicated in the next table. The total and average number of live-born children, not reportable pregnancies, are given.

TABLE 40.—TOTAL AND AVERAGE NUMBER OF LIVE-BORN CHILDREN BORNE BY MARRIED MOTHERS HAVING EITHER A LIVE BIRTH OR A STILLBIRTH IN 1911, CLASSIFIED BY NATIVITY AND AGE OF MOTHER.

| AGE OF MOTHER AT BIRTH OF CHILD IN 1911. | ALL MARRIED MOTHERS. | | | NATIVE MARRIED MOTHERS. | | | FOREIGN MARRIED MOTHERS. | | |
|---|---|---|---|---|---|---|---|---|---|
| | Total. | Live-born children. | | Total. | Live-born children. | | Total. | Live-born children. | |
| | | Number. | Average. | | Number. | Average. | | Number. | Average. |
| All ages | 1,465 | 5,363 | 3.7 | 801 | 2,600 | 3.2 | 664 | 2,763 | 4.2 |
| Under 20 years | 81 | 96 | 1.2 | 62 | 70 | 1.1 | 19 | 26 | 1.4 |
| 20 to 24 years | 456 | 908 | 2.0 | 258 | 483 | 1.9 | 198 | 425 | 2.1 |
| 25 to 29 years | 389 | 1,261 | 3.2 | 196 | 536 | 2.7 | 193 | 725 | 3.8 |
| 30 to 39 years | 459 | 2,480 | 5.4 | 240 | 1,188 | 5.0 | 219 | 1,292 | 5.9 |
| 40 years and over | 80 | 618 | 7.7 | 45 | 323 | 7.2 | 35 | 295 | 8.4 |

The next table shows all losses of pregnancy sustained by 628 mothers and the rate of loss per 1,000 births for mothers having different numbers of births or reportable pregnancies. For all mothers it was 188.4. "Loss," as here used, means the sum of infant deaths (or deaths in first year) and stillbirths.

TABLE 41.—AGGREGATE NUMBER OF BIRTHS, LOSSES, AND RATE OF LOSS PER 1,000 BIRTHS, ACCORDING TO NUMBER OF BIRTHS PER MOTHER.

| NUMBER OF BIRTHS PER MOTHER. | Aggregate number of births. | Aggregate number of losses. | Rate of loss per 1,000 births. |
|---|---|---|---|
| Total | 5,617 | 1,058 | 188.4 |
| 1 | 335 | 53 | 158.6 |
| 2 | 554 | 87 | 157.0 |
| 3 | 648 | 113 | 174.4 |
| 4 | 748 | 109 | 145.7 |
| 5 | 740 | 133 | 179.7 |
| 6 | 576 | 119 | 206.6 |
| 7 | 574 | 104 | 181.2 |
| 8 | 432 | 102 | 236.1 |
| 9 | 324 | 65 | 200.6 |
| 10 or more | 686 | 173 | 252.2 |

The influence of the economic factor on infant mortality among the babies born prior to 1911 can not be determined with exactness, as no inquiry was made concerning earnings of the father when the other children were born. But it is believed that his earnings during the year following the birth of the 1911 baby can be regarded as an index of the economic standing of the family for some time past. In individual cases, of course, revolutionary changes in the family's income may have occurred, but for the great mass of people in the group considered it is not likely that within such a short space of time as that covered by the child-bearing period of the women considered—most of whom had not had numerous pregnancies—marked changes had taken place. If these known earnings are accepted as an index, the following variations are found to occur in the infant mortality rate for all the babies of whom a record was secured:

TABLE 42.—INFANT MORTALITY RATE FOR ALL CHILDREN OF MARRIED MOTHERS INCLUDED IN THIS INVESTIGATION, DISTRIBUTED ACCORDING TO THE FATHER'S EARNINGS.

| FATHER'S ANNUAL EARNINGS. | Infant mortality rate. | FATHER'S ANNUAL EARNINGS. | Infant mortality rate. |
|---|---|---|---|
| Under $521 | 197.3 | $780 to $899 | 168.4 |
| $521 to $624 | 193.1 | $900 to $1,199 | 142.3 |
| $625 to $779 | 163.1 | $1,200 and over | 102.2 |

The infant mortality rate for the babies whose fathers earn under $521 is almost twice as great as for those born into families in the most prosperous group. These figures strengthen the conclusion reached in the study of the babies born in 1911, namely that the economic factor is of far-reaching importance in determining the baby's chance of life.

# GENERAL TABLES.

# GENERAL TABLES.

TABLE I.—DISTRIBUTION OF BIRTHS ACCORDING TO NATIONALITY OF MOTHER, BY SECTION OF CITY AND WARD.

| SECTION OF CITY AND WARD. | Births to all mothers.[1] | Births to native mothers. | BIRTHS TO FOREIGN MOTHERS. | | | | | | | | |
|---|---|---|---|---|---|---|---|---|---|---|---|
| | | | Total. | Slovaks, Poles, etc. | Croatians, Servians, etc. | Italians. | Germans. | Magyars. | British. | Syrians and Greeks. | Hebrew. |
| All sections | 1,551 | 860 | 691 | 394 | 76 | 75 | 53 | 38 | 33 | 12 | 10 |
| Down town | 87 | 69 | 18 | | | 2 | 3 | | 7 | 4 | 2 |
| Ward 1 | 42 | 36 | 6 | | | | 2 | | 3 | | 1 |
| Ward 2 | 20 | 14 | 6 | | | | 1 | | 4 | 1 | |
| Ward 3 | 11 | 6 | 5 | | | 2 | | | | 2 | 1 |
| Ward 4 | 14 | 13 | 1 | | | | | | | 1 | |
| Kernville | 106 | 100 | 6 | | | 1 | 2 | | 2 | | 1 |
| Ward 5 | 34 | 33 | 1 | | | 1 | | | | | |
| Ward 6 | 72 | 67 | 5 | | | | 2 | | 2 | | 1 |
| Hornerstown—Ward 7 | 118 | 107 | 11 | | | 5 | 3 | | 2 | | 1 |
| Roxbury—Ward 8 | 90 | 83 | 7 | 4 | | | | | 3 | | |
| Conemaugh Borough | 142 | 78 | 64 | 18 | | 41 | 3 | | 1 | 1 | |
| Ward 9 | 75 | 48 | 27 | 1 | | 24 | 1 | | | 1 | |
| Ward 10 | 67 | 30 | 37 | 17 | | 17 | 2 | | 1 | | |
| Woodvale—Ward 11 | 113 | 25 | 88 | 49 | 11 | 6 | 14 | 6 | 1 | | 1 |
| Prospect—Ward 12 | 57 | 33 | 24 | | | 17 | 3 | | 4 | | |
| Peelorville—Ward 13 | 20 | 18 | 2 | | | | 1 | | | | 1 |
| Minersville—Ward 14 | 77 | 18 | 59 | 52 | | | 3 | | 2 | | 2 |
| Cambria City | 330 | 31 | 299 | 204 | 59 | | 5 | 21 | 4 | 4 | 2 |
| Ward 15 | 105 | 7 | 98 | 65 | 22 | | 1 | 6 | | 2 | 2 |
| Ward 16 | 225 | 24 | 201 | 139 | 37 | | 4 | 15 | 4 | 2 | |
| Moxham—Ward 17 | 169 | 133 | 36 | 21 | | 1 | 4 | 4 | 4 | 2 | |
| Morrellville | 204 | 135 | 69 | 42 | 6 | 1 | 11 | 5 | 3 | 1 | |
| Ward 18 | 89 | 44 | 45 | 30 | 6 | | 7 | | 2 | | |
| Ward 19 | 55 | 45 | 10 | 4 | | 1 | 2 | 2 | 1 | | |
| Ward 20 | 60 | 46 | 14 | 8 | | | 2 | 3 | | 1 | |
| Coopersdale—Ward 21 | 38 | 30 | 8 | 4 | | 1 | 1 | 2 | | | |

[1] Includes both legitimate and illegitimate births.

TABLE II.—DISTRIBUTION OF BIRTHS, LIVE BIRTHS, STILLBIRTHS, AND DEATHS IN FIRST YEAR, ACCORDING TO NATIVITY OF MOTHER, BY SECTION OF CITY AND WARD.

| SECTION OF CITY AND WARD. | ALL MOTHERS.[1] | | | | NATIVE MOTHERS.[1] | | | | FOREIGN MOTHERS.[1] | | | |
|---|---|---|---|---|---|---|---|---|---|---|---|---|
| | All births. | Live births. | Stillbirths. | Deaths in first year. | All births. | Live births. | Stillbirths. | Deaths in first year. | All births. | Live births. | Stillbirths. | Deaths in first year. |
| All sections | 1,551 | 1,463 | 88 | 196 | 860 | 815 | 45 | 85 | 691 | 648 | 43 | 111 |
| Down town | 87 | 80 | 7 | 4 | 69 | 63 | 6 | 4 | 18 | 17 | 1 | ..... |
| Ward 1 | 42 | 40 | 2 | 2 | 36 | 34 | 2 | 2 | 6 | 6 | ..... | ..... |
| Ward 2 | 20 | 17 | 3 | 1 | 14 | 12 | 2 | 1 | 6 | 5 | 1 | ..... |
| Ward 3 | 11 | 10 | 1 | ..... | 6 | 5 | 1 | ..... | 5 | 5 | ..... | ..... |
| Ward 4 | 14 | 13 | 1 | 1 | 13 | 12 | 1 | 1 | 1 | 1 | ..... | ..... |
| Kernville | 106 | 104 | 2 | 6 | 100 | 98 | 2 | 5 | 6 | 6 | ..... | 1 |
| Ward 5 | 34 | 34 | ..... | 3 | 33 | 33 | ..... | 2 | 1 | 1 | ..... | 1 |
| Ward 6 | 72 | 70 | 2 | 3 | 67 | 65 | 2 | 3 | 5 | 5 | ..... | ..... |
| Hornerstown—Ward 7 | 118 | 109 | 9 | 17 | 107 | 100 | 7 | 16 | 11 | 9 | 2 | 1 |
| Roxbury—Ward 8 | 90 | 85 | 5 | 10 | 83 | 79 | 4 | 8 | 7 | 6 | 1 | 2 |
| Conemaugh Borough | 142 | 136 | 6 | 16 | 78 | 75 | 3 | 6 | 64 | 61 | 3 | 10 |
| Ward 9 | 75 | 72 | 3 | 10 | 48 | 46 | 2 | 3 | 27 | 26 | 1 | 7 |
| Ward 10 | 67 | 64 | 3 | 6 | 30 | 29 | 1 | 3 | 37 | 35 | 2 | 3 |
| Woodvale—Ward 11 | 113 | 107 | 6 | 29 | 25 | 24 | 1 | 6 | 88 | 83 | 5 | 23 |
| Prospect—Ward 12 | 57 | 55 | 2 | 11 | 33 | 33 | ..... | 8 | 24 | 22 | 2 | 3 |
| Peelorville—Ward 13 | 20 | 18 | 2 | 1 | 18 | 16 | 2 | 1 | 2 | 2 | ..... | ..... |
| Minersville—Ward 14 | 77 | 72 | 5 | 9 | 18 | 17 | 1 | 3 | 59 | 55 | 4 | 6 |
| Cambria City | 330 | 310 | 20 | 55 | 31 | 29 | 2 | 4 | 299 | 281 | 18 | 51 |
| Ward 15 | 105 | 98 | 7 | 20 | 7 | 6 | 1 | 1 | 98 | 92 | 6 | 19 |
| Ward 16 | 225 | 212 | 13 | 35 | 24 | 23 | 1 | 3 | 201 | 189 | 12 | 32 |
| Moxham—Ward 17 | 169 | 157 | 12 | 14 | 133 | 124 | 9 | 10 | 36 | 33 | 3 | 4 |
| Morrellville | 204 | 194 | 10 | 16 | 135 | 129 | 6 | 10 | 69 | 65 | 4 | 6 |
| Ward 18 | 89 | 85 | 4 | 8 | 44 | 43 | 1 | 4 | 45 | 42 | 3 | 4 |
| Ward 19 | 55 | 52 | 3 | 5 | 45 | 42 | 3 | 3 | 10 | 10 | ..... | 2 |
| Ward 20 | 60 | 57 | 3 | 3 | 46 | 44 | 2 | 3 | 14 | 13 | 1 | ..... |
| Coopersdale—Ward 21 | 38 | 36 | 2 | 8 | 30 | 28 | 2 | 4 | 8 | 8 | ..... | 4 |

[1] Includes both married and unmarried mothers.

TABLE III.—DISTRIBUTION OF BIRTHS TO NATIVE AND FOREIGN MARRIED MOTHERS AND NUMBER AND PER CENT OF BIRTHS IN EACH GROUP TO THOSE GAINFULLY EMPLOYED, BY SECTION OF CITY.

| SECTION OF CITY. | BIRTHS TO MARRIED MOTHERS. | | | | | | | | |
|---|---|---|---|---|---|---|---|---|---|
| | All. | | | Native. | | | Foreign. | | |
| | Total. | Gainfully employed. | | Total. | Gainfully employed. | | Total. | Gainfully employed. | |
| | | Number. | Per cent.[1] | | Number. | Per cent.[1] | | Number. | Per cent.[1] |
| All sections | 1,517 | 281 | 18.5 | 828 | 26 | 3.1 | 689 | 255 | 37.0 |
| Down town | 86 | 4 | 4.7 | 68 | 2 | 2.9 | 18 | 2 | ........ |
| Kernville | 104 | 3 | 2.9 | 98 | 3 | 3.1 | 6 | ........ | ........ |
| Hornerstown | 112 | 1 | .9 | 101 | 1 | 1.0 | 11 | ........ | ........ |
| Roxbury | 85 | 1 | 1.2 | 78 | 1 | 1.3 | 7 | ........ | ........ |
| Conemaugh Borough | 143 | 40 | 28.0 | 78 | 4 | 5.1 | 65 | 36 | 55.4 |
| Woodvale | 110 | 50 | 45.5 | 23 | 2 | ........ | 87 | 48 | 55.2 |
| Prospect | 52 | 6 | 11.5 | 28 | 2 | ........ | 24 | 4 | ........ |
| Peelorville | 19 | 1 | ........ | 17 | 1 | ........ | 2 | ........ | ........ |
| Minersville | 75 | 23 | 30.7 | 17 | 1 | ........ | 58 | 22 | 37.9 |
| Cambria City | 329 | 121 | 36.8 | 31 | 1 | ........ | 298 | 120 | 40.3 |
| Moxham | 167 | 18 | 10.8 | 131 | 2 | 1.5 | 36 | 16 | ........ |
| Morrellville | 197 | 11 | 5.6 | 128 | 6 | 4.7 | 69 | 5 | 7.2 |
| Coopersdale | 38 | 2 | ........ | 30 | ........ | ........ | 8 | 2 | ........ |

[1] Not shown when base is less than 50.

TABLE IV.—DISTRIBUTION OF BIRTHS TO MARRIED MOTHERS ACCORDING TO ATTENDANT AT BIRTH AND TO NATIVITY OF MOTHER, BY SECTION OF CITY AND WARD.

| SECTION OF CITY AND WARD. | ATTENDANT AT BIRTH | | | | | | | | | | | |
|---|---|---|---|---|---|---|---|---|---|---|---|---|
| | All married mothers. | | | | Native married mothers. | | | | Foreign married mothers. | | | |
| | All births. | Physician. | Midwife. | Other or none. | All births. | Physician. | Midwife. | Other or none. | All births. | Physician. | Midwife. | Other or none. |
| All sections | 1,517 | 877 | 605 | 35 | 828 | 743 | 83 | 2 | 689 | 134 | 522 | 33 |
| Down town | 86 | 80 | 6 | ..... | 68 | 66 | 2 | ..... | 18 | 14 | 4 | ..... |
| Ward 1 | 42 | 41 | 1 | ..... | 36 | 36 | ..... | ..... | 6 | 5 | 1 | ..... |
| Ward 2 | 20 | 19 | 1 | ..... | 14 | 14 | ..... | ..... | 6 | 5 | 1 | ..... |
| Ward 3 | 10 | 8 | 2 | ..... | 5 | 5 | ..... | ..... | 5 | 3 | 2 | ..... |
| Ward 4 | 14 | 12 | 2 | ..... | 13 | 11 | 2 | ..... | 1 | 1 | ..... | ..... |
| Kernville | 104 | 94 | 10 | ..... | 98 | 91 | 7 | ..... | 6 | 3 | 3 | ..... |
| Ward 5 | 34 | 32 | 2 | ..... | 33 | 32 | 1 | ..... | 1 | ..... | 1 | ..... |
| Ward 6 | 70 | 62 | 8 | ..... | 65 | 59 | 6 | ..... | 5 | 3 | 2 | ..... |
| Hornerstown—Ward 7 | 112 | 93 | 18 | 1 | 101 | 89 | 11 | 1 | 11 | 4 | 7 | ..... |
| Roxbury—Ward 8 | 85 | 78 | 7 | ..... | 78 | 73 | 5 | ..... | 7 | 5 | 2 | ..... |
| Conemaugh Borough | 143 | 72 | 70 | 1 | 78 | 66 | 11 | 1 | 65 | 6 | 59 | ..... |
| Ward 9 | 75 | 47 | 28 | ..... | 48 | 44 | 4 | ..... | 27 | 3 | 24 | ..... |
| Ward 10 | 68 | 25 | 42 | 1 | 30 | 22 | 7 | 1 | 38 | 3 | 35 | ..... |
| Woodvale—Ward 11 | 110 | 32 | 71 | 7 | 23 | 18 | 5 | ..... | 87 | 14 | 66 | 7 |
| Prospect—Ward 12 | 52 | 31 | 21 | ..... | 28 | 23 | 5 | ..... | 24 | 8 | 16 | ..... |
| Peelorville—Ward 13 | 19 | 15 | 4 | ..... | 17 | 13 | 4 | ..... | 2 | 2 | ..... | ..... |
| Minersville—Ward 14 | 75 | 24 | 47 | 4 | 17 | 13 | 4 | ..... | 58 | 11 | 43 | 4 |
| Cambria City | 329 | 53 | 255 | 21 | 31 | 26 | 5 | ..... | 298 | 27 | 250 | 21 |
| Ward 15 | 105 | 11 | 88 | 6 | 7 | 4 | 3 | ..... | 98 | 7 | 85 | 6 |
| Ward 16 | 224 | 42 | 167 | 15 | 24 | 22 | 2 | ..... | 200 | 20 | 165 | 15 |
| Moxham—Ward 17 | 167 | 140 | 26 | 1 | 131 | 123 | 8 | ..... | 36 | 17 | 18 | 1 |
| Morrellville | 197 | 133 | 64 | ..... | 128 | 113 | 15 | ..... | 69 | 20 | 49 | ..... |
| Ward 18 | 87 | 46 | 41 | ..... | 42 | 36 | 6 | ..... | 45 | 10 | 35 | ..... |
| Ward 19 | 55 | 48 | 7 | ..... | 45 | 42 | 3 | ..... | 10 | 6 | 4 | ..... |
| Ward 20 | 55 | 39 | 16 | ..... | 41 | 35 | 6 | ..... | 14 | 4 | 10 | ..... |
| Coopersdale—Ward 21 | 38 | 32 | 6 | ..... | 30 | 29 | 1 | ..... | 8 | 3 | 5 | ..... |

TABLE V.—DISTRIBUTION OF LIVE BIRTHS AND OF DEATHS DURING FIRST YEAR, ACCORDING TO NUMBER OF PERSONS AND NUMBER OF ROOMS PER FAMILY.

| PERSONS PER FAMILY (NOT INCLUDING BABY). | | All live-born babies. | NUMBER OF BABIES WHO WERE BORN ALIVE AND NUMBER OF SUCH BABIES WHO DIED DURING FIRST YEAR IN HOMES HAVING— | | | | | | | | | | |
|---|---|---|---|---|---|---|---|---|---|---|---|---|---|
| | | | 1 room. | 2 rooms. | 3 rooms. | 4 rooms. | 5 rooms. | 6 rooms. | 7 rooms. | 8 rooms. | 9 rooms. | 10 rooms and over. | Unknown number of rooms. |
| Total | Births | 1,463 | 33 | 165 | 147 | 526 | 222 | 233 | 38 | 43 | 22 | 12 | 22 |
| | Deaths | 196 | 3 | 29 | 24 | 79 | 20 | 20 | 6 | 6 | 4 | 2 | 3 |
| 2 | Births | 24 | 3 | 7 | 4 | 6 | 2 | | | | | | 2 |
| | Deaths | 19 | 1 | 5 | 4 | 6 | 1 | | | | | | 2 |
| 3 | Births | 275 | 14 | 46 | 35 | 96 | 29 | 37 | 4 | 6 | 1 | | 7 |
| | Deaths | 31 | | 5 | 4 | 12 | 2 | 3 | 3 | 2 | | | |
| 4 | Births | 234 | 7 | 44 | 20 | 83 | 40 | 23 | 4 | 5 | 2 | 2 | 4 |
| | Deaths | 30 | 1 | 12 | 5 | 9 | 2 | | | | | 1 | |
| 5 | Births | 229 | | 27 | 24 | 88 | 31 | 43 | 4 | 5 | 1 | 1 | 5 |
| | Deaths | 22 | | 1 | 6 | 9 | 1 | 4 | | 1 | | | |
| 6 | Births | 182 | 2 | 21 | 17 | 56 | 37 | 34 | 5 | 7 | 2 | | 1 |
| | Deaths | 18 | | 4 | | 8 | 2 | 3 | | 1 | | | |
| 7 | Births | 164 | 2 | 10 | 20 | 50 | 32 | 30 | 9 | 6 | 3 | 1 | 1 |
| | Deaths | 15 | | 1 | 2 | 6 | 1 | 3 | 1 | | 1 | | |
| 8 | Births | 107 | 2 | 5 | 14 | 37 | 16 | 18 | 4 | 6 | 2 | 3 | |
| | Deaths | 17 | | | 2 | 6 | 3 | 1 | 2 | 1 | 1 | 1 | |
| 9 | Births | 79 | 2 | 2 | 6 | 27 | 13 | 13 | 6 | 2 | 4 | 4 | |
| | Deaths | 8 | 1 | | | 2 | 2 | 1 | | | 2 | | |
| 10 | Births | 58 | 1 | 1 | 2 | 26 | 7 | 15 | 1 | 1 | 3 | | 1 |
| | Deaths | 15 | | | 1 | 11 | 2 | 1 | | | | | |
| 11 | Births | 36 | | 1 | 1 | 16 | 3 | 10 | | 3 | 2 | | |
| | Deaths | 4 | | 1 | | 1 | 1 | 1 | | | | | |
| 12 | Births | 21 | | 1 | 1 | 10 | 2 | 6 | | 1 | | | |
| | Deaths | 5 | | | | 2 | 1 | 1 | | 1 | | | |
| 13 | Births | 20 | | | 1 | 13 | 4 | | | | 1 | 1 | |
| | Deaths | 4 | | | | 3 | 1 | | | | | | |
| 14 | Births | 8 | | | 1 | 5 | 2 | | | | | | |
| | Deaths | 2 | | | | 1 | 1 | | | | | | |
| 15 | Births | 6 | | | | 3 | 2 | | | | | | 1 |
| | Deaths | 1 | | | | | | | | | | | 1 |
| 16 | Births | 4 | | | | 4 | | | | | | | |
| | Deaths | 2 | | | | 2 | | | | | | | |
| 17 | Births | 3 | | | | 1 | | 1 | | 1 | | | |
| | Deaths | | | | | | | | | | | | |
| 18 | Births | 5 | | | 1 | 1 | | 1 | 1 | | 1 | | |
| | Deaths | 1 | | | | 1 | | | | | | | |
| 19 | Births | 2 | | | | 2 | | | | | | | |
| | Deaths | | | | | | | | | | | | |
| 20 | Births | 3 | | | | 1 | 1 | 1 | | | | | |
| | Deaths | 1 | | | | | | 1 | | | | | |
| 22 | Births | 1 | | | | | | 1 | | | | | |
| | Deaths | 1 | | | | | | 1 | | | | | |
| 23 | Births | 1 | | | | 1 | | | | | | | |
| | Deaths | | | | | | | | | | | | |
| Not reported | Births | 1 | | | | | 1 | | | | | | |
| | Deaths | | | | | | | | | | | | |

TABLE VI.—DISTRIBUTION OF BIRTHS, LIVE BIRTHS, STILLBIRTHS, AND OF DEATHS DURING FIRST YEAR, ACCORDING TO NATIONALITY (DETAILED) OF MOTHER.

| NATIONALITY OF MOTHER. | All births. | Live births. | Still-births. | Deaths during first year. |
|---|---|---|---|---|
| All mothers | 1,551 | 1,463 | 88 | 196 |
| Native mothers | 860 | 815 | 45 | 85 |
| Foreign mothers | 691 | 648 | 43 | 111 |
| Slovak, Polish, etc | 394 | 367 | 27 | 65 |
| Slovak | 276 | 258 | 18 | 48 |
| Polish | 108 | 100 | 8 | 14 |
| Bohemian | 2 | 2 | | |
| Ruthenian or Russniak | 7 | 6 | 1 | 3 |
| Danish | 1 | 1 | | |
| Croatian, Servian, etc | 76 | 72 | 4 | 19 |
| Croatian | 34 | 32 | 2 | 8 |
| Servian | 39 | 37 | 2 | 10 |
| Krainer | 3 | 3 | | 1 |
| Italian | 75 | 71 | 4 | 13 |
| German | 53 | 47 | 6 | 6 |
| Magyar | 38 | 38 | | 4 |
| British | 33 | 31 | 2 | 4 |
| English | 12 | 12 | | 2 |
| Irish | 13 | 13 | | 2 |
| Scotch | 4 | 3 | 1 | |
| Welsh | 4 | 3 | 1 | |
| Syrian and Greek | 12 | 12 | | |
| Syrian | 10 | 10 | | |
| Greek | 2 | 2 | | |
| Hebrew | 10 | 10 | | |

TABLE VII.—DISTRIBUTION OF BIRTHS, LIVE BIRTHS, STILLBIRTHS, AND OF DEATHS DURING FIRST YEAR, ACCORDING TO ATTENDANT AT BABY'S BIRTH AND NATIONALITY OF MOTHER.

| ATTENDANT AT BABY'S BIRTH AND NATIONALITY OF MOTHER. | All births. | Live births. | Stillbirths. | Deaths in first year. |
|---|---|---|---|---|
| All mothers | 1,551 | 1,463 | 88 | 196 |
| Physician | 928 | 866 | 62 | 87 |
| Midwife | 588 | 562 | 26 | 101 |
| Other | 14 | 14 | | 5 |
| None | 21 | 21 | | 3 |
| Native mothers | 860 | 815 | 45 | 85 |
| Physician | 774 | 730 | 44 | 68 |
| Midwife | 84 | 83 | 1 | 15 |
| Other | 2 | 2 | | 2 |
| Foreign mothers | 691 | 648 | 43 | 111 |
| Physician | 154 | 136 | 18 | 19 |
| Midwife | 504 | 479 | 25 | 86 |
| Other | 12 | 12 | | 3 |
| None | 21 | 21 | | 3 |
| Slovak, Polish, etc | 394 | 367 | 27 | 65 |
| Physician | 45 | 36 | 9 | 10 |
| Midwife | 340 | 322 | 18 | 54 |
| Other | 2 | 2 | | 1 |
| None | 7 | 7 | | |
| Croatian, Servian, etc | 76 | 72 | 4 | 19 |
| Physician | 31 | 28 | 3 | 2 |
| Midwife | 22 | 21 | 1 | 12 |
| Other | 9 | 9 | | 2 |
| None | 14 | 14 | | 3 |
| Italian | 75 | 71 | 4 | 13 |
| Physician | 4 | 4 | | 1 |
| Midwife | 71 | 67 | 4 | 12 |
| German | 53 | 47 | 6 | 6 |
| Physician | 27 | 23 | 4 | 3 |
| Midwife | 26 | 24 | 2 | 3 |
| Magyar | 38 | 38 | | 4 |
| Physician | 7 | 7 | | 1 |
| Midwife | 31 | 31 | | 3 |
| British | 33 | 31 | 2 | 4 |
| Physician | 29 | 27 | 2 | 2 |
| Midwife | 3 | 3 | | 2 |
| Other | 1 | 1 | | |
| Syrian and Greek | 12 | 12 | | |
| Physician | 3 | 3 | | |
| Midwife | 9 | 9 | | |
| Hebrew | 10 | 10 | | |
| Physician | 8 | 8 | | |
| Midwife | 2 | 2 | | |

TABLE VIII.—DISTRIBUTION OF DEATHS OF INFANTS AT SPECIFIED AGE, ACCORDING TO CAUSE OF DEATH OF INFANT AND NATIVITY OF MOTHER.

| CAUSE OF DEATH OF INFANT AND NATIVITY OF MOTHER. | Total deaths under 1 year of age. | AGE AT DEATH. Less than 1 week. | | | | 1 week but less than 1 month. | | | | 1 month but less than 1 year. | | | | | |
|---|---|---|---|---|---|---|---|---|---|---|---|---|---|---|---|
| | | Total. | 1 day or less. | 2 days. | 3 to 6 days. | Total. | 1 week but less than 2. | 2 weeks but less than 3. | 3 weeks but less than 1 month. | Total. | 1 month but less than 2. | 2 months but less than 3. | 3 months but less than 6. | 6 months but less than 9. | 9 months and over. |
| All causes | 196 | 45 | 30 | 4 | 11 | 29 | 14 | 7 | 8 | 122 | 18 | 16 | 42 | 31 | 15 |
| Native mothers | 85 | 25 | 18 | 3 | 4 | 9 | 2 | 1 | 6 | 51 | 9 | 7 | 18 | 12 | 5 |
| Foreign mothers | 111 | 20 | 12 | 1 | 7 | 20 | 12 | 6 | 2 | 71 | 9 | 9 | 24 | 19 | 10 |
| Diarrhea and enteritis | 52 | 1 | .... | .... | 1 | 5 | .... | 3 | 2 | 46 | 5 | 4 | 17 | 15 | 5 |
| Native mothers | 17 | 1 | .... | .... | 1 | .... | .... | .... | .... | 16 | 3 | 1 | 5 | 5 | 2 |
| Foreign mothers | 35 | .... | .... | .... | .... | 5 | .... | 3 | 2 | 30 | 2 | 3 | 12 | 10 | 3 |
| Respiratory diseases | 50 | .... | .... | .... | .... | 3 | 3 | .... | .... | 47 | 7 | 4 | 15 | 13 | 8 |
| Native mothers | 19 | .... | .... | .... | .... | .... | .... | .... | .... | 19 | 2 | 2 | 8 | 5 | 2 |
| Foreign mothers | 31 | .... | .... | .... | .... | 3 | 3 | .... | .... | 28 | 5 | 2 | 7 | 8 | 6 |
| Premature births | 24 | 21 | 19 | .... | 2 | 3 | 3 | .... | .... | .... | .... | .... | .... | .... | .... |
| Native mothers | 11 | 11 | 11 | .... | .... | .... | .... | .... | .... | .... | .... | .... | .... | .... | .... |
| Foreign mothers | 13 | 10 | 8 | .... | 2 | 3 | 3 | .... | .... | .... | .... | .... | .... | .... | .... |
| Congenital debility or malformation | 19 | 10 | 7 | 1 | 2 | 6 | 2 | 3 | 1 | 3 | 1 | 2 | .... | .... | .... |
| Native mothers | 5 | 4 | 3 | .... | 1 | 1 | .... | .... | 1 | .... | .... | .... | .... | .... | .... |
| Foreign mothers | 14 | 6 | 4 | 1 | 1 | 5 | 2 | 3 | .... | 3 | 1 | 2 | .... | .... | .... |
| Injuries at birth | 7 | 7 | 3 | 2 | 2 | .... | .... | .... | .... | .... | .... | .... | .... | .... | .... |
| Native mothers | 6 | 6 | 3 | 2 | 1 | .... | .... | .... | .... | .... | .... | .... | .... | .... | .... |
| Foreign mothers | 1 | 1 | .... | .... | 1 | .... | .... | .... | .... | .... | .... | .... | .... | .... | .... |
| Other or not reported | 44 | 6 | 1 | 1 | 4 | 12 | 6 | 1 | 5 | 26 | 5 | 6 | 10 | 3 | 2 |
| Native mothers | 27 | 3 | 1 | 1 | 1 | 8 | 2 | 1 | 5 | 16 | 4 | 4 | 5 | 2 | 1 |
| Foreign mothers | 17 | 3 | .... | .... | 3 | 4 | 4 | .... | .... | 10 | 1 | 2 | 5 | 1 | 1 |

TABLE IX.—DISTRIBUTION OF BABIES ALIVE AT BEGINNING OF EACH MONTH FROM FIRST TO NINTH, ACCORDING TO TYPE OF FEEDING DURING EACH MONTH; NUMBER CONTINUING SUCH DIET UNTIL FOLLOWING MONTH; NUMBER CHANGING TO OTHER SPECIFIED TYPE OF FEEDING; NUMBER OF DEATHS IN EACH GROUP IN FIRST YEAR AND ALSO DEATHS AT BEGINNING OF NEXT MONTH.

| TYPE OF FEEDING. | ALIVE AT BEGINNING OF SPECIFIED MONTH. | | | ON SAME DIET AT BEGINNING OF NEXT MONTH. | | | CHANGED TO MIXED DIET AT BEGINNING OF NEXT MONTH. | | | CHANGED TO ARTIFICIAL DIET AT BEGINNING OF NEXT MONTH. | | | CHANGED TO BREAST EXCLUSIVELY AT BEGINNING OF NEXT MONTH. | | | Dead at beginning of next month. |
|---|---|---|---|---|---|---|---|---|---|---|---|---|---|---|---|---|
| | Total. | Lived first year. | Died in first year. | Total. | Lived first year. | Died in first year. | Total. | Lived first year. | Died in first year. | Total. | Lived first year. | Died in first year. | Total. | Lived first year. | Died in first year. | |
| First month | 1,463 | 1,267 | 196 | 1,267 | 1,164 | 103 | 43 | 39 | 4 | 78 | 63 | 15 | 1 | 1 | | 74 |
| Breast exclusively | 1,333 | 1,193 | 140 | 1,180 | 1,095 | 85 | 43 | 39 | 4 | 72 | 59 | 13 | | | | 38 |
| Mixed | 43 | 36 | 7 | 34 | 32 | 2 | | | | 5 | 4 | 1 | | | | 3 |
| Artificial exclusively | 55 | 38 | 17 | 53 | 37 | 16 | | | | 1 | | 1 | 1 | 1 | | 1 |
| No feeding, infant died at once | 32 | | 32 | | | | | | | | | | | | | 32 |
| Second month | 1,389 | 1,267 | 122 | 1,306 | 1,213 | 93 | 24 | 21 | 3 | 40 | 32 | 8 | 1 | 1 | | 18 |
| Breast exclusively | 1,181 | 1,096 | 85 | 1,111 | 1,051 | 60 | 23 | 20 | 3 | 32 | 25 | 7 | | | | 15 |
| Mixed | 77 | 71 | 6 | 74 | 68 | 6 | 1 | 1 | | 2 | 2 | | | | | |
| Artificial exclusively | 131 | 100 | 31 | 121 | 94 | 27 | | | | 6 | 5 | 1 | 1 | 1 | | 3 |
| Third month | 1,371 | 1,267 | 104 | 1,228 | 1,145 | 83 | 83 | 81 | 2 | 43 | 40 | 3 | 1 | 1 | | 16 |
| Breast exclusively | 1,112 | 1,052 | 60 | 986 | 940 | 46 | 80 | 78 | 2 | 37 | 34 | 3 | | | | 9 |
| Mixed | 98 | 89 | 9 | 92 | 84 | 8 | 3 | 3 | | 2 | 2 | | | | | 1 |
| Artificial exclusively | 161 | 126 | 35 | 150 | 121 | 29 | | | | 4 | 4 | | 1 | 1 | | 6 |
| Fourth month | 1,355 | 1,267 | 88 | 1,211 | 1,148 | 63 | 87 | 84 | 3 | 36 | 32 | 4 | 3 | 3 | | 18 |
| Breast exclusively | 987 | 941 | 46 | 868 | 835 | 33 | 85 | 82 | 3 | 27 | 24 | 3 | | | | 7 |
| Mixed | 175 | 165 | 10 | 166 | 159 | 7 | 2 | 2 | | 1 | 1 | | 3 | 3 | | 3 |
| Artificial exclusively | 193 | 161 | 32 | 177 | 154 | 23 | | | | 8 | 7 | 1 | | | | 8 |
| Fifth month | 1,337 | 1,267 | 70 | 1,203 | 1,159 | 44 | 83 | 80 | 3 | 32 | 28 | 4 | | | | 19 |
| Breast exclusively | 871 | 838 | 33 | 780 | 760 | 20 | 68 | 65 | 3 | 15 | 13 | 2 | | | | 8 |
| Mixed | 253 | 243 | 10 | 227 | 220 | 7 | 15 | 15 | | 8 | 8 | | | | | 3 |
| Artificial exclusively | 213 | 186 | 27 | 196 | 179 | 17 | | | | 9 | 7 | 2 | | | | 8 |

TABLE IX.—DISTRIBUTION OF BABIES ALIVE AT BEGINNING OF EACH MONTH FROM FIRST TO NINTH, ACCORDING TO TYPE OF FEEDING DURING EACH MONTH; NUMBER CONTINUING SUCH DIET UNTIL FOLLOWING MONTH; NUMBER CHANGING TO OTHER SPECIFIED TYPE OF FEEDING; NUMBER OF DEATHS IN EACH GROUP IN FIRST YEAR AND ALSO DEATHS AT BEGINNING OF NEXT MONTH—Continued.

| TYPE OF FEEDING. | ALIVE AT BEGINNING OF SPECIFIED MONTH. | | | ON SAME DIET AT BEGINNING OF NEXT MONTH. | | | CHANGED TO MIXED DIET AT BEGINNING OF NEXT MONTH. | | | CHANGED TO ARTIFICIAL DIET AT BEGINNING OF NEXT MONTH. | | | CHANGED TO BREAST EXCLUSIVELY AT BEGINNING OF NEXT MONTH. | | | Dead at beginning of next month. |
|---|---|---|---|---|---|---|---|---|---|---|---|---|---|---|---|---|
| | Total. | Lived first year. | Died in first year. | Total. | Lived first year. | Died in first year. | Total. | Lived first year. | Died in first year. | Total. | Lived first year. | Died in first year. | Total. | Lived first year. | Died in first year. | |
| Sixth month | 1,318 | 1,267 | 51 | 1,108 | 1,064 | 44 | 160 | 158 | 2 | 45 | 45 | | | | | 5 |
| Breast exclusively | 780 | 760 | 20 | 616 | 598 | 18 | 148 | 147 | 1 | 15 | 15 | | | | | 1 |
| Mixed | 310 | 300 | 10 | 287 | 279 | 8 | 12 | 11 | 1 | 10 | 10 | | | | | 1 |
| Artificial exclusively | 228 | 207 | 21 | 205 | 187 | 18 | | | | 20 | 20 | | | | | 3 |
| Seventh month | 1,313 | 1,267 | 46 | 1,166 | 1,130 | 36 | 112 | 110 | 2 | 27 | 27 | | | | | 8 |
| Breast exclusively | 616 | 598 | 18 | 502 | 489 | 13 | 98 | 96 | 2 | 13 | 13 | | | | | 3 |
| Mixed | 447 | 437 | 10 | 429 | 420 | 9 | 14 | 14 | | 3 | 3 | | | | | 1 |
| Artificial exclusively | 250 | 232 | 18 | 235 | 221 | 14 | | | | 11 | 11 | | | | | 4 |
| Eighth month | 1,305 | 1,267 | 38 | 1,141 | 1,119 | 22 | 95 | 94 | 1 | 55 | 54 | 1 | | | | 14 |
| Breast exclusively | 502 | 489 | 13 | 395 | 388 | 7 | 91 | 90 | 1 | 11 | 11 | | | | | 5 |
| Mixed | 541 | 530 | 11 | 516 | 507 | 9 | 4 | 4 | | 19 | 19 | | | | | 2 |
| Artificial exclusively | 262 | 248 | 14 | 230 | 224 | 6 | | | | 25 | 24 | 1 | | | | 7 |
| Ninth month | 1,291 | 1,267 | 24 | 1,003 | 989 | 14 | 158 | 158 | | 121 | 120 | 1 | | | | 9 |
| Breast exclusively | 395 | 388 | 7 | 220 | 217 | 3 | 140 | 140 | | 32 | 31 | 1 | | | | 3 |
| Mixed | 611 | 601 | 10 | 551 | 543 | 8 | 18 | 18 | | 40 | 40 | | | | | 2 |
| Artificial exclusively | 285 | 278 | 7 | 232 | 229 | 3 | | | | 49 | 49 | | | | | 4 |

TABLE X.—DISTRIBUTION OF BIRTHS TO MARRIED WAGE-EARNING MOTHERS, ACCORDING TO HUSBAND'S ANNUAL EARNINGS AND NATIVITY AND EARNINGS OF MOTHER.

| NATIVITY AND ANNUAL EARNINGS OF MARRIED MOTHER. | Total births. | BIRTHS TO MARRIED WAGE-EARNING MOTHER WITH HUSBAND EARNING ANNUALLY— | | | | | | |
|---|---|---|---|---|---|---|---|---|
| | | Under $521. | $521 to $624. | $625 to $779. | $780 to $899. | $900 to $1,199. | $1,200 and over. | Ample.[1] |
| All wage-earning mothers | 281 | 112 | 57 | 51 | 25 | 14 | 1 | 21 |
| Under $53 | 20 | 6 | 5 | 1 | 4 | 1 | ...... | 3 |
| $53 to $103 | 57 | 23 | 12 | 11 | 7 | 3 | ...... | 1 |
| $104 to $207 | 89 | 46 | 16 | 19 | 3 | 3 | ...... | 2 |
| $208 to $311 | 60 | 23 | 16 | 12 | 4 | 3 | 1 | 1 |
| $312 and over | 46 | 14 | 8 | 8 | 7 | 2 | ...... | 7 |
| Not reported | 9 | ...... | ...... | ...... | ...... | 2 | ...... | 7 |
| Native wage-earning mothers | 26 | 9 | 3 | 4 | 6 | 1 | ...... | 3 |
| Under $53 | 6 | 2 | 1 | ...... | 2 | 1 | ...... | ...... |
| $53 to $103 | 5 | 2 | 1 | 2 | ...... | ...... | ...... | ...... |
| $104 to $207 | 5 | 1 | 1 | 2 | 1 | ...... | ...... | ...... |
| $208 to $311 | 4 | 3 | ...... | ...... | 1 | ...... | ...... | ...... |
| $312 and over | 3 | 1 | ...... | ...... | 2 | ...... | ...... | ...... |
| Not reported | 3 | ...... | ...... | ...... | ...... | ...... | ...... | 3 |
| Foreign wage-earning mothers | 255 | 103 | 54 | 47 | 19 | 13 | 1 | 18 |
| Under $53 | 14 | 4 | 4 | 1 | 2 | ...... | ...... | 3 |
| $53 to $103 | 52 | 21 | 11 | 9 | 7 | 3 | ...... | 1 |
| $104 to $207 | 84 | 45 | 15 | 17 | 2 | 3 | ...... | 2 |
| $208 to $311 | 56 | 20 | 16 | 12 | 3 | 3 | 1 | 1 |
| $312 and over | 43 | 13 | 8 | 8 | 5 | 2 | ...... | 7 |
| Not reported | 6 | ...... | ...... | ...... | ...... | 2 | ...... | 4 |

[1] See note on page 45.

TABLE XI.—DISTRIBUTION OF RESULTS OF REPORTABLE PREGNANCIES (LIVE BIRTHS AND STILLBIRTHS) AND MISCARRIAGES, ACCORDING TO NUMBER PER MOTHER AND NATIVITY OF MOTHER.

| NUMBER OF REPORTABLE PREGNANCIES PER MOTHER AND NATIVITY OF MOTHER. | REPORTABLE PREGNANCIES AND RESULTS THEREOF. | | | | | | | | | | | | MISCARRIAGES IN ADDITION TO REPORTABLE PREGNANCIES. | | |
|---|---|---|---|---|---|---|---|---|---|---|---|---|---|---|---|
| | | | | | Live births. | | | | | Stillbirths. | | | | Number of mothers reporting miscarriages. | |
| | | | | | | | Deaths in first year. | | | | | | | | |
| | Total pregnancies. | Total births. | Excess due to plural births. | Number of mothers. | Number. | Number of mothers having live births. | Number. | Number of mothers having babies die. | Infant mortality rate. | Number of stillbirths. | Number of mothers having stillbirths. | Per cent of all births. | Number of miscarriages reported. | Total mothers. | Per cent of all mothers. |
| All married mothers | 5,554 | 5,617 | 63 | 1,491 | 5,363 | 1,465 | 804 | 509 | 149.9 | 254 | 194 | 4.5 | 191 | 130 | 8.7 |
| 1 | 339 | 343 | 4 | 339 | 322 | 318 | 35 | 34 | 108.7 | 21 | 21 | 6.1 | 8 | 8 | 2.4 |
| 2 | 566 | 576 | 10 | 283 | 544 | 279 | 59 | 54 | 108.5 | 32 | 28 | 5.6 | 23 | 16 | 5.7 |
| 3 | 642 | 650 | 8 | 214 | 626 | 214 | 92 | 75 | 147.0 | 24 | 23 | 3.7 | 26 | 18 | 8.4 |
| 4 | 744 | 752 | 8 | 186 | 723 | 186 | 78 | 64 | 107.9 | 29 | 21 | 3.9 | 22 | 18 | 9.7 |
| 5 | 735 | 740 | 5 | 147 | 704 | 147 | 103 | 67 | 146.3 | 36 | 31 | 4.9 | 20 | 14 | 9.5 |
| 6 | 564 | 568 | 4 | 94 | 546 | 93 | 88 | 60 | 161.2 | 22 | 13 | 3.9 | 23 | 14 | 14.9 |
| 7 | 581 | 586 | 5 | 83 | 555 | 83 | 78 | 48 | 140.5 | 31 | 22 | 5.3 | 27 | 15 | 18.1 |
| 8 | 432 | 437 | 5 | 54 | 426 | 54 | 95 | 42 | 223.0 | 11 | 7 | 2.5 | 15 | 9 | 16.7 |
| 9 | 297 | 299 | 2 | 33 | 283 | 33 | 41 | 20 | 144.9 | 16 | 11 | 5.4 | 13 | 8 | (1) |
| 10 or more | 654 | 666 | 12 | 58 | 634 | 58 | 135 | 45 | 212.9 | 32 | 17 | 4.8 | 14 | 10 | 17.2 |
| Native | 2,717 | 2,744 | 27 | 816 | 2,600 | 801 | 294 | 206 | 113.1 | 144 | 115 | 5.2 | 136 | 92 | 11.3 |
| 1 | 234 | 236 | 2 | 234 | 224 | 222 | 17 | 17 | 75.9 | 12 | 12 | 5.1 | 7 | 7 | 3.0 |
| 2 | 346 | 351 | 5 | 173 | 327 | 170 | 25 | 23 | 76.5 | 24 | 21 | 6.8 | 18 | 13 | 7.5 |
| 3 | 333 | 338 | 5 | 111 | 322 | 111 | 38 | 31 | 118.0 | 16 | 16 | 4.7 | 21 | 15 | 13.5 |
| 4 | 376 | 377 | 1 | 94 | 362 | 94 | 36 | 31 | 99.4 | 15 | 13 | 4.0 | 13 | 10 | 10.6 |
| 5 | 325 | 326 | 1 | 65 | 302 | 65 | 26 | 21 | 86.1 | 24 | 19 | 7.4 | 13 | 10 | 15.4 |
| 6 | 222 | 222 | ........ | 37 | 216 | 37 | 34 | 22 | 157.4 | 6 | 5 | 2.7 | 17 | 9 | (1) |
| 7 | 266 | 267 | 1 | 38 | 250 | 38 | 25 | 18 | 100.0 | 17 | 11 | 6.4 | 25 | 13 | (1) |
| 8 | 184 | 187 | 3 | 23 | 184 | 23 | 29 | 17 | 157.6 | 3 | 2 | 1.6 | 8 | 5 | (1) |
| 9 | 117 | 118 | 1 | 13 | 109 | 13 | 14 | 7 | 128.4 | 9 | 6 | 7.6 | 4 | 3 | (1) |
| 10 or more | 314 | 322 | 8 | 28 | 304 | 28 | 50 | 19 | 164.5 | 18 | 10 | 5.6 | 10 | 7 | (1) |

| | | | | | | | | | | | | | | | |
|---|---|---|---|---|---|---|---|---|---|---|---|---|---|---|---|
| Foreign | 2,837 | 2,873 | 36 | 675 | 2,763 | 664 | 510 | 303 | 184.6 | 110 | 79 | 3.8 | 55 | 38 | 5.6 |
| 1 | 105 | 107 | 2 | 105 | 98 | 96 | 18 | 17 | 183.7 | 9 | 9 | 8.4 | 1 | 1 | 1.0 |
| 2 | 220 | 225 | 5 | 110 | 217 | 109 | 34 | 31 | 156.7 | 8 | 7 | 3.6 | 5 | 3 | 2.7 |
| 3 | 309 | 312 | 3 | 103 | 304 | 103 | 54 | 44 | 177.6 | 8 | 7 | 2.6 | 5 | 3 | 2.9 |
| 4 | 368 | 375 | 7 | 92 | 361 | 92 | 42 | 33 | 116.3 | 14 | 8 | 3.7 | 9 | 8 | 8.7 |
| 5 | 410 | 414 | 4 | 82 | 402 | 82 | 77 | 46 | 191.5 | 12 | 12 | 2.9 | 7 | 4 | 4.9 |
| 6 | 342 | 346 | 4 | 57 | 330 | 56 | 54 | 38 | 163.6 | 16 | 8 | 4.6 | 6 | 5 | 8.8 |
| 7 | 315 | 319 | 4 | 45 | 305 | 45 | 53 | 30 | 173.8 | 14 | 11 | 4.4 | 2 | 2 | (1) |
| 8 | 248 | 250 | 2 | 31 | 242 | 31 | 66 | 25 | 272.7 | 8 | 5 | 3.2 | 7 | 4 | (1) |
| 9 | 180 | 181 | 1 | 20 | 174 | 20 | 27 | 13 | 155.2 | 7 | 5 | 3.9 | 9 | 5 | (1) |
| 10 or more | 340 | 344 | 4 | 30 | 330 | 30 | 85 | 26 | 257.6 | 14 | 7 | 4.1 | 4 | 3 | (1) |

[1] Not shown when base is less than 50.

TABLE XII.—DISTRIBUTION OF RESULTS OF REPORTABLE PREGNANCIES (LIVE BIRTHS AND STILLBIRTHS) AND MISCARRIAGES, ACCORDING TO NUMBER PER MOTHER AND AGE OF MOTHER AT EACH PREGNANCY

| NUMBER OF REPORTABLE PREGNANCIES AND AGE OF MOTHER AT BIRTH OF BABY BORN IN 1911. | REPORTABLE PREGNANCIES. | | | | LIVE BIRTHS. | | BABIES DYING IN FIRST YEAR. | | | STILLBIRTHS. | | | MISCARRIAGES. | | |
|---|---|---|---|---|---|---|---|---|---|---|---|---|---|---|---|
| | Total. | Resulting births. | | Number of mothers. | Number. | Number of mothers. | Number. | Number of mothers. | Infant mortality rate. | Number. | Number of mothers. | Per cent of all births. | Number reported. | Mothers reporting. | |
| | | Number. | Excess over pregnancies.[1] | | | | | | | | | | | Number. | Per cent of all mothers. |
| All married mothers | 5,554 | 5,617 | 63 | 1,491 | 5,363 | 1,465 | 804 | 509 | 149.9 | 254 | 194 | 4.5 | 191 | 130 | 8.7 |
| Under 20 years | 107 | 108 | 1 | 89 | 96 | 81 | 12 | 11 | 125.0 | 12 | 12 | 11.1 | | | |
| 20 to 24 years | 933 | 946 | 13 | 461 | 908 | 456 | 140 | 115 | 154.2 | 38 | 29 | 4.0 | 19 | 18 | 3.9 |
| 25 to 29 years | 1,316 | 1,329 | 13 | 395 | 1,261 | 389 | 185 | 132 | 146.7 | 68 | 55 | 5.1 | 46 | 27 | 6.8 |
| 30 to 39 years | 2,570 | 2,595 | 25 | 466 | 2,480 | 459 | 382 | 207 | 154.0 | 115 | 84 | 4.4 | 95 | 66 | 14.2 |
| 40 years and over | 628 | 639 | 11 | 80 | 618 | 80 | 85 | 44 | 137.5 | 21 | 14 | 3.3 | 31 | 19 | 23.8 |
| Average age: 28 years. | | | | | | | | | | | | | | | |
| 1 reportable pregnancy | 339 | 343 | 4 | 339 | 322 | 318 | 35 | 34 | 108.7 | 21 | 21 | 6.1 | 8 | 8 | 2.4 |
| Under 20 years | 74 | 75 | 1 | 74 | 67 | 66 | 8 | 7 | 119.4 | 8 | 8 | 10.7 | | | |
| 20 to 24 years | 178 | 179 | 1 | 178 | 176 | 175 | 18 | 18 | 102.3 | 3 | 3 | 1.7 | 3 | 3 | 1.7 |
| 25 to 29 years | 57 | 58 | 1 | 57 | 54 | 53 | 4 | 4 | 74.1 | 4 | 4 | 6.9 | 3 | 3 | 5.3 |
| 30 to 39 years | 30 | 31 | 1 | 30 | 25 | 24 | 5 | 5 | (2) | 6 | 6 | (2) | 2 | 2 | (2) |
| Average age: 23 years. | | | | | | | | | | | | | | | |
| 2 reportable pregnancies | 566 | 576 | 10 | 283 | 544 | 279 | 59 | 54 | 108.5 | 32 | 28 | 5.6 | 23 | 16 | 5.7 |
| Under 20 years | 24 | 24 | | 12 | 21 | 12 | 3 | 3 | (2) | 3 | 3 | (2) | | | |
| 20 to 24 years | 312 | 317 | 5 | 156 | 302 | 154 | 42 | 37 | 139.1 | 15 | 13 | 4.7 | 6 | 6 | 3.8 |
| 25 to 29 years | 148 | 151 | 3 | 74 | 141 | 73 | 9 | 9 | 63.8 | 10 | 9 | 6.6 | 5 | 3 | 4.1 |
| 30 to 39 years | 78 | 80 | 2 | 39 | 76 | 38 | 5 | 5 | 65.8 | 4 | 3 | 5.0 | 12 | 7 | (2) |
| 40 years and over | 4 | 4 | | 2 | 4 | 2 | | | | | | | | | |
| Average age: 25 years. | | | | | | | | | | | | | | | |
| 3 reportable pregnancies | 642 | 650 | 8 | 214 | 626 | 214 | 92 | 75 | 147.0 | 24 | 23 | 3.7 | 26 | 18 | 8.4 |
| Under 20 years | 9 | 9 | | 3 | 8 | 3 | 1 | 1 | (2) | 1 | 1 | (2) | | | |
| 20 to 24 years | 221 | 234 | 3 | 77 | 227 | 77 | 40 | 31 | 176.2 | 7 | 6 | 3.0 | 7 | 6 | 7.8 |
| 25 to 29 years | 285 | 288 | 3 | 95 | 277 | 95 | 41 | 33 | 148.0 | 11 | 11 | 3.8 | 14 | 7 | 7.4 |
| 30 to 39 years | 108 | 110 | 2 | 36 | 105 | 36 | 8 | 8 | 76.2 | 5 | 5 | 4.5 | 4 | 4 | (2) |
| 40 years and over | 9 | 9 | | 3 | 9 | 3 | 2 | 2 | (2) | | | | 1 | 1 | (2) |
| Average age: 26 years. | | | | | | | | | | | | | | | |

| | | | | | | | | | | | | | | | |
|---|---|---|---|---|---|---|---|---|---|---|---|---|---|---|---|
| 4 reportable pregnancies | 744 | 752 | 8 | 186 | 723 | 186 | 78 | 64 | 107.9 | 29 | 21 | 3.9 | 22 | 18 | 9.7 |
| 20 to 24 years | 156 | 160 | 4 | 39 | 148 | 39 | 28 | 21 | 189.2 | 12 | 6 | 7.5 | 3 | 3 | (2) |
| 25 to 29 years | 300 | 301 | 1 | 75 | 290 | 75 | 26 | 23 | 89.7 | 11 | 10 | 3.7 | 10 | 6 | 8.0 |
| 30 to 39 years | 252 | 255 | 3 | 63 | 249 | 63 | 21 | 17 | 84.3 | 6 | 5 | 2.4 | 6 | 6 | 9.5 |
| 40 years and over | 36 | 36 | | 9 | 36 | 9 | 3 | 3 | (2) | | | | 3 | 3 | (2) |
| Average age: 29 years. | | | | | | | | | | | | | | | |
| 5 reportable pregnancies | 735 | 740 | 5 | 147 | 704 | 147 | 103 | 67 | 146.3 | 36 | 31 | 4.9 | 20 | 14 | 9.5 |
| 20 to 24 years | 50 | 50 | | 10 | 49 | 10 | 9 | 7 | 183.7 | 1 | 1 | 2.0 | | | |
| 25 to 29 years | 280 | 283 | 3 | 56 | 266 | 56 | 51 | 31 | 191.7 | 17 | 15 | 6.0 | 6 | 4 | 7.1 |
| 30 to 39 years | 375 | 377 | 2 | 75 | 361 | 75 | 40 | 27 | 110.8 | 16 | 14 | 4.2 | 12 | 8 | 10.7 |
| 40 years and over | 30 | 30 | | 6 | 28 | 6 | 3 | 2 | (2) | 2 | 1 | (2) | 2 | 2 | (2) |
| Average age: 30 years. | | | | | | | | | | | | | | | |
| 6 reportable pregnancies | 564 | 568 | 4 | 94 | 546 | 93 | 88 | 60 | 161.2 | 22 | 13 | 3.9 | 23 | 14 | 14.9 |
| 20 to 24 years | 6 | 6 | | 1 | 6 | 1 | 3 | 1 | (2) | | | | | | |
| 25 to 29 years | 132 | 133 | 1 | 22 | 127 | 21 | 23 | 17 | 181.1 | 6 | 1 | 4.5 | 6 | 3 | (2) |
| 30 to 39 years | 360 | 362 | 2 | 60 | 347 | 60 | 54 | 36 | 155.6 | 15 | 11 | 4.1 | 13 | 9 | 15.0 |
| 40 years and over | 66 | 67 | 1 | 11 | 66 | 11 | 8 | 6 | 121.2 | 1 | 1 | 1.5 | 4 | 2 | (2) |
| Average age: 33 years. | | | | | | | | | | | | | | | |
| 7 reportable pregnancies | 581 | 586 | 5 | 83 | 555 | 83 | 78 | 48 | 140.5 | 31 | 22 | 5.3 | 27 | 15 | 18.1 |
| 25 to 29 years | 98 | 99 | 1 | 14 | 90 | 14 | 23 | 13 | 255.6 | 9 | 5 | 10.0 | 2 | 1 | (2) |
| 30 to 39 years | 392 | 395 | 3 | 56 | 377 | 56 | 45 | 28 | 119.4 | 18 | 15 | 4.6 | 19 | 11 | 19.6 |
| 40 years and over | 91 | 92 | 1 | 13 | 88 | 13 | 10 | 7 | 113.6 | 4 | 2 | 4.3 | 6 | 3 | (2) |
| Average age: 34 years. | | | | | | | | | | | | | | | |
| 8 reportable pregnancies | 432 | 437 | 5 | 54 | 426 | 54 | 95 | 42 | 223.0 | 11 | 7 | 2.5 | 15 | 9 | 16.7 |
| 25 to 29 years | 16 | 16 | | 2 | 16 | 2 | 8 | 2 | (2) | | | | | | |
| 30 to 39 years | 408 | 413 | 5 | 51 | 403 | 51 | 87 | 40 | 215.9 | 10 | 6 | 2.4 | 15 | 9 | 17.6 |
| 40 years and over | 8 | 8 | | 1 | 7 | 1 | | | | 1 | 1 | (2) | | | |
| Average age: 35 years. | | | | | | | | | | | | | | | |
| 9 reportable pregnancies | 297 | 299 | 2 | 33 | 283 | 33 | 41 | 20 | 144.9 | 16 | 11 | 5.4 | 13 | 8 | 24.2 |
| 30 to 39 years | 207 | 208 | 1 | 23 | 195 | 23 | 32 | 15 | 164.1 | 13 | 8 | 6.3 | 5 | 4 | (2) |
| 40 years and over | 90 | 91 | 1 | 10 | 88 | 10 | 9 | 5 | 102.3 | 3 | 3 | 3.3 | 8 | 4 | (2) |
| Average age: 37 years. | | | | | | | | | | | | | | | |
| 10 or more reportable pregnancies | 654 | 666 | 12 | [3] 58 | 634 | 58 | 135 | 45 | 212.9 | 32 | 17 | 4.8 | 14 | 10 | 17.2 |
| 30 to 39 years | 360 | 364 | 4 | 33 | 342 | 33 | 85 | 26 | 248.5 | 22 | 11 | 6.0 | 7 | 6 | (2) |
| 40 years and over | 294 | 302 | 8 | 25 | 292 | 25 | 50 | 19 | 171.2 | 10 | 6 | 3.3 | 7 | 4 | (2) |
| Average age: 39 years. | | | | | | | | | | | | | | | |

[1] Excess of births over pregnancies due to plural births.
[2] Rate not computed because of small base.
[3] Includes 21 having 10 pregnancies; 16 having 11; 11 having 12; 6 having 13; 3 having 14; 1 having 16.

TABLE XIII.—DISTRIBUTION OF RESULTS OF REPORTABLE PREGNANCIES (LIVE BIRTHS AND STILLBIRTHS) AND MISCARRIAGES, ACCORDING TO NUMBER PER MOTHER AND HUSBAND'S EARNINGS.

| SPECIFIED NUMBER OF PREGNANCIES FOR ALL MARRIED MOTHERS AND ANNUAL EARNINGS OF HUSBAND. | REPORTABLE PREGNANCIES. | | | | LIVE BIRTHS. | | BABIES DYING IN FIRST YEAR. | | | STILLBIRTHS. | | | MISCARRIAGES. | | |
|---|---|---|---|---|---|---|---|---|---|---|---|---|---|---|---|
| | Total. | Resulting births. | | Number of mothers. | Number. | Number of mothers. | Number. | Infant mortality rate.[1] | Number of mothers. | Number. | Number of mothers. | Per cent of all births.[1] | Number reported. | Mothers reporting. | |
| | | Number. | Excess over pregnancies. | | | | | | | | | | | Number. | Per cent of all mothers. |
| All reportable pregnancies | 5,554 | 5,617 | 63 | 1,491 | 5,363 | 1,465 | 804 | 149.9 | 509 | 254 | 194 | 4.5 | 191 | 130 | 8.7 |
| Husband earns: | | | | | | | | | | | | | | | |
| Under $521 | 938 | 946 | 8 | 233 | 902 | 227 | 178 | 197.3 | 110 | 44 | 31 | 4.7 | 27 | 17 | 7.31 |
| $521 to $624 | 691 | 700 | 9 | 174 | 668 | 173 | 129 | 193.1 | 75 | 32 | 25 | 4.6 | 22 | 14 | 8.0 |
| $625 to $779 | 816 | 826 | 10 | 229 | 797 | 227 | 130 | 163.1 | 88 | 29 | 21 | 3.5 | 21 | 15 | 6.6 |
| $780 to $899 | 611 | 616 | 5 | 166 | 588 | 163 | 99 | 168.4 | 61 | 28 | 23 | 4.5 | 30 | 19 | 11.4 |
| $900 to $1,199 | 574 | 581 | 7 | 146 | 548 | 143 | 78 | 142.3 | 48 | 33 | 24 | 5.7 | 25 | 18 | 12.3 |
| $1,200 and over | 196 | 199 | 3 | 50 | 186 | 49 | 30 | 161.3 | 18 | 13 | 9 | 6.5 | 8 | 6 | 12.0 |
| Ample[2] | 1,728 | 1,749 | 21 | 493 | 1,674 | 483 | 160 | 95.6 | 109 | 75 | 61 | 4.3 | 58 | 41 | 8.3 |
| 1 reportable pregnancy | 339 | 343 | 4 | 339 | 322 | 318 | 35 | 108.7 | 34 | 21 | 21 | 6.1 | 8 | 8 | 2.4 |
| Husband earns: | | | | | | | | | | | | | | | |
| Under $521 | 48 | 48 | ... | 48 | 43 | 43 | 11 | ... | 11 | 5 | 5 | ... | ... | ... | ... |
| $521 to $624 | 23 | 23 | ... | 23 | 22 | 22 | 2 | ... | 2 | 1 | 1 | ... | 1 | 1 | ... |
| $625 to $779 | 46 | 48 | 2 | 46 | 46 | 44 | 6 | ... | 5 | 2 | 2 | ... | 2 | 2 | ... |
| $780 to $899 | 35 | 35 | ... | 35 | 32 | 32 | 3 | ... | 3 | 3 | 3 | ... | ... | ... | ... |
| $900 to $1,199 | 38 | 39 | 1 | 38 | 36 | 35 | 4 | ... | 4 | 3 | 3 | ... | ... | ... | ... |
| $1,200 and over | 13 | 13 | ... | 13 | 13 | 13 | 1 | ... | 1 | ... | ... | ... | ... | ... | ... |
| Ample[2] | 136 | 137 | 1 | 136 | 130 | 129 | 8 | 61.5 | 8 | 7 | 7 | 5.1 | 5 | 5 | ... |
| 2 reportable pregnancies | 566 | 576 | 10 | 283 | 544 | 279 | 59 | 108.5 | 54 | 32 | 28 | 5.6 | 23 | 16 | 5.7 |
| Husband earns: | | | | | | | | | | | | | | | |
| Under $521 | 62 | 64 | 2 | 31 | 62 | 31 | 11 | 176.4 | 11 | 2 | 2 | 3.1 | ... | ... | ... |
| $521 to $624 | 72 | 74 | 2 | 36 | 68 | 36 | 8 | 177.6 | 6 | 6 | 6 | 8.1 | 3 | 1 | ... |
| $625 to $779 | 110 | 111 | 1 | 55 | 108 | 55 | 17 | 157.4 | 16 | 3 | 3 | 2.7 | 2 | 2 | 4.4 |
| $780 to $899 | 56 | 56 | ... | 28 | 53 | 28 | 9 | 169.8 | 7 | 3 | 3 | 5.4 | 4 | 2 | ... |
| $900 to $1,199 | 46 | 46 | ... | 23 | 41 | 23 | 2 | ... | 2 | 5 | 5 | ... | 4 | 4 | ... |
| $1,200 and over | 16 | 16 | ... | 8 | 14 | 7 | 1 | ... | 1 | 2 | 1 | ... | 1 | 1 | ... |
| Ample[2] | 204 | 209 | 5 | 102 | 198 | 99 | 11 | 55.6 | 11 | 11 | 8 | 5.3 | 9 | 6 | 5.9 |

| | | | | | | | | | | | | | | | |
|---|---|---|---|---|---|---|---|---|---|---|---|---|---|---|---|
| 3 reportable pregnancies | 642 | 650 | 8 | 214 | 626 | 214 | 92 | 147.0 | 75 | 24 | 23 | 3.7 | 26 | 18 | 8.4 |
| Husband earns: | | | | | | | | | | | | | | | |
| Under $521 | 114 | 115 | 1 | 38 | 110 | 38 | 27 | 245.5 | 23 | 5 | 4 | 4.3 | 5 | 3 | ...... |
| $521 to $624 | 102 | 104 | 2 | 34 | 101 | 34 | 16 | 158.4 | 13 | 3 | 3 | 1.9 | 1 | 1 | ...... |
| $625 to $779 | 84 | 84 | ...... | 28 | 82 | 28 | 13 | 158.5 | 11 | 2 | 2 | 2.4 | 3 | 2 | ...... |
| $780 to $899 | 87 | 87 | ...... | 29 | 83 | 29 | 6 | 72.3 | 6 | 4 | 4 | 4.6 | 5 | 4 | ...... |
| $900 to $1,199 | 57 | 58 | 1 | 19 | 55 | 19 | 11 | 200.0 | 8 | 3 | 3 | 5.2 | 7 | 3 | ...... |
| $1,200 and over | 6 | 7 | 1 | 2 | 7 | 2 | 1 | ...... | 1 | ...... | ...... | ...... | ...... | ...... | ...... |
| Ample[2] | 192 | 195 | 3 | 64 | 188 | 64 | 18 | 95.7 | 13 | 7 | 7 | 3.6 | 5 | 5 | 7.8 |
| 4 reportable pregnancies | 744 | 752 | 8 | 186 | 723 | 186 | 78 | 107.9 | 64 | 29 | 21 | 3.9 | 22 | 18 | 9.7 |
| Husband earns: | | | | | | | | | | | | | | | |
| Under $521 | 104 | 104 | ...... | 26 | 101 | 26 | 13 | 128.7 | 9 | 3 | 2 | 1.9 | 4 | 2 | ...... |
| $521 to $624 | 88 | 89 | 1 | 22 | 86 | 22 | 10 | 116.3 | 9 | 3 | 1 | 3.4 | 2 | 2 | ...... |
| $625 to $779 | 136 | 137 | 1 | 34 | 129 | 34 | 19 | 147.3 | 15 | 8 | 6 | 5.8 | 3 | 2 | ...... |
| $780 to $899 | 96 | 97 | 1 | 24 | 95 | 24 | 13 | 136.8 | 12 | 2 | 1 | 2.1 | 3 | 3 | ...... |
| $900 to $1,199 | 56 | 58 | 2 | 14 | 55 | 14 | 4 | 72.7 | 2 | 3 | 1 | 5.2 | 2 | 2 | ...... |
| $1,200 and over | 40 | 41 | 1 | 10 | 39 | 10 | 5 | ...... | 4 | 2 | 2 | ...... | 2 | 2 | ...... |
| Ample[2] | 224 | 226 | 2 | 56 | 218 | 56 | 14 | 64.2 | 13 | 8 | 8 | 3.5 | 6 | 5 | 8.9 |
| 5 reportable pregnancies | 735 | 740 | 5 | 147 | 704 | 147 | 103 | 146.3 | 67 | 36 | 31 | 4.9 | 20 | 14 | 9.5 |
| Husband earns: | | | | | | | | | | | | | | | |
| Under $521 | 130 | 131 | 1 | 26 | 125 | 26 | 21 | 168.0 | 12 | 6 | 6 | 4.6 | 3 | 3 | ...... |
| $521 to $624 | 90 | 91 | 1 | 18 | 85 | 18 | 20 | 235.3 | 12 | 6 | 5 | 6.6 | 3 | 1 | ...... |
| $625 to $779 | 100 | 100 | ...... | 20 | 99 | 20 | 18 | 181.8 | 13 | 1 | 1 | 1.0 | 3 | 2 | ...... |
| $780 to $899 | 110 | 110 | ...... | 22 | 106 | 22 | 13 | 122.6 | 8 | 4 | 4 | 3.6 | 3 | 2 | ...... |
| $900 to $1,199 | 65 | 66 | 1 | 13 | 60 | 13 | 6 | 100.0 | 5 | 6 | 4 | 10.0 | ...... | ...... | ...... |
| $1,200 and over | 30 | 30 | ...... | 6 | 26 | 6 | 10 | ...... | 6 | 4 | 3 | ...... | 2 | 1 | ...... |
| Ample[2] | 210 | 212 | 2 | 42 | 203 | 42 | 15 | 73.9 | 11 | 9 | 8 | 4.2 | 6 | 5 | ...... |
| 6 reportable pregnancies | 564 | 568 | 4 | 94 | 546 | 93 | 88 | 161.2 | 60 | 22 | 13 | 3.9 | 23 | 14 | 14.9 |
| Husband earns: | | | | | | | | | | | | | | | |
| Under $521 | 132 | 132 | ...... | 22 | 124 | 21 | 26 | 209.7 | 14 | 8 | 3 | 6.1 | 2 | 2 | ...... |
| $521 to $624 | 60 | 60 | ...... | 10 | 59 | 10 | 9 | 152.5 | 8 | 1 | 1 | 1.7 | 6 | 2 | ...... |
| $625 to $779 | 114 | 115 | 1 | 19 | 110 | 19 | 14 | 127.3 | 11 | 5 | 2 | 4.3 | 3 | 2 | ...... |
| $780 to $899 | 48 | 48 | ...... | 8 | 48 | 8 | 7 | ...... | 6 | ...... | ...... | ...... | 4 | 2 | ...... |
| $900 to $1,199 | 72 | 74 | 2 | 12 | 70 | 12 | 12 | 171.4 | 9 | 4 | 3 | 5.4 | 4 | 3 | ...... |
| $1,200 and over | 12 | 12 | ...... | 2 | 11 | 2 | 3 | ...... | 1 | 1 | 1 | ...... | ...... | ...... | ...... |
| Ample[2] | 126 | 127 | 1 | 21 | 124 | 21 | 17 | 137.1 | 11 | 3 | 3 | 2.4 | 4 | 3 | ...... |

[1] Not shown when base is less than 50.

[2] See note on page 45.

TABLE XIII.—DISTRIBUTION OF RESULTS OF REPORTABLE PREGNANCIES (LIVE BIRTHS AND STILLBIRTHS) AND MISCARRIAGES, ACCORDING TO NUMBER PER MOTHER AND HUSBAND'S EARNINGS—Continued.

| SPECIFIED NUMBER OF PREGNANCIES FOR ALL MARRIED MOTHERS AND ANNUAL EARNINGS OF HUSBAND. | REPORTABLE PREGNANCIES. | | | | LIVE BIRTHS. | | BABIES DYING IN FIRST YEAR. | | | STILLBIRTHS. | | | MISCARRIAGES. | | |
|---|---|---|---|---|---|---|---|---|---|---|---|---|---|---|---|
| | Total. | Resulting births. | | Number of mothers. | Number. | Number of mothers. | Number. | Infant mortality rate.[1] | Number of mothers. | Number. | Number of mothers. | Per cent of all births.[1] | Number reported. | Mothers reporting. | |
| | | Number. | Excess over pregnancies. | | | | | | | | | | | Number. | Per cent of all mothers. |
| 7 reportable pregnancies | 581 | 586 | 5 | 83 | 555 | 83 | 78 | 140.5 | 48 | 31 | 22 | 5.3 | 27 | 15 | 78.1 |
| Husband earns: | | | | | | | | | | | | | | | |
| Under $521 | 91 | 92 | 1 | 13 | 88 | 13 | 13 | 147.7 | 8 | 4 | 4 | 4.3 | 4 | 2 | |
| $521 to $624 | 56 | 56 | | 8 | 51 | 8 | 15 | 294.1 | 6 | 5 | 4 | 8.9 | 1 | 1 | |
| $625 to $779 | 98 | 101 | 3 | 14 | 97 | 14 | 16 | 164.9 | 9 | 4 | 3 | 4.0 | | | |
| $780 to $899 | 35 | 35 | | 5 | 32 | 5 | 6 | | 5 | 3 | 2 | | 3 | 1 | |
| $900 to $1,199 | 84 | 84 | | 12 | 79 | 12 | 7 | 88.6 | 5 | 5 | 2 | 6.0 | 5 | 3 | |
| $1,200 and over | 21 | 22 | 1 | 3 | 22 | 3 | 1 | | 1 | | | | 2 | 1 | |
| Ample[2] | 196 | 196 | | 8 2 | 186 | 28 | 20 | 107.5 | 14 | 10 | 7 | 5.1 | 12 | 7 | |
| 8 reportable pregnancies | 432 | 437 | 5 | 54 | 426 | 54 | 95 | 223.0 | 42 | 11 | 7 | 2.5 | 15 | 9 | 16.7 |
| Husband earns: | | | | | | | | | | | | | | | |
| Under $521 | 120 | 120 | | 15 | 117 | 15 | 31 | 265.0 | 12 | 3 | 2 | 2.5 | 5 | 2 | |
| $521 to $624 | 96 | 98 | 2 | 12 | 94 | 12 | 22 | 234.0 | 10 | 4 | 2 | 4.1 | 1 | 1 | |
| $625 to $779 | 40 | 41 | 1 | 5 | 41 | 5 | 11 | | 4 | | | | 2 | 1 | |
| $780 to $899 | 48 | 49 | 1 | 6 | 46 | 6 | 11 | | 5 | 3 | 2 | | 5 | 3 | |
| $900 to $1,199 | 24 | 24 | | 3 | 24 | 3 | 6 | | 3 | | | | 1 | 1 | |
| $1,200 and over | 16 | 16 | | 2 | 16 | 2 | 3 | | 2 | | | | 1 | 1 | |
| Ample[2] | 88 | 89 | 1 | 11 | 88 | 11 | 11 | 125.0 | 6 | 1 | 1 | 1.1 | | | |
| 9 reportable pregnancies | 297 | 299 | 2 | 33 | 283 | 33 | 41 | 144.9 | 20 | 16 | 11 | 5.4 | 13 | 8 | |
| Husband earns: | | | | | | | | | | | | | | | |
| Under $521 | 81 | 82 | 1 | 9 | 80 | 9 | 15 | 187.5 | 6 | 2 | 2 | 2.4 | 3 | 2 | |
| $521 to $624 | 72 | 72 | | 8 | 70 | 8 | 10 | 142.9 | 6 | 2 | 1 | 2.8 | 3 | 3 | |
| $625 to $779 | 18 | 18 | | 2 | 15 | 2 | | | | 3 | 1 | | 1 | 1 | |
| $780 to $899 | 18 | 19 | 1 | 2 | 17 | 2 | 5 | | 2 | 2 | 2 | | | | |
| $900 to $1,199 | 18 | 18 | | 2 | 18 | 2 | 2 | | 2 | | | | | | |
| $1,200 and over | 18 | 18 | | 2 | 16 | 2 | | | | 2 | 1 | | | | |
| Ample[2] | 72 | 72 | | 8 | 67 | 8 | 9 | 134.3 | 4 | 5 | 4 | 6.9 | 6 | 2 | |

| | | | | | | | | | | | | | | | |
|---|---|---|---|---|---|---|---|---|---|---|---|---|---|---|---|
| 10 or more reportable pregnancies | 654 | 366 | 12 | 58 | 634 | 58 | 135 | 212.9 | 45 | 32 | 17 | 4.8 | 14 | 10 | 17.2 |
| Husband earns: | | | | | | | | | | | | | | | |
| Under $521 | 56 | 58 | 2 | 5 | 52 | 5 | 10 | 192.3 | 4 | 6 | 1 | 10.3 | 1 | 1 | ........ |
| $521 to $624 | 32 | 33 | 1 | 3 | 32 | 3 | 17 | ........ | 3 | 1 | 1 | ........ | 1 | 1 | ........ |
| $625 to $779 | 70 | 71 | 1 | 6 | 70 | 6 | 16 | 228.6 | 4 | 1 | 1 | 1.4 | 2 | 1 | ........ |
| $780 to $899 | 78 | 80 | 2 | 7 | 76 | 7 | 26 | 342.1 | 7 | 4 | 2 | 5.0 | 3 | 2 | ........ |
| $900 to $1,199 | 114 | 114 | ........ | 10 | 110 | 10 | 24 | 218.2 | 8 | 4 | 3 | 3.5 | 2 | 2 | ........ |
| $1,200 and over | 24 | 24 | ........ | 2 | 22 | 2 | 5 | ........ | 1 | 2 | 1 | 8.3 | ........ | ........ | ........ |
| Ample[2] | 280 | 286 | 6 | 25 | 272 | 25 | 37 | 136.0 | 18 | 14 | 8 | 4.9 | 5 | 3 | ........ |

[1] Not shown when base is less than 50.

[2] See note on page 45.

TABLE XIV.—DISTRIBUTION ACCORDING TO NUMBER OF PREGNANCIES AND AGE GROUPS OF MARRIED MOTHERS CLASSIFIED BY NATIVITY.

| MOTHER'S AGE AND NUMBER OF REPORTABLE PREGNANCIES. | ALL MOTHERS. | | NATIVE MOTHERS. | | FOREIGN MOTHERS. | |
|---|---|---|---|---|---|---|
| | Number. | Per cent. | Number. | Per cent. | Number. | Per cent. |
| Total pregnancies | 1,491 | 100.0 | 816 | 100.0 | 675 | 100.0 |
| 1 | 339 | 22.7 | 234 | 28.7 | 105 | 15.6 |
| 2 | 283 | 19.0 | 173 | 21.2 | 110 | 16.3 |
| 3 | 214 | 14.4 | 111 | 13.6 | 103 | 15.3 |
| 4 | 186 | 12.5 | 94 | 11.5 | 92 | 13.6 |
| 5 | 147 | 9.8 | 65 | 8.0 | 82 | 12.1 |
| 6 | 94 | 6.3 | 37 | 4.5 | 57 | 8.4 |
| 7 | 83 | 5.6 | 38 | 4.7 | 45 | 6.7 |
| 8 | 54 | 3.6 | 23 | 2.8 | 31 | 4.6 |
| 9 | 33 | 2.2 | 13 | 1.6 | 20 | 3.0 |
| 10 and over | 58 | 3.9 | 28 | 3.4 | 30 | 4.4 |
| Under 20 years, total pregnancies | 89 | 100.0 | 66 | 100.0 | 23 | 100.0 |
| 1 | 74 | 83.1 | 55 | 83.3 | 19 | 82.6 |
| 2 | 12 | 13.5 | 10 | 15.2 | 2 | 8.7 |
| 3 | 3 | 3.4 | 1 | 1.5 | 2 | 8.7 |
| 20 to 24 years, total pregnancies | 461 | 100.0 | 261 | 100.0 | 200 | 100.0 |
| 1 | 178 | 38.6 | 114 | 43.7 | 64 | 32.0 |
| 2 | 156 | 33.8 | 86 | 33.0 | 70 | 35.0 |
| 3 | 77 | 16.7 | 42 | 16.1 | 35 | 17.5 |
| 4 | 39 | 8.5 | 14 | 5.4 | 25 | 12.5 |
| 5 | 10 | 2.2 | 4 | 1.5 | 6 | 3.0 |
| 6 | 1 | .2 | 1 | 0.4 | | |
| 25 to 29 years, total pregnancies | 395 | 100.0 | 199 | 100.0 | 196 | 100.0 |
| 1 | 57 | 14.5 | 45 | 22.6 | 12 | 6.1 |
| 2 | 74 | 18.7 | 46 | 23.1 | 28 | 14.3 |
| 3 | 95 | 24.1 | 40 | 20.1 | 55 | 28.1 |
| 4 | 75 | 19.0 | 40 | 20.1 | 35 | 17.9 |
| 5 | 56 | 14.2 | 17 | 8.5 | 39 | 19.9 |
| 6 | 22 | 5.6 | 7 | 3.6 | 15 | 7.7 |
| 7 | 14 | 3.5 | 4 | 2.0 | 10 | 5.1 |
| 8 | 2 | 4 | | | 2 | 1.0 |
| 30 to 39 years, total pregnancies | 466 | 100.0 | 245 | 100.0 | 221 | 100.0 |
| 1 | 30 | 6.4 | 20 | 8.2 | 10 | 4.5 |
| 2 | 39 | 8.4 | 29 | 11.8 | 10 | 4.5 |
| 3 | 36 | 7.7 | 25 | 10.2 | 11 | 5.0 |
| 4 | 63 | 13.5 | 33 | 13.5 | 30 | 13.6 |
| 5 | 75 | 16.1 | 40 | 16.3 | 35 | 15.8 |
| 6 | 60 | 12.9 | 24 | 9.8 | 36 | 16.3 |
| 7 | 56 | 12.0 | 28 | 11.4 | 28 | 12.7 |
| 8 | 51 | 10.9 | 23 | 9.4 | 28 | 12.7 |
| 9 | 23 | 4.9 | 8 | 3.3 | 15 | 6.8 |
| 10 and over | 33 | 7.1 | 15 | 6.1 | 18 | 8.1 |
| 40 years and over, total pregnancies | 80 | 100.0 | 45 | 100.0 | 35 | 100.0 |
| 2 | 2 | 2.5 | 2 | 4.4 | | |
| 3 | 3 | 3.8 | 3 | 6.7 | | |
| 4 | 9 | 11.3 | 7 | 15.6 | 2 | 5.7 |
| 5 | 6 | 7.5 | 4 | 8.9 | 2 | 5.7 |
| 6 | 11 | 13.8 | 5 | 11.1 | 6 | 17.1 |
| 7 | 13 | 16.3 | 6 | 13.3 | 7 | 20.0 |
| 8 | 1 | 1.3 | | | 1 | 2.9 |
| 9 | 10 | 12.5 | 5 | 11.1 | 5 | 14.3 |
| 10 and over | 25 | 31.3 | 13 | 28.9 | 12 | 34.3 |

TABLE XV.—DISTRIBUTION OF MARRIED MOTHERS BY LOSSES SUSTAINED, ACCORDING TO NATIVITY OF MOTHER AND NUMBER OF POSSIBLE LOSSES.

| NUMBER OF BIRTHS OR POSSIBLE LOSSES AND NATIVITY OF MOTHER. | Number of mothers. | DISTRIBUTION OF MOTHERS ACCORDING TO NUMBER OF LOSSES. | | | | | | | |
|---|---|---|---|---|---|---|---|---|---|
| | | 1 loss. | 2 losses. | 3 losses. | 4 losses. | 5 losses. | 6 losses. | 8 losses. | 10 or more losses. |
| All mothers | 1,491 | 399 | 121 | 60 | 24 | 13 | 8 | 1 | 2 |
| 1 birth | 335 | 53 | ...... | ...... | ...... | ...... | ...... | ...... | ...... |
| 2 births | 277 | 67 | 10 | ...... | ...... | ...... | ...... | ...... | ...... |
| 3 births | 216 | 73 | 14 | 4 | ...... | ...... | ...... | ...... | ...... |
| 4 births | 187 | 55 | 13 | 8 | 1 | ...... | ...... | ...... | ...... |
| 5 births | 148 | 48 | 19 | 11 | 1 | 2 | ...... | ...... | ...... |
| 6 births | 96 | 44 | 13 | 8 | 2 | 1 | 2 | ...... | ...... |
| 7 births | 82 | 22 | 19 | 10 | 2 | ...... | 1 | ...... | ...... |
| 8 births | 54 | 18 | 8 | 10 | 4 | 2 | 2 | ...... | ...... |
| 9 births | 36 | 9 | 10 | 5 | 1 | 1 | 2 | ...... | ...... |
| 10 or more births | 60 | 10 | 15 | 4 | 13 | 7 | 1 | 1 | 2 |
| Native mothers | 816 | 199 | 59 | 19 | 5 | 6 | 1 | 1 | ...... |
| 1 birth | 232 | 29 | ...... | ...... | ...... | ...... | ...... | ...... | ...... |
| 2 births | 170 | 36 | 5 | ...... | ...... | ...... | ...... | ...... | ...... |
| 3 births | 111 | 35 | 7 | 1 | ...... | ...... | ...... | ...... | ...... |
| 4 births | 98 | 33 | 6 | 3 | ...... | ...... | ...... | ...... | ...... |
| 5 births | 65 | 19 | 10 | 4 | ...... | ...... | ...... | ...... | ...... |
| 6 births | 38 | 19 | 7 | 1 | ...... | 1 | ...... | ...... | ...... |
| 7 births | 37 | 10 | 8 | 3 | ...... | ...... | 1 | ...... | ...... |
| 8 births | 21 | 8 | 5 | 3 | ...... | ...... | ...... | ...... | ...... |
| 9 births | 15 | 4 | 4 | 3 | 1 | ...... | ...... | ...... | ...... |
| 10 or more births | 29 | 6 | 7 | 1 | 4 | 5 | ...... | 1 | ...... |
| Foreign mothers | 675 | 200 | 62 | 41 | 19 | 7 | 7 | ...... | 2 |
| 1 birth | 103 | 24 | ...... | ...... | ...... | ...... | ...... | ...... | ...... |
| 2 births | 107 | 31 | 5 | ...... | ...... | ...... | ...... | ...... | ...... |
| 3 births | 105 | 38 | 7 | 3 | ...... | ...... | ...... | ...... | ...... |
| 4 births | 89 | 22 | 7 | 5 | 1 | ...... | ...... | ...... | ...... |
| 5 births | 83 | 29 | 9 | 7 | 1 | 2 | ...... | ...... | ...... |
| 6 births | 58 | 25 | 6 | 7 | 2 | ...... | 2 | ...... | ...... |
| 7 births | 45 | 12 | 11 | 7 | 2 | ...... | ...... | ...... | ...... |
| 8 births | 33 | 10 | 3 | 7 | 4 | 2 | 2 | ...... | ...... |
| 9 births | 21 | 5 | 6 | 2 | ...... | 1 | 2 | ...... | ...... |
| 10 or more births | 31 | 4 | 8 | 3 | 9 | 2 | 1 | ...... | 2 |

# APPENDIXES.

## APPENDIX I.

### STATEMENTS OF MOTHERS.

The statements appended herewith are taken from the testimony of the mothers whose babies were included in the investigation. They, like photographs of random spots, illustrate instances where hard work and a limited income are coexistent with marked loss of infant life. They are offered not as medical or scientific testimony, but because of the natural interest in the mother's viewpoint on these intimate matters. A closer contact with a few individual cases can not but serve to humanize and make more realistic a mass of figures on similar and related topics.

Mother aged 34 years; 9 pregnancies in 17 years; 7 live born; 2 stillborn; no miscarriages reported; 3 deaths in first year, viz, aged 9 weeks, strangled on milk; aged 1 year, pneumonia; aged 6 months, pneumonia; 3 children living at time of agent's visit. In poor health. Has had sunstroke. Worries. Torn at birth of one child. Has lacked medical attention. Father has miner's consumption.

Mother aged 36 years; 10 pregnancies in 12 years; 6 live born; 1 stillborn; 3 miscarriages reported; one death in first year, viz, 4 hours, hemorrhage; 5 children living at time of agent's visit. Formerly toll keeper and had to lift heavy gate during earlier pregnancies. Housework since marriage excessive. Always has instrument deliveries. Home fair. Father skilled mill hand.

Mother aged 38 years; 12 pregnancies in 17 years; 11 live born; 1 miscarriage reported; 3 deaths the first year, viz, 3 weeks, prematurity; 3 months, pneumonia; 3 weeks, unknown; 7 children living at time of agent's visit. During pregnancy resulting in premature birth, in a state of worry and excitement owing to frequent fights in neighborhood. During pregnancy resulting in miscarriage she overexerted self doing heavy laundry work, lifting boilers, etc. Home fair.

Mother aged 35 years; 11 pregnancies in 15 years; 8 live born; 3 miscarriages reported; 3 deaths in first year, viz, aged 10 days, yellow jaundice; 10 days, cause unknown; 6 months, spinal meningitis; 4 children alive at time of agent's visit. Had to do excessive work during pregnancies, as sweeping, washing, lifting tubs, carrying water, etc.

Mother aged 25 years; 7 pregnancies in 6 years; 3 live born; 4 stillborn; 2 deaths the first year, viz, aged 11 days, cause unknown; aged 2 days, cause unknown; 1 child alive at time of agent's visit. Physician stated mother was overworked during pregnancies, therefore during pregnancy resulting in birth of healthy baby in 1911 she was extra careful of self. Fair home. Father skilled mill worker.

Mother aged 34 years; 4 pregnancies in 5 years; all live born; 1 death the first year, viz, aged 11 months, spinal meningitis; 3 children alive at time of agent's visit. Doctor stated period of gestation only 8½ months for each pregnancy. Always miserable during pregnancies. Can not eat. Feet and legs swell. Children fed and cared for intelligently. Home good.

Mother aged 41 years; 12 pregnancies in 22 years; 12 live born; 1 death the first year, viz, aged 3 weeks, spasms; 11 children alive at time of agent's visit. Baby of 1911 poorly developed and in poor health at 1 year of age. When 6 months old was given soup, milk, coffee, and crackers; at 9 months, sauerkraut, cabbage, pie, and everything. Dirty house. Father machinist in mill.

Mother aged 37 years; 12 pregnancies in 15 years; 8 live born; 4 miscarriages reported; 1 death the first year, viz, aged 1 month, cause unknown; 6 children alive at time of agent's visit. Hard worked and worried during pregnancies. Laundry and char work in addition to home duties, but manages to give babies only breast milk during first year.

Mother aged 31 years; 10 pregnancies in 10 years; 8 live born; 2 stillborn; 4 deaths the first year, viz, aged 7 days, 2 days, 1 day, 12 hours, cause unknown; 4 children alive at time of agent's visit. Doctor says not strong enough to bear babies to term or to have healthy children.

Mother aged 32 years; 7 pregnancies in 11 years; 5 live born; 2 stillborn; one death the first year, viz, aged 2 months, mother says from nervous shock and fright from passing trains. Baby died a day or so after family moved to house along railroad track; 3 children alive at time of agent's visit.

Mother aged 27 years; 6 pregnancies in 10 years; 6 live born; 3 deaths the first year, viz, all aged few weeks, cause unknown; 3 children alive at time of agent's visit. Babies who died all born before marriage, when mother was a servant and had to leave them to be artificially fed and poorly cared for when she went to work.

Mother aged 30 years; 9 pregnancies in 14 years; 6 live born; 3 stillborn; no deaths the first year; 3 children alive at time of agent's visit During one pregnancy resulting in stillbirth felt strain of struggle she made to separate fighting lodgers; during another resulting in stillbirth she had fall on ice; and during the third her work had been excessive.

Mother aged 41 years; 13 pregnancies in 22 years; 13 live born; 7 deaths the first year, viz, aged 1 year, 1 year, 2 days, 1 month, few minutes, 6 weeks, 8 weeks, causes unknown; 4 children alive at time of agent's visit. No member of family has ever attended school. They own a lot in a miserable unpaved alley, on which they have built houses 3 deep. They have a dirty cow shed there and sell milk in open receptacles. No sewer connection; yard privy; but they have city water. Save father's earnings and live on milk sales. Never has a doctor or midwife at child birth—manages alone. Began to do her housework two days after birth of 1911 baby.

Mother aged 26 years; 6 pregnancies in 5 years; 5 live born; 1 stillborn; 3 deaths in first year, viz, aged 15 minutes, one-half day, 3 days; 1 child alive at time of agent's visit. The 1911 baby alive and in poor health at 1 year of age. Was given table food in addition to breast milk from 4 months of age.

Mother aged 31 years; 6 pregnancies in 9 years; 6 live born; 2 deaths the first year, viz, aged a few months, croup; a few months, bronchitis and pneumonia; two others at 14 months, each of bronchitis and pneumonia; 2 children alive at time of agent's visit. Father has tuberculosis. Poor, insanitary home. Total income, $500 a year.

Mother aged 33 years; 4 pregnancies in 8 years; 3 live born; 1 miscarriage reported; 1 death the first year, viz, aged 4 months, pneumonia; 2 children alive at time of agent's visit. Does excessive work in own home in addition to char work. The 1911 baby was only one to die in first year. Deserted by husband early in that pregnancy. This pregnancy period was one of worry and mental and physical strain to support her family, and when baby was born she had no milk and gave him condensed milk from birth.

Mother aged 30 years; 11 pregnancies in 12 years; all live born; 5 deaths the first year, of which 2 were from pneumonia; 6 children alive at time of agent's visit. Frail, hard worked, and worried over money matters. Kitchen is living room and a "dark hole in basement." Ventilation of home bad; sleeping-room window always shut "tight." Baby born in 1911 died of pneumonia at age of 9 months.

Mother aged 34 years; 6 pregnancies in 10 years; 6 live born; 5 deaths in first year; causes thereof unknown. The 1911 baby was aged 2 months at death; 1 child alive at time of agent's visit. Says she has never had enough to eat since marriage and that breast milk always leaves her two weeks after childbirth. Poor, dirty, close house. Father a teamster who spends considerable portion of wages in drink.

Mother aged 20 years; 1 pregnancy, resulting in a live-born child who died at the age of 9 months of cholera infantum. Her only child born over one year after husband's desertion; latter claims she is syphilitic. She comes from feeble-minded family whose history is matter of State record. Her grandfather acquitted of killing his son on account of mental condition. Her mother and sister and latter's 18-months-old baby all officially pronounced feeble-minded. Family of loose morals. The baby born in 1911 weaned from breast at age of 4 months and died of cholera infantum at age of 9 months.

Mother aged 30 years; 9 pregnancies in 11 years; 8 live births; 1 miscarriage reported; 3 deaths in first year, viz, aged 3 months, pneumonia; aged 8 months, malarial fever and rheumatism; and the baby born in 1911 weaned from breast when 6 weeks of age, died at age of 9½ months of gastroenteritis; 5 children alive at time of agent's visit. During pregnancy resulting in miscarriage two months after conception, lived on second floor and had to carry heavy wash up and down from yard.

Mother aged 27 years; 3 pregnancies in 3 years, all live births; 2 died in first year, viz, aged 15 days of cause unknown to mother, and other born in 1911, of hereditary syphilis, according to death certificate. Poor, dirty home. Father a steel-mill laborer at $10 a week. One child alive at time of agent's visit.

Mother aged 35 years; 6 births in 12 years; 4 live births and 2 stillbirths. All live born died in first year, viz, aged 6 weeks, bronchitis; aged 13 days, bronchitis; aged 2 days, weak from birth; aged 4 hours, inanition, the last being the 1911 baby. Had another child the following year and she and her husband were so anxious that at least one child should live that she consulted physician concerning its care. Upon his advice she gave up her 20 boarders immediately after child's birth and devoted all her time to it. Thinks she did not stop her hard work soon enough; says she has always worked too hard, keeping boarders in this country and cutting wood and carrying it and water on her back in the old country. Also says the carrying of water, coal, and cases of beer in this country is great strain on her. Father furious because all babies die; wore red necktie to funeral of last to show his disrespect for wife who can only produce children that die. A type of woman who would follow, and profit by, instruction in prenatal care.

Mother aged 25 years; 3 pregnancies in 3 years; all live births; 2 died in first year, viz, aged 1 day, cause unknown; aged 11 months (born in 1911), pneumonia; 1 child alive at time of agent's visit. Father a steel-mill hand. Damp, badly ventilated home, outside toilet.

Mother aged 27 years; 8 children; 1 before marriage and 7 in the 11-year period since marriage at the age of 16. All live births; 3 deaths under 1 year of age, viz, aged 8 months, unknown cause, "stomach turned black"; 3-months old, same statement as for 8-months old child; aged 11 months, ileocolitis. This last born in 1911, was breast fed only three months and then given condensed milk to supplement breast-milk feeding. Four children alive at time of agent's visit. Boarders. Fairly good home. Father a steel-mill hand.

Mother aged 25 years; 2 pregnancies in 8 years; both live-born children, of whom one died, aged 2 days, cause unknown. Mother says neither doctor nor midwife present at birth; that husband "caught" baby at 3 a. m., and she was up and doing regular work at 6 a. m. One child alive at time of agent's visit. Thirteen boarders. Family sleeps in kitchen, which is also used as dining and living room for boarders. Water supply in yard, and privy in yard used by several families. Father works in coal mine.

Mother aged 34 years; 8 pregnancies in 16 years; all live-born children, all but 2 of whom died in first 2 weeks of life from unknown causes, except the last, whose death was certified as from ileocolitis; 2 children alive at time of agent's visit. Never has doctor or midwife at childbirth. Very ignorant. Father a laborer in steel mill.

Mother aged 28 years; 3 pregnancies in 3 years, resulting in 4 live births; 2 (twins) died in their first year, aged 1 month and 4 months, of inanition and malnutrition, respectively; they were never breast fed; condensed milk from birth; 2 children alive at time of agent's visit. Six boarders. Poor, dirty home. City water in yard, also dry privy. Father a steel-mill hand.

Mother aged 36 years; 12 pregnancies in 17 years; all live births; 3 died first year, viz, aged 9 days, born sickly with big head; 9 months, bowel trouble; 10 months, bowel trouble; 9 children alive at time of agent's visit. Began to feed the 1911 baby, who died last, on raw cows' milk from the age of 2 months because she went out to do laundry work and cleaning in the home of a physician and the baby had to be fed in her absence. Bought milk from neighboring cow shed. Combined housework for her large family and outside work a great strain on mother. Dirty home. Father works in mine.

Mother aged 31 years; 10 births in 14 years, 1 being stillbirth. Every live-born child of this woman died in 1 year or less, as follows: Age 4 months, cough; 3 months, cough; 1 year, unknown; 1 year, unknown (the last two were insured for $26 each;

one baby died before company delivered policy); the others died at ages of 3 months, 4 months, 1 year, 3 months, and 10 weeks, respectively, of causes unknown to mother, who said all had "sores on body." Certificate gives scrofula as cause of death of baby born in 1911. The first 2 children were born and died in Europe. Attending midwife in Johnstown says father has syphilis. Both parents, however, claim to be healthy; father drinks, came to United States 2 years ahead of wife. Had worked in cigar factory from age of 13 until she came to United States. Her own mother had worked in same place 30 years. She never stays in bed over 3 days when a child is born. Father a car-shop rigger.

Mother aged 25 years; only 1 pregnancy; mother married 2 years. Baby born alive with "sores on body"; died aged 4 months; she says "wasted away"; certificate states ileocolitis. Weaned from breast when 3 weeks old because she had typhoid. Hard worker, but has dirty home and never opens a window. Water and privy in yard. Father a steel-mill hand.

Mother aged 20 years. First and only pregnancy resulted in live-born child who died, aged 6 months, of convulsions. Weaned from breast, aged 4 months, because her milk left her on account of hard work. Baby on condensed milk till 5 months old, then given bread, cakes, apples, etc. Five boarders. Home neither clean nor well ventilated. Father a steel-mill worker.

Mother aged 22 years; only 1 pregnancy; a live-born child that died in July, aged 7 months, of cholera infantum. Milk and crackers added to breast feeding at age of 5 months. Again pregnant when baby was 6 months old, but continued nursing baby until its death, 1 month later. Unclean 1-room home; yard hydrant and privy for use of this and other families. Father works in coal mine.

Mother aged 38; 13 pregnancies in 17 years, 11 live births and 2 premature stillbirths. Only 2 children living at time of agent's visit. The second to eighth, the eleventh, and the thirteenth children died of bowel trouble at ages ranging from 3 weeks to 4 months. Only cause of death she can give is that "food did not agree with them." Believed in feeding babies and gave them everything anybody told her to give them; begins at 1 month to give them bread, potatoes, egg, crackers, etc. For last baby that died she got a goat and gave the baby its milk; goat got sick, but she persisted in giving the baby its milk until the goat went dry. Directed the feeding of her daughter's baby until its death at 3 months of age. On account of many children she has had, the neighbors consider her an authority on baby care. Slovenly home. Dry privy in yard. Father a stable hand.

#### MOTHERS WHO HAD STILLBORN CHILDREN IN 1911.

Mother aged 23 years; 2 live births and 1 stillbirth in 4 years. Stillbirth followed a fall down cellar steps while carrying coal when 6 months pregnant; 2 children alive at time of agent's visit. Father works in coal mine.

Mother aged 24 years; 3 pregnancies in 5 years, 2 live births and 1 stillbirth, which physician said was due to excessive work on sewing machine during pregnancy. Both live-born children alive at time of agent's visit. Father a steel-mill hand. Good home.

Mother aged 30 years; no live births; 2 miscarriages and 1 stillbirth from August, 1910, to November, 1911; periods of gestation 5, 4, and 6 months, respectively. Cause of losses unknown. When 21 years old had operation for prolapsis. Always tired and weak during pregnancies. Father a steel-mill worker. Home good.

Mother aged 39 years; 9 pregnancies in 19 years; 5 live births; 2 stillbirths; 2 miscarriages reported. Gives overwork and worry as cause of miscarriages and 1 stillbirth and a fall as cause in the other stillbirth; 4 children alive at time of agent's visit. Father laborer in steel mill. Home good.

Mother aged 27 years; 3 pregnancies in 8 years; 2 live births (in 1903 and 1905) and 1 stillbirth (in 1911); 2 children alive at time of agent's visit. In 1908 had fall which caused internal misplacements; never had treatment for same; during 1911 pregnancy had convulsions from uremic poisoning. She has kidney trouble. Fair living conditions. Father a mill hand.

Mother aged 30 years; 2 pregnancies in 2 years; no live births. First a miscarriage after 4½ months' gestation, said to be due to fall; second, after 7 months' gestation, attributed to indigestion. Father a machinist in steel mill. Home clean. Dry privy and well are in yard.

Mother aged 37 years; 10 pregnancies in 16 years; first, seventh, eighth, and ninth children were live born; the others stillborn. All the live born died, as follows: Age 3 months, scarlet fever; 2 months, scarlet fever; 6 months, "boils on stomach"; 6 weeks, cause unknown. Has no idea of causes of stillbirths; very ignorant. Keeps boarders. Father a laborer in steel mill.

Mother aged 31 years; 5 pregnancies in 8 years; 4 live born; 1 (the last) premature stillborn from an unknown cause. All the live-born children died under 6 months of age, viz, 6 months old, summer complaint; 2 months, summer complaint; 2 weeks, unknown cause, but was half black and had sores on stomach; 1 day old, cause unknown. Keeps boarders. Home bad. Father a laborer in steel mill.

Mother aged 28 years; 5 pregnancies in 3 years; 4 live births, the last a stillbirth; all live born died of unknown causes at ages of 10 months, 3 weeks, 2 weeks, and 2 weeks, respectively. First baby bottle fed from birth; could not nurse him on account of having "neck full of boils." Has had hospital treatment for womb trouble. Father a steel-mill worker. Insanitary home.

Mother aged 23 years; 4 pregnancies in 3 years; 1 live birth and 3 stillbirths. The live-born baby, who died at age of 3 months of unknown cause, had "scabs on face." She is a charwoman, who thinks that "possibly" she works too hard. While pregnant always has fear babies will be born dead. Does not feel good after big day's work done during pregnancy. Father a steel-mill hand. Poor home conditions.

## APPENDIX II.

### DETAILED DESCRIPTION OF METHOD USED FOR COMPUTING INFANT MORTALITY RATE FOR THIS REPORT, AND COMPARISON WITH CONVENTIONAL METHOD.

In this study the infant mortality rate is obtained by comparing the number of babies born alive in Johnstown in 1911 with the number of those same babies who died before they were a year old, omitting, as was necessary in a detailed study where approximations were not allowed, those babies whose parents could not be located by the bureau's agents. This method gives an exact and absolute infant mortality rate of 134 per thousand for this limited group of babies.

Obviously, this method can not practically be used to obtain the infant mortality rate for large groups of population, year by year. Where there is a constant flow of population, cities, States, or communities can not trace the place of birth of infants dying within their respective areas or follow each child born within their boundaries if it moves away. It is impossible to know the life history of each child born in the area considered in a given year and to determine, as has been done for this intensive study of a small and definite group, how many babies per 1,000 live born in a given area actually do die under 1 year of age.

The established method of obtaining an infant mortality rate is to compare the live births in a given area during a single calendar year with the infant deaths (that is, deaths of babies under 1 year of age) occurring during that same year. Of course, the babies dying in that year are not all born in the same year nor in that same area, and of those born in the given calendar year not all who die under 12 months of age die in the calendar year of their birth. But this is the only feasible method as yet discovered for approximating an infant mortality rate for large areas, and it is sufficiently accurate for practical and comparative purposes; that is, for approximating the relative rank of different cities, States, and countries with respect to infant mortality.

The infant mortality rates of the various States and also of cities of at least 50,000 population within the registration area [1] of the United States for the year 1910 are shown in the following table, taken from a bulletin of the Federal Census Bureau.[2] All the rates in this table are computed by the established method.

---

[1] The Bureau of the Census designates as the registration area the area comprising States in which the registration laws are of suitable character and sufficiently well enforced to insure at least approximately complete (i. e., at least 90 per cent) returns of births and deaths. In addition to such States it includes certain cities in nonregistration States in which the returns are made with equal effectiveness under local ordinances.

[2] Bulletin 109, Mortality Statistics: 1910. Government Printing Office, Washington, 1912.

Population, Registered Births, Deaths of Infants under 1 Year of Age, and Infant Mortality Rates for Registration States and Registration Cities having a Population of at Least 50,000 in 1910.

| AREA. | Population in 1910. | Births.[1] | Deaths[2] of infants under 1 year of age. | |
|---|---|---|---|---|
| | | | Number. | Per 1,000 births.[3] |
| REGISTRATION STATES. | | | | |
| Connecticut | 1,114,756 | 27,291 | 3,476 | 127 |
| Maine | 742,371 | 15,578 | 2,108 | 135 |
| Massachusetts | 3,366,416 | 86,765 | 11,377 | 131 |
| Michigan | 2,810,173 | 63,566 | 7,912 | 124 |
| New Hampshire | 430,572 | 9,385 | 1,373 | 146 |
| Pennsylvania | 7,665,111 | 202,631 | 28,377 | 140 |
| Rhode Island | 542,610 | [4] 6,595 | [4] 1,111 | [4] 168 |
| Vermont | 355,956 | 7,343 | 791 | 168 |
| REGISTRATION CITIES OF 50,000 POPULATION OR OVER IN 1910. | | | | |
| Connecticut: | | | | |
| Bridgeport | 102,054 | 2,976 | 367 | 123 |
| Hartford | 98,915 | 2,411 | 286 | 119 |
| New Haven | 133,605 | 3,772 | 406 | 108 |
| Waterbury | 73,141 | 2,150 | 320 | 149 |
| Washington, D. C | 331,069 | 7,016 | 1,068 | 152 |
| Portland, Me | 58,571 | 1,163 | 167 | 144 |
| Massachusetts: | | | | |
| Boston | 670,585 | 17,760 | 2,246 | 126 |
| Brockton | 56,878 | 1,359 | 134 | 99 |
| Cambridge | 104,839 | 2,462 | 293 | 119 |
| Fall River | 119,295 | 4,591 | 854 | 186 |
| Holyoke | 57,730 | 1,702 | 362 | 213 |
| Lawrence | 85,892 | 3,165 | 529 | 167 |
| Lowell | 106,294 | 2,630 | 607 | 231 |
| Lynn | 89,336 | 2,218 | 216 | 97 |
| New Bedford | 96,652 | 3,873 | 685 | 177 |
| Somerville | 77,236 | 1,728 | 174 | 101 |
| Springfield | 88,926 | 2,438 | 302 | 124 |
| Worcester | 145,986 | 3,918 | 536 | 137 |
| Michigan: | | | | |
| Detroit | 465,766 | 11,960 | 2,138 | 179 |
| Grand Rapids | 112,571 | 2,693 | 329 | 122 |
| Saginaw | 50,510 | 897 | 130 | 145 |
| Manchester, N. H | 70,063 | 1,939 | 375 | 193 |
| New York, N. Y | 4,766,883 | 129,316 | 6,159 | 125 |
| Bronx Borough | 430,980 | 10,926 | 11,047 | 96 |
| Brooklyn Borough | 1,634,351 | 43,128 | 5,063 | 117 |
| Manhattan Borough | 2,331,542 | 66,112 | 8,900 | 135 |
| Queens Borough | 284,041 | 7,095 | 865 | 122 |
| Richmond Borough | 85,969 | 2,055 | 284 | 138 |
| Pennsylvania: | | | | |
| Allentown | 51,913 | 1,406 | 202 | 144 |
| Altoona | 52,127 | 1,392 | 100 | 110 |
| Erie | 66,525 | 1,713 | 197 | 115 |
| Harrisburg | 64,186 | 1,308 | 169 | 129 |
| Johnstown | 55,482 | 1,628 | 268 | 165 |
| Philadelphia | 1,549,008 | 38,666 | 5,334 | 138 |
| Pittsburgh | 533,905 | 15,059 | 2,259 | 150 |
| Reading | 96,071 | 2,370 | 336 | 142 |
| Scranton | 129,867 | 3,512 | 520 | 148 |
| Wilkes-Barre | 67,105 | 1,840 | 269 | 146 |
| Rhode Island: | | | | |
| Pawtucket | 51,622 | (5) | 191 | (5) |
| Providence | 224,326 | (5) | 827 | (5) |

1 Provisional figures; exclusive of stillbirths.
2 Exclusive of stillbirths.
3 Based on provisional figures for births.
4 The figures for Rhode Island are exclusive of Providence and Pawtucket.
5 Returns of births not received from State board in time for inclusion.

It will be seen by this table that Johnstown is among the 10 cities of more than 50,000 population which had an infant mortality rate for 1910 in excess of 150 per 1,000 births. These 10 cities and their respective rates are as follows: Lowell, Mass., 231; Holyoke, Mass., 213; Manchester, N. H., 193; Fall River, Mass., 186; Detroit, Mich., 179; New Bedford, Mass., 177; Lawrence, Mass., 167; Johnstown, Pa., 165; Washington, D. C., 152; and Pittsburgh, Pa., 150.

It should be borne in mind that the absolute infant mortality rate of 134, computed for the group of babies included in this investigation, that is, for those born in Johnstown in 1911, can not be compared with any of the approximate rates in the foregoing table, since the basis of computation is entirely different. But the method used in this report seemed to be the only practicable one for our purpose, namely, to measure the infant mortality rate in different districts of the city where the babies are subjected to varying conditions.

# APPENDIX III.

## THE MILK SUPPLY.

[A study by the Dairy Division, United States Department of Agriculture, May 23 to June 16, 1913. Conducted by L. B. Cook, C. E. Clement, and B. J. Davis.]

Between the dates of May 23 and June 16, 1913, the Dairy Division, United States Department of Agriculture, made a study and survey of the milk supply of Johnstown, Pa. This study consisted of a chemical and bacteriological examination of samples and an inspection of the sources of supply. The Government score card was used for all inspection work. This work showed that about 4,000 gallons of milk were consumed daily in the city, or an average of a little over one-half pint per capita. About two-thirds of this milk is shipped over the Baltimore & Ohio and the Pennsylvania Railroads, but by far the most over the Baltimore & Ohio. The sources of the milk supply may easily be divided into city cow dairies, farmer milk dealers, dairy farms, city milk plants, and stores. Each of these will be discussed separately.

### CITY COW DAIRIES.

About 150 cows are kept within the city limits. Most of these dairies are owned by foreigners and consist of two or three cows. The city dairies produced about 150 to 200 gallons of the city's milk supply. These dairies are very filthy and the sanitary conditions bad. The health of the cows is somewhat questionable, because the majority are stabled in small stables throughout the year. These stables are so small and the cows so crowded in that in some stables they have to take turns in lying down. The stables frequently have no means of ventilation or lighting except one or two small openings in the sides of the building. Most of the stables were located near contaminating surroundings, such as manure piles and outside closets.

The food for the cows in many of these dairies was fermented and in a bad condition, due to its being a wet mixture which was prepared far in advance of feeding.

The utensils were very poor in construction, most of them having open seams and in a condition impossible to clean properly. The pails were of the common cheap open type. In nearly all cases city water was used for all purposes.

The cows were not in as bad a condition as they might have been with regard to cleanliness, although very little bedding was used, but the manure as a rule was not left standing in the stable, which accounts partly for the condition of the cows.

The uncleanliness of the stable was marked, and usually no credit was given under this heading. Very few whitewashed stables were found, while cobwebs, dirt, and dust abounded nearly everywhere.

The manure was removed to a box or pile near the stable. Some of these boxes were covered, but many were not.

These city dairies had no milk houses. As soon as the milk was milked it was taken to the house, strained, and delivered to the customers, who were usually the neighbors.

The milk utensils were often found dirty and being used for many other purposes. It is very doubtful if many of these milk pails are ever thoroughly scalded. After being washed they were kept almost any place, but were seldom put in a good place free from contaminating surroundings.

The milking was usually done by the women, who wore very dirty clothes and often milked with wet and filthy hands. No pretense was made to clean the cows or use a damp cloth.

The milk was not cooled, but sold while warm at 8 cents per quart. Most of the consumers who bought this milk had no ice or refrigerators, therefore it remained warm for some time or until consumed. Sometimes the milk was placed in earthen jars and set on the cellar bottom, but as a rule no effort was made at cooling. The milk was sold twice a day.

The average score for the 48 city dairies visited was 26.34 points. The highest was 43.50 and the lowest 16.75—12 scored below 20, 23 between 20 and 30, and 12 in the thirties, with 1 above 40.

### FARMER MILK DEALERS.

By farmer milk dealers is meant those farmers who retail their own milk and possibly buy a little from other farms. There are about 26 such dealers in the city and they handle about 1,000 gallons of the city's milk supply. Some of these dairies were the source of the city's best milk. The average score of these dairies was 39.43. Most of this milk is hauled from 3 to 5 miles to the city, then peddled upon the street. These dealers bottle very little milk, and most of it is drawn from a faucet. They use covered wagons and some peddle garden truck—like flowers, onions, etc.—on the same wagon.

The cows, as a rule, seemed to be in good health, but very few had ever been tuberculin tested. The barns were of the sort typical of that section of the country, with a stone wall on one side and an overhanging shed on the other, which meant that the stables were dark, as light could only enter at the ends. The basement was used for all the farm animals, as horses, pigs, cows, chickens, etc., and the cow stable was not separated from the rest. The general construction was only fair. A few cement floors, tight walls, ceilings, etc., were found.

The ventilation was poor and conditions as to the cleanliness of the stable very bad. In many of the stables at this time of the year the manure was not removed daily and oftentimes it was piled near the stable. In general the cows could be well rated as to cleanliness, as they were outdoors both day and night.

At some of these farms milk houses were found, but many used the cellar of the house for handling and cooling the milk. These milk rooms were often used for the storage of other things and were not as clean as they should be. Some strained the milk at the stable, but many removed it to the milk room for straining.

Many of the utensils were of poor construction and were not thoroughly washed. The milk dealers usually scalded the pails and had a place to keep them after being washed. No covered pails or special milking suits were found and only one milk cooler. Most of the milkers milk with a dry hand, but do not clean the cows or use a damp cloth. Most of these farms had excellent water facilities, having running water at a temperature of from 50° to 55° F. This was used for washing utensils and cooling the milk.

The cooling was done by setting the 5-gallon cans in a trough of running water, but oftentimes the milk was not stirred, therefore the cooling was delayed. Some of these dairymen used ice on the farms and on the wagons.

The lowest score of these farmer milk dealers was 22.40 and the highest was 53.50. There were 4 farms scoring in the twenties, 8 in the thirties, 13 in the forties, and 1 above 50.

### DAIRY FARMS.

Under this heading is meant the farms that ship or draw milk to the dealers. Some of these farms sold cream in the summer and milk in the winter. Two hundred and twenty-one of such farms were visited and their average score was 36.06, which was a little lower than the farmer dealer. Some of these farms were fairly good, but most of them were poor in their facilities and methods of handling milk. In general, these farms were like the farm dealers, but many were much worse. Very few had any milk houses, but handled the milk in the cellar or set the cans in some trough of running water. These farmers oftentimes had to carry their milk several miles over very bad roads to the railroad station where it was shipped to Johnstown. Very few covered pails or milk coolers were being used.

The lowest score for these farms was 22.50, while the highest was 70.6. Of these farms 52.9 per cent scored between 30 and 40.

*Transportation.*—Most of this milk was shipped over the Baltimore & Ohio Railroad from points between Somerset, Pa., and Johnstown. The milk was placed on the uncovered platform at the receiving station, then placed in baggage cars for transportation. No refrigerator cars were used. The total railroad haul on this line is about 40 miles. When the milk reaches Johnstown it is at a temperature of about 65° F., depending on the outside temperature. It is then unloaded onto an uncovered platform, and if the dealer does not take it away at once it is left in the sun to get still warmer. One day after taking temperatures on arrival of the train, the inspectors returned in one and one-half hours and found about one-half of the milk still in the sun and the temperature of the milk was then about 15° warmer, or at a temperature of about 85° to 90° F.

Some of the milk shipped over the Pennsylvania Railroad comes a longer distance, but no refrigerator cars are used for the Johnstown supply and about the same conditions exist.

### CITY MILK PLANTS.

There are about 15 city milk dealers. These dealers have their milk shipped in or hauled on wagons. The two large dealers in Johnstown handle about one-half of the city's milk supply.

The small dealers have no milk plant, as they take the milk as delivered from the farm and peddle it direct. Most of them have a refrigerator for storage of any milk left over. They bottle very little, and a few use ice.

The two large milk companies pasteurize and bottle all of their retail trade. One of these dairies has four creameries outside of Johnstown from which it draws some of its supply when needed. These plants are located at Indiana, Martinsburg, Woodbury, and New Enterprise, Pa. These plants do a considerable cream and ice cream business; some of them also pasteurize the milk before it is shipped to Johnstown, where it may be repasteurized and is bottled.

The sanitary conditions in these plants were found to be poor and no ice was used on the wagons. Apparently, from the bacterial results, the pasteurizing did very little, if any, good. The flash method was used at a temperature of about 165° F., and after pasteurizing the milk was exposed to much contamination.

The average score of all of these plants was 39.37. Some of the plants received a higher score than they really deserved, because they had no real plant but only a refrigerator and a place to wash the utensils, the milk not being brought to the plant.

The milk cans as returned to the farmer were in a very bad condition, as these plants do not properly wash them. Some of them rinse the cans, while others do not even do that; consequently when the farmer receives the cans they have sour milk in them and very bad odors. With a farmer's limited means at hand it is nearly impossible to get these cans in proper condition to again ship sweet milk in them.

One creamery at Friedens, Pa., ships about 100 gallons of milk direct to some of the small city dealers and stores.

### STORES HANDLING MILK.

A great many of the stores sell milk. Some of these buy bottled milk, while others buy direct from the farmer and sell dipped or faucet milk. Most of this milk is sold as an accommodation to customers. Many of these stores have ice boxes or refrigerators to keep the milk cold. However, some of the stores have no facilities for keeping the milk at a low temperature and the cans or bottles are allowed to sit on the floor until all the milk is sold. These stores do not wash the cans or bottles. Much of this store milk is open to considerable contamination from dust, dirt, and flies.

The average score of the stores handling bulk milk was 46.11. The highest was 72.75, and the lowest 12.30.

### BACTERIOLOGICAL AND CHEMICAL RESULTS.

Samples for this work were taken at as many sources as possible. The samples taken at the city cow dairies gave a low bacteria count, due to the sample being taken immediately after milking. In all, 163 samples of milk were examined, 115 being from producers and 48 from dealers. The maximum bacteria count was 319 million per cubic centimeter, and the minimum count was 3,650 bacteria per cubic centimeter. This sample was taken from one of the city cow dairies and it was fresh milk direct from the cow.

The average count of all samples was 1,699,587 bacteria per cubic centimeter. Two samples were sour when taken at the railroad station.

7 samples, or 4.2 per cent, were under 50,000 bacteria per cubic centimeter.

6 samples, or 3.6 per cent, were between 50,000 and 100,000 bacteria per cubic centimeter.

31 samples, or 19 per cent, were between 100,000 and 500,000 bacteria per cubic centimeter.

22 samples, or 13.5 per cent, were between 500,000 and 1,000,000 bacteria per cubic centimeter.

45 samples, or 27.6 per cent, were between 1,000,000 and 10,000,000 bacteria per cubic centimeter.

44 samples, or 27 per cent, were between 10,000,000 and 50,000,000 bacteria per cubic centimeter.

8 samples, or 4.9 per cent, were over 50,000,000 bacteria per cubic centimeter.

This table shows that 59.5 per cent of the samples contained over 1,000,000 bacteria per cubic centimeter.

The fat was only determined on 161 samples, and the average per cent was found to be 3.58. The minimum per cent was 1.2 and the maximum 5.

14 samples, or 8.7 per cent, contained below 3 per cent fat.

108 samples, or 66.1 per cent, contained between 3 and 4 per cent fat.

39 samples, or 25.1 per cent, contained 4 per cent fat or above.

The total solids was determined on 93 samples with an average of 11.68.

## GENERAL SUMMARY.

The bacterial results and the inspection work show that the milk sold in Johnstown, Pa., is very poor. The scores are low and most of the milk has a bacteria count in the millions. This is easily explained by the fact that the city does no milk inspection work, therefore the general methods and ideas in use do not tend for clean milk. The general idea is that if milk is not sour it must be all right; then where the milk is pasteurized no particular pains are taken with its care. Our results show that pasteurizing did very little if any good. On the farms and in the city no particular methods or care are used to keep the bacteria count low.

1. There are 48 dairies in the city with an average score of only 26.84 out of a possible 100. On the whole, the city dairies were vile from a sanitary standpoint. While the bacteria counts taken on this milk were fairly low it must be remembered that milk produced at these places is delivered warm to the consumer; this milk is sold in the poorer sections, where there is usually no way to keep it cold until it is used, so that before it is finally consumed the bacteria count is probably extremely high.

2. The dairymen who operated farms and sold the milk from their own farms were in average condition for uninspected dairies. Their average score was 39.43 out of a possible 100.

3. Transportation facilities are very crude and there is an entire lack of care in handling the milk from the farm to the city.

4. The facilities for handling the milk in the city are very poor; many dealers have no equipment or means of refrigerating the milk or handling it properly. The average score of the city dairies was 39.37 out of a possible 100. There were only two plants inspected which were in fairly presentable condition. Pasteurization as carried on at the present time in Johnstown is a farce. This is shown by the fact that 52 farmers shipping milk to one of the dairies averaged 1,419,961 bacteria per cubic centimeter when the milk arrived at Johnstown, while samples taken from the milk supply handled by this dairy showed an average count of 18,337,500 bacteria per cubic centimeter, indicating that the milk was much worse after it had been "pasteurized" than it was before. Another large dairy did a little better, but the results obtained there showed a very incomplete pasteurizing process. Twenty-eight dairymen supplying milk to the latter dairy averaged 30,410,071 bacteria per cubic centimeter when the milk arrived at Johnstown, while the finished product as put out by the dairy averaged 3,150,083 bacteria per cubic centimeter.

5. A large amount of dipped milk is sold both from the wagons and from stores in Johnstown at the present time. Such a practice is at best insanitary, but carried on as it is in Johnstown it is a positive menace.

6. Bacteria counts showed that the milk averaged 1,699,587 and that 59.5 per cent of the samples showed over a million bacteria per cubic centimeter.

7. Aside from the bacteriological condition of the milk it was found to be in many cases lacking in the required food elements. Of 44 samples taken from milk dealers 29.5 per cent were found to be below the State standard for butter fat, while of 118 samples taken from producers, 22.9 per cent were found to be below the State standard for butter fat.

RESULTS OF THE INSPECTION WORK DONE IN JOHNSTOWN, PA.

| Score. | City cow dairies. | Farm milk dealers. | Dairy farms. | City milk plants. | Stores. |
|---|---|---|---|---|---|
| 0 to 10 | ........ | ........ | ........ | 1 | 2 |
| 10 to 20 | 12 | ........ | 43 | ........ | ........ |
| 20 to 30 | 23 | 4 | 117 | 4 | ........ |
| 30 to 40 | 12 | 8 | 55 | 4 | 1 |
| 40 to 50 | 1 | 13 | 3 | 2 | 4 |
| 50 to 60 | ........ | 1 | 1 | ........ | ........ |
| 60 to 70 | ........ | ........ | 2 | ........ | 1 |
| 70 to 80 | ........ | ........ | ........ | ........ | ........ |
| 80 to 90 | ........ | ........ | ........ | ........ | ........ |
| 90 to 100 | ........ | ........ | ........ | ........ | ........ |
| Total[1] | 48 | 26 | 221 | 11 | 8 |
| Average score | 26.34 | 39.43 | 36.06 | 39.37 | 46.11 |

[1] In all, 314.

PLATE A



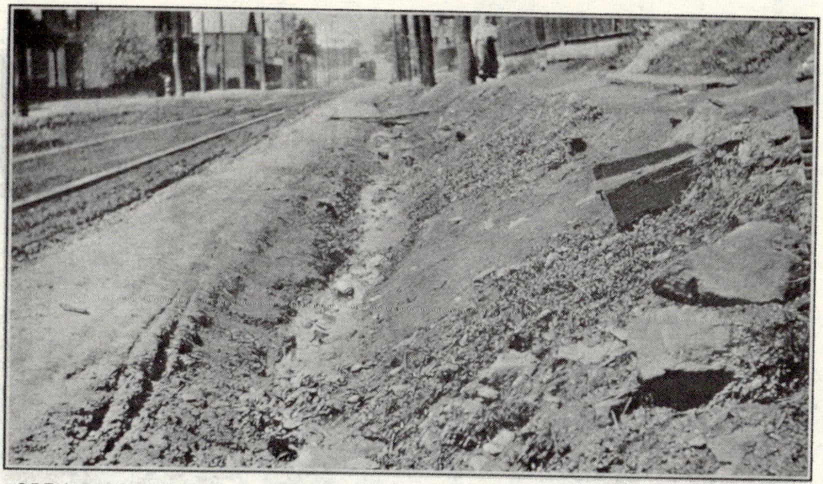

OPEN DITCH ALONG WOODVALE AVENUE, WHICH RECEIVES ALL KINDS OF HOUSE DRAINAGE.

This ditch is cleaned out by heavy rains, but within a few days becomes offensive again. This important street in Woodvale is unpaved and without sidewalks.

PLATE B

Infant Mortality: Johnstown, Pa., 1913.

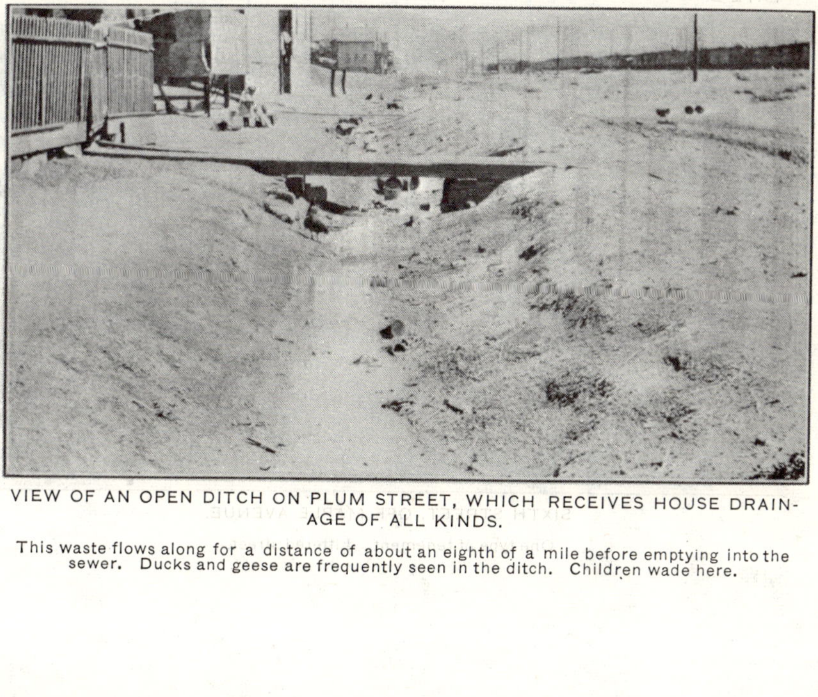

VIEW OF AN OPEN DITCH ON PLUM STREET, WHICH RECEIVES HOUSE DRAINAGE OF ALL KINDS.

This waste flows along for a distance of about an eighth of a mile before emptying into the sewer. Ducks and geese are frequently seen in the ditch. Children wade here.

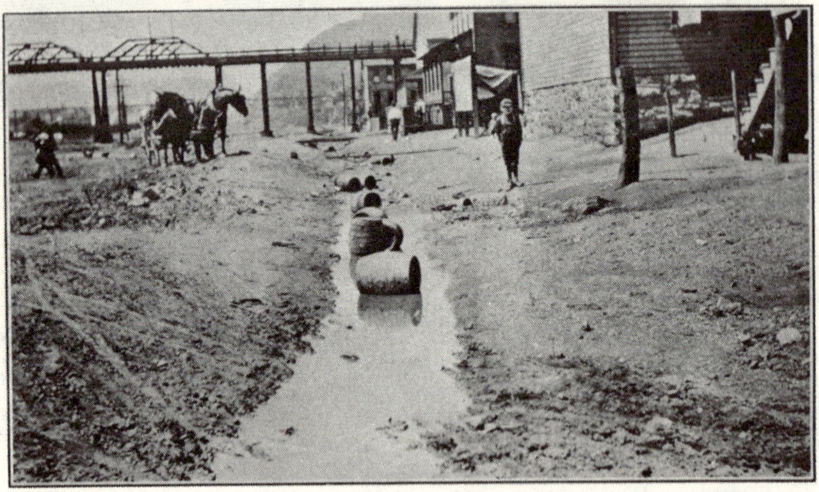

ANOTHER VIEW OF PLUM STREET.

Open sewer ditch, a convenient dumping place for empty beer kegs, etc.



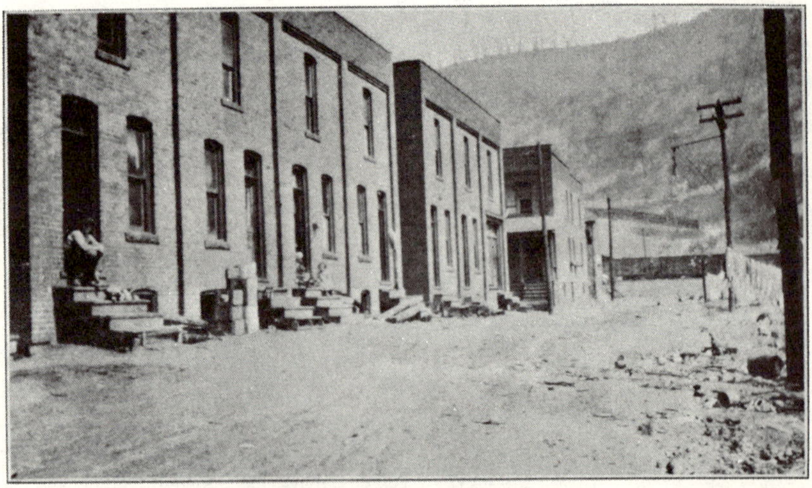

SIXTH STREET, OFF MAPLE AVENUE.

One type of tenement. Littered street.

PLATE E Infant Mortality: Johnstown, Pa., 1913.

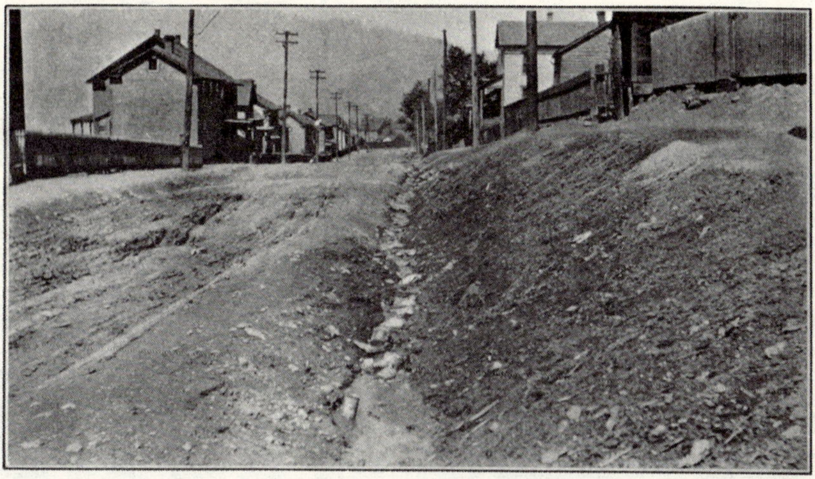

AN OPEN DITCH ALONG NEW STREET, PROSPECT.

Private pipes into this ditch are numerous. Here the waste flows along until it enters a sewer at the right of the fence near the center of the background.

PLATE F Infant Mortality: Johnstown, Pa., 1913.

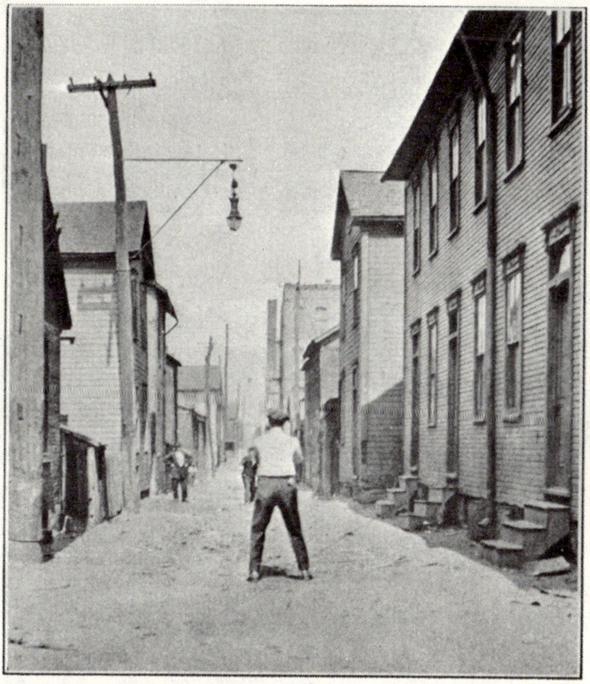

LOWER PART OF BRADLEY ALLEY, WHICH RUNS ALMOST THE ENTIRE LENGTH OF CAMBRIA CITY.

Main or front entrances to abutting houses shown. Unpaved. Width, 19 feet 10 inches.

PLATE G

Infant Mortality: Johnstown, Pa., 1913.

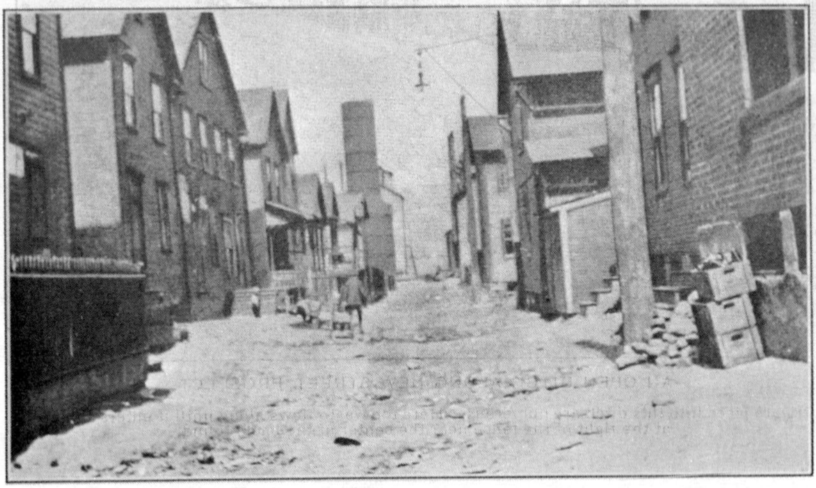

UPPER END OF BRADLEY ALLEY, CAMBRIA CITY.

(See preceding picture.)

PLATE H

Infant Mortality: Johnstown, Pa., 1913.

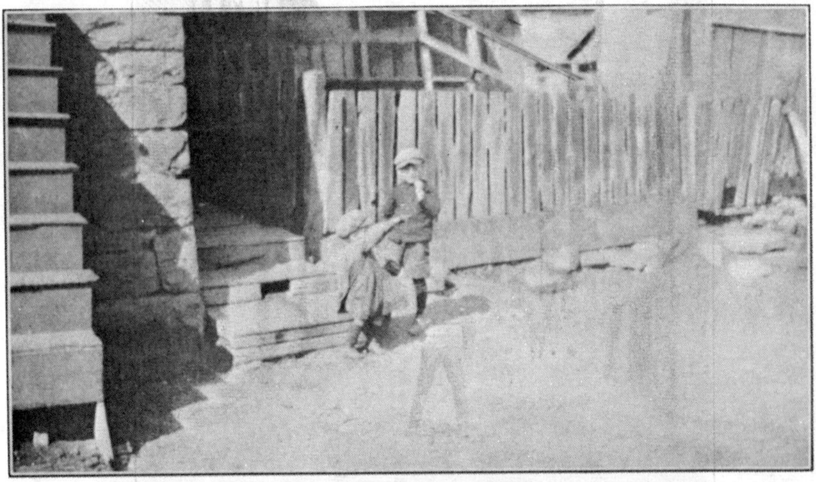

A FRONT YARD ON CONNELLY AVENUE, MINERSVILLE.

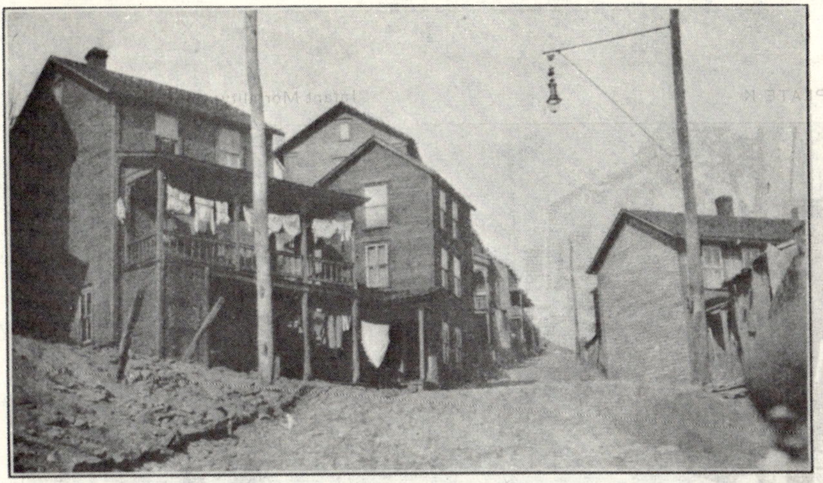

A VIEW OF KELLEY ALLEY OR GARVEY PLACE IN MINERSVILLE.

Houses to the left of the picture are of flimsy construction. Drainage from the large house flows into the street.



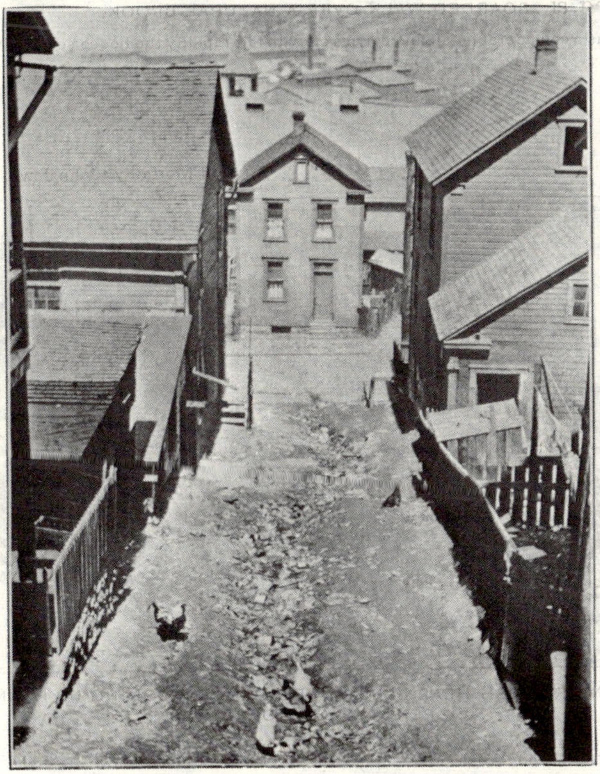

ONE OF SEVERAL LITTLE ALLEYS OF CONEMAUGH BOROUGH LEADING DOWN THE HILL FROM HUBER STREET.

Waste water from the houses not absorbed by the soil trickles down the depression noted in the center.

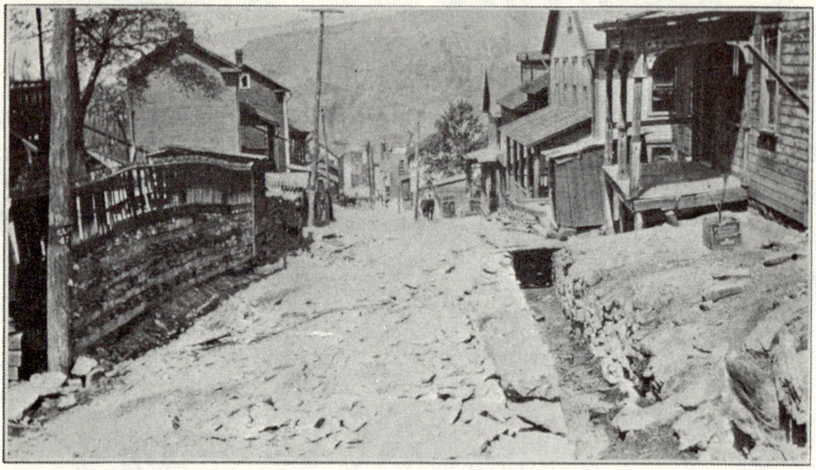

HORRICK STREET, CONEMAUGH BOROUGH, NEAR CITY LIMITS; LOOSELY BOARDED WALK OVER A NATURAL BROOK.

The brook has a considerable fall and carries off with fair rapidity the house sewage it receives.



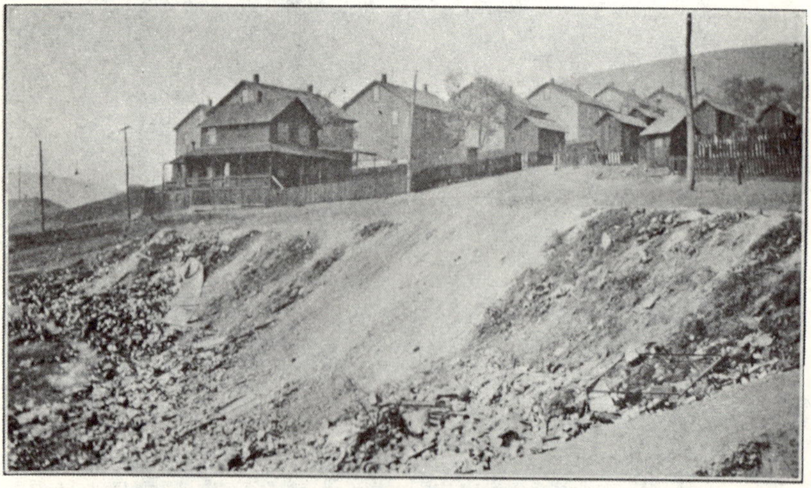

AN ASH AND RUBBISH HEAP BELOW PEELORVILLE, LOOKING UP FROM THE PENNSYLVANIA DEPOT.

Company houses shown in the picture.

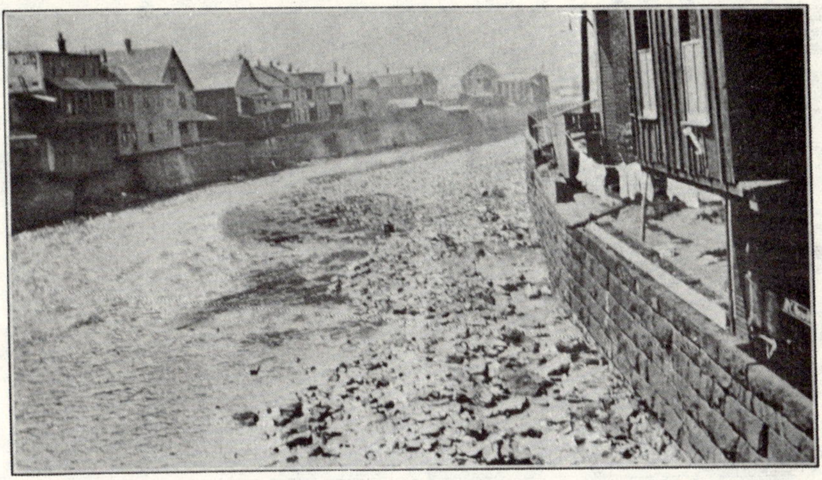

THE CONEMAUGH RIVER, TAKEN FROM WALNUT STREET BRIDGE NEAR THE PENNSYLVANIA RAILROAD DEPOT.

Because of the low stage of water usual in the warm months, sewage is exposed on the stones and rocks.



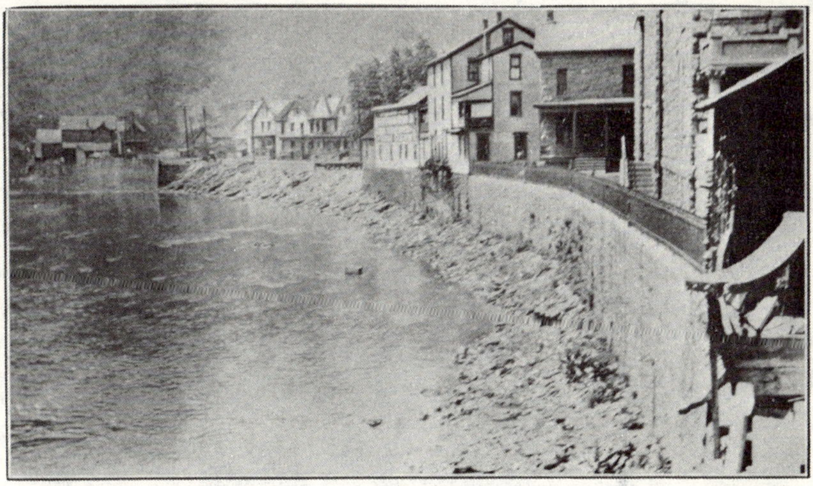

VIEW OF STONY CREEK, LOOKING WEST, TAKEN FROM FRANKLIN STREET BRIDGE.

Discharge of sewage through some of the outlets in the wall trickles down the wall for a distance of perhaps 6 feet before reaching the water. At low stage of the river the deposits on the stones below become very offensive.

PLATE O



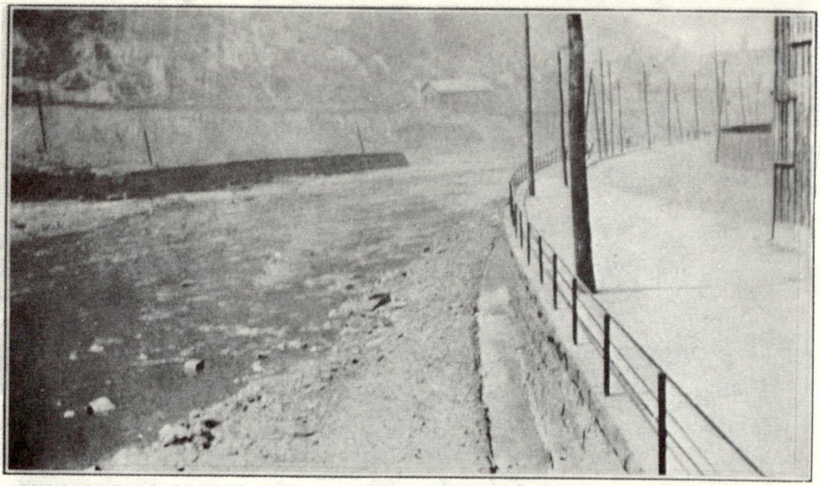

THE CONEMAUGH RIVER.

View from foot of bridge at end of Johns Street, just above the point where the Conemaugh and Stony Creek meet. The sewer drainage settles in the ditch alongside the retaining wall for perhaps 150 feet before reaching the sluggish current of the river itself. When the ditch becomes clogged it is dug out, and the contents thrown on the dry bed between the ditch and the river must remain there until washed into the middle of the stream by high water.

PLATE P

Infant Mortality: Johnstown, Pa., 1913.

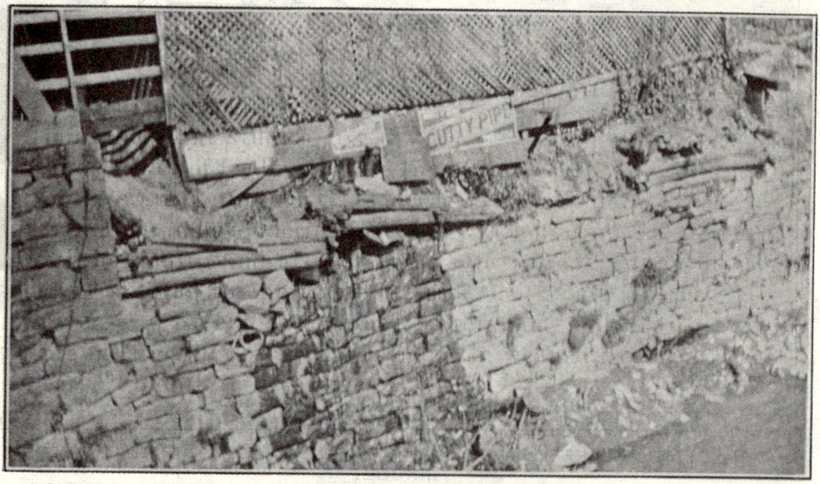

A CLOSER VIEW OF THE DISCHARGE FROM A SEWER OUTLET SET IN THE RETAINING WALL ALONG STONY CREEK.

Taken at extreme east end of the Haynes Street footbridge, where odors from the stream are especially offensive. Note that the sewage does not enter the water directly but in a way liable to promote nuisance.

PLATE Q



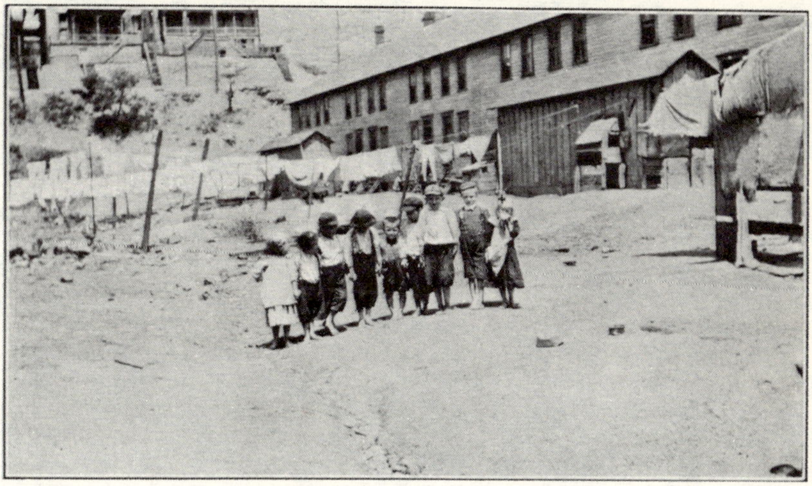

TEN-FAMILY TENEMENT, PLUM STREET, WOODVALE. OUTDOOR TOILETS OPPOSITE FRONT DOORS.

PLATE R

Infant Mortality: Johnstown, Pa., 1913.

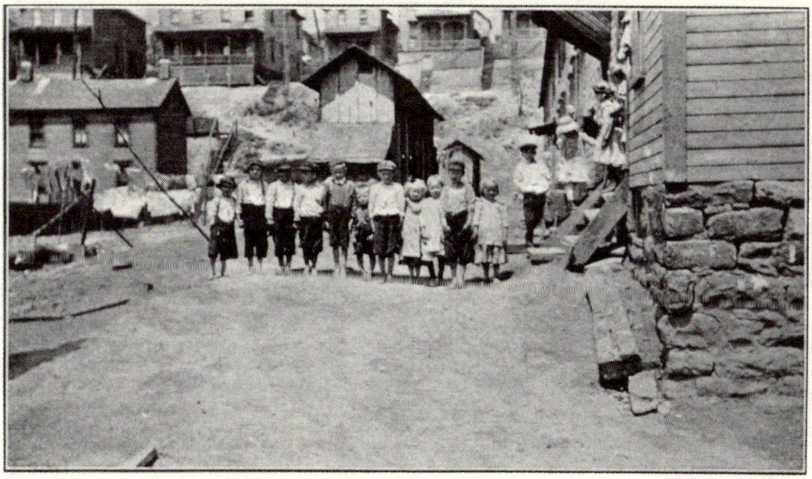

A CLOSER VIEW OF THE SAME PLUM STREET, WOODVALE, TENEMENTS AND TOILETS.

The steep hill toward the back leads to Woodvale Avenue.

U. S. DEPARTMENT OF LABOR
CHILDREN'S BUREAU
JULIA C. LATHROP, Chief

# MATERNAL MORTALITY

## FROM ALL CONDITIONS CONNECTED WITH CHILDBIRTH

## IN THE UNITED STATES AND CERTAIN OTHER COUNTRIES

BY

GRACE L. MEIGS, M. D.

---

MISCELLANEOUS SERIES No. 6
Bureau Publication No. 19

WASHINGTON
GOVERNMENT PRINTING OFFICE
1917

# CONTENTS.

## LETTER OF TRANSMITTAL.

U. S. DEPARTMENT OF LABOR,
CHILDREN'S BUREAU,
*Washington, September 25, 1916.*

SIR: I transmit herewith a report entitled "Maternal Mortality from all Conditions Connected with Childbirth in the United States and Certain Other Countries," by Dr. Grace L. Meigs, in charge of the hygiene division of this bureau. This report has been prepared because the bureau's studies of infant mortality in towns and rural districts reveal a connection between maternal and infant welfare so close that it becomes plain that infancy can not be protected without the protection of maternity.

In this study Dr. Meigs undertakes to do no more than to assemble and interpret figures already published by the United States Bureau of the Census and by the statistical authorities of various foreign countries, and to state accepted scientific views as to the proper care of maternity. She points out clearly that maternal mortality is in great measure preventable, that no available figures show a decrease in the United States in recent years, and that certain other countries now exhibit more favorable rates. This report reveals an unconscious neglect due to age-long ignorance and fatalism. It is earnestly believed that whenever the public realizes the facts it will awake to action and that adequate provision for maternal and infant welfare will become an integral part of all plans for public health protection.

The generous assistance of the United States Bureau of the Census in the preparation of this report is gratefully acknowledged.

Dr. Meigs desires that special mention be made of the assistance of Miss Emma Duke, head of the statistical division of the Children's Bureau, and of Miss Viola Paradise, research assistant in the division of hygiene.

Respectfully submitted.

JULIA C. LATHROP,
*Chief of Bureau.*

Hon. WILLIAM B. WILSON,
*Secretary of Labor.*

## MATERNAL MORTALITY FROM ALL CONDITIONS CONNECTED WITH CHILDBIRTH.

### SUMMARY.

In 1913 in this country at least 15,000 women, it is estimated, died from conditions caused by childbirth; about 7,000 of these died from childbed fever, a disease proved to be almost entirely preventable, and the remaining 8,000 from diseases now known to be to a great extent preventable or curable. Physicians and statisticians agree that these figures are a great underestimate.

In 1913 the death rate per 100,000 population from all conditions caused by childbirth was little lower than that from typhoid fever; this rate would be almost quadrupled if only the group of the population which can be affected, women of childbearing age, were considered.

In 1913 childbirth caused more deaths among women 15 to 44 years old than any disease except tuberculosis.

The death rate due to this cause is almost twice as high in the colored as in the white population.

Only 2 of a group of 15 important foreign countries show higher rates from this cause than the rate in the registration area of the United States. The rates of 3 countries, Sweden, Norway, and Italy, which are notably low, show that low rates for these diseases are attainable.

The death rates from childbirth and from childbed fever for the registration area of this country apparently are not falling to any great extent; during the 13 years from 1900 to 1913 they have shown no demonstrable decrease. These years have been marked by a revolution in the control of certain other preventable diseases, such as typhoid, diphtheria, and tuberculosis. During that time the typhoid rate has been cut in half, the rate from tuberculosis markedly reduced, and the rate from diphtheria reduced to less than one-half. During this period there has been a decrease in the death rate from childbirth per 1,000 live births in England and Wales, Ireland, Japan, New Zealand, and Switzerland.

These facts point to the need in this country and in foreign countries of higher standards of care for women at the time of childbirth.

The low standards at present existing in this country result chiefly from two causes: (1) General ignorance of the dangers connected with childbirth and of the need for proper hygiene and skilled care in order to prevent them; (2) difficulty in the provision of adequate care due to special problems characteristic of this country. Such problems vary greatly in the city and in the rural districts. In the country inaccessibility of any skilled care is a chief factor.

Improvement will come about only through a general realization of the necessity for better care at childbirth. If women demand better care, physicians will provide it, medical colleges will furnish better training in obstetrics, and communities will realize the vital importance of community measures to insure good care for all classes of women.

# PART I. GENERAL DISCUSSION.

## STATISTICS RELATING TO CHILDBIRTH IN THE UNITED STATES AND IN CERTAIN FOREIGN COUNTRIES.

### Introduction.

For the last two decades civilized countries have been absorbed in the problem of preventing the enormous and needless waste of human life represented by their infant death rates. The importance of this problem has been felt more keenly in the last two years in the countries now at war; in these countries the efforts toward saving the lives of babies have redoubled since the war began. Side by side with this problem, another, which is only of late finding its true place, is that of the protection of the lives and health of mothers during their pregnancy and confinement. This is a question so closely bound up with that of the prevention of infant mortality that the two can not be separated.

It is now realized that a large proportion of the deaths of babies occur in the first days and weeks of life, and that these deaths can be prevented only through proper care of the mother before and at the birth of her baby. It is also realized that breast feeding through the greater part of the first year of the baby's life is the chief protection from all diseases; and that mothers are much more likely to be able to nurse their babies successfully if they receive proper care before, at, and after childbirth. Moreover, in the progress of work for the prevention of infant mortality it has become ever clearer that all such work is useful only in so far as it helps the mother to care better for her baby. It must be plain, then, to what a degree the sickness or death of the mother lessens the chances of the baby for life and health.

This question has also another side. Each death at childbirth is a serious loss to the country. The women who die from this cause are lost at the time of their greatest usefulness to the State and to their families; and they give their lives in carrying out a function which must be regarded as the most important in the world.

Questions then of the most vital interest to the whole Nation are these: How are the lives of the mothers in this country and other countries being protected? To what degree are the diseases caused by pregnancy and childbirth preventable? If preventable, how far are they being prevented in this country? Has there been the same great decrease in the last few years in sickness and death from these causes as that which has marked the great campaigns against other preventable diseases such as typhoid, tuberculosis, or diphtheria? How do the conditions in the United States compare with those in other countries?

In the following report the attempt has been made to derive answers to these questions from the official records of this country and of foreign countries.

**Are the diseases caused by pregnancy and confinement preventable diseases?**

These diseases[1] fall naturally into two groups, which differ considerably as to the degree to which they are preventable:

1. Childbed fever, or puerperal septicemia (an infection arising in connection with miscarriage or confinement), which is to a great degree a preventable disease.

2. All other diseases and complications caused by pregnancy and confinement, including conditions varying very much in the degree to which they can be prevented or cured.

*Puerperal septicemia (childbed fever).*—The fact is now well known that puerperal septicemia, or childbed fever, is in reality a wound infection, similar to such an infection after an accident or an operation, and that it can be prevented by the same measures of cleanliness and asepsis which are used so universally in modern surgery to prevent infection. The proof of the nature of this disease is one of the tremendous results of the scientific discoveries which were made in the latter part of the nineteenth century.

During the early part of that century childbed fever was one of the greatest hospital scourges known. It occurred also in private practice; but in hospitals where there was great opportunity for the spreading of infection the death rate from this disease was appalling. The average death rate in hospitals in all countries was 3 to 4 per cent of all women confined; sometimes it reached 10 to 20 per cent and even over 50 per cent during short periods of epidemics.[2] In the face of this terrific mortality many obstetrical hospitals were closed. Commissions were appointed to investigate the cause of these epidemics, and medical congresses devoted sessions to the discussion of the problem. In 1843 Oliver Wendell Holmes, and in 1847 Semmelweiss, published articles stating the theory that this fever was similar to a wound infection and was due chiefly to the carrying of infectious material on the hands of attendants from one case to another. The

---

[1] Throughout this report when reference is made to causes of death the term "childbirth" will be used as synonymous with "all diseases caused by pregnancy and confinement"; and each of these terms will be used as being the sum of the two groups, "puerperal septicemia" and "all other diseases caused by pregnancy and confinement." It will be noted that diseases of the breast during lactation are included in the latter group. For a fuller discussion of these causes of death, and the titles of the International List of Causes of Death to which they correspond, see p. 29.

[2] Williams, J. W. "Obstetrics and animal experimentation." Defense of Research Pamphlet XVIII, Amer. Med. Assn., Chicago, 1911, pp. 5-19.

same ideas had been published much earlier but had not received attention.

At the time of the publications of Holmes and Semmelweiss it was not known that the infection of wounds is caused by the action of bacteria or germs. This discovery followed the pioneer discovery of living bacteria causing fermentation, made by Pasteur about 1863, which has revolutionized all surgery and preventive medicine.

In 1867 Lister began to apply to surgery the work of Pasteur; he taught that wound infection at operation could be prevented by the destruction of bacteria through disinfection or antisepsis. Though these methods have been supplemented in later years by the better methods of absolute surgical cleanliness or asepsis, they represented at that time a great advance.

About 1875 Lister's methods began to be generally accepted and applied in hospitals to the prevention of infection at childbirth. This movement gained great support in 1879 when Pasteur proved definitely that childbed fever is caused by bacteria.

Gradually the methods of antisepsis or disinfection and later the better methods of asepsis were accepted in obstetrical hospitals; and at the same time the mortality, once so high, dropped enormously. At present the death rate from puerperal septicemia among cases delivered in hospitals is extremely low. Williams says: "At the present time it is safe to say that in well-regulated hospitals the mortality from puerperal infection is less than 0.25 per cent. This is in great contrast with the average mortality of 3 to 4 per cent observed [in hospitals] throughout the world prior to the introduction of antiseptic methods, and means that only 1 woman now dies as compared with 15 or 20 formerly."[1]

This experience in hospitals has proved definitely that puerperal septicemia is to a very large degree preventable. One fact, however, complicates the whole question and makes it impossible to say that the disease is in all cases absolutely preventable, namely, that a very small number of cases develops even under conditions of the best hospital or private care, when every method for avoiding infection has been used. This fact has led to much controversy. In general obstetricians of the greatest experience believe that a small number of cases of infection after childbirth may develop from bacteria which were already in the body of the patient before confinement; but that in the main such cases are of mild severity and that only a few fatal cases are due to this cause. Another point which must be borne in mind is that, in a certain number of cases, women may infect themselves through improper hygiene during pregnancy or just before or at confinement. Therefore the teaching of proper hygiene is an essential part of the work for the prevention of infection.

[1] Williams, J. W. Supra cit., p. 19.

To sum up, experience has shown that by far the major part of all serious cases of infection at childbirth may be prevented by the application of such principles of hygiene and of strict surgical cleanliness as are now established beyond question.

*All other diseases caused by pregnancy and confinement.*—The diseases and complications included under this heading are those given on page 30 as being included under "Other puerperal accidents of pregnancy and labor."

A definite statement such as that made above regarding the preventability of puerperal septicemia can not be made about this second group of diseases, which includes many different conditions. However, it is a fact well proved in practice that a large number of these complications can be prevented through proper hygiene and supervision during pregnancy and through skilled care at labor. Certain other complications which can not be prevented can be detected before serious harm is done, and treatment can be given which will save the mother's life. We can see this more clearly if we consider as examples two of the most important complications.

Puerperal albuminuria and convulsions, called also eclampsia, or toxemia of pregnancy, is a disease which occurs most frequently during pregnancy but may occur at or following confinement. It is a relatively frequent complication among women bearing their first children. When fully established its chief symptoms are convulsions and unconsciousness. In the early stages of the disease the symptoms are slight puffiness of the face, hands, and feet; headache; albumen in the urine; and usually a rise in blood pressure. Very often proper treatment and diet at the beginning of such early symptoms may prevent the development of the disease; but in many cases where the disease is well established before the physician is consulted, the woman and baby can not be saved by any treatment. In the prevention of deaths from this cause it is essential, therefore, that each woman, especially each woman bearing her first child, should know what she can do, by proper hygiene and diet, to prevent the disease; that she should know the meaning of these early symptoms if they arise, so that she may seek at once the advice of her doctor; and that she should have regular supervision during pregnancy, with examination of the urine at intervals.

Some obstruction to labor in the small size or abnormal shape of the pelvic canal causes many deaths of mothers included in the class "other accidents of labor" and also many stillbirths. If such difficulty is discovered before labor, proper treatment will in almost all cases insure the life of mother and child; if it is not discovered until labor has begun, or perhaps until it has continued for many hours, the danger to both is greatly increased. Every woman, therefore, should have during pregnancy—and above all during her first pregnancy—an examination in which measurements are made to enable the physician to judge whether or not there will be any obstruction to labor. A case in which a complication of this kind is found requires the greatest skill and experience in treatment,[1] but with such treatment the life and health of the mother are almost always safe.

These two examples will suffice. In the same way it could be shown, with regard to all the other complications of pregnancy and labor, that those which can not be prevented can be treated successfully in most cases if detected in time.

It can be regarded, then, as a generally accepted fact that all illness and death connected with childbearing is, to a certain and large degree, preventable, through the application of the scientific knowledge which is now well established. The next questions are, How far are these diseases being prevented in the United States? How many deaths do they cause each year? What are the death rates from these causes, and are they decreasing or increasing? The statistics gathered by the United States Bureau of the Census have been studied for answers to these questions.

There are other equally important questions to which these figures will not give answers. In addition to the number of deaths and death rates, it is important to know how much illness is caused by the diseases of pregnancy and confinement. How many women do they disable for months or years? Undoubtedly the health of these mothers affects enormously the welfare of their children. Unfortunately such questions can not be answered; puerperal septicemia is not a reportable disease in this country as it is in many others. We can only remember that for each woman who died there are surely many who were ill for days, weeks, or months, but who finally recovered.

The following pages give a brief summary of the data, published by the United States Bureau of the Census, dealing with deaths from childbirth. These are discussed in further detail in other sections of the report.

**Reliability of data.**

The statement is frequently made that all statistics on this subject are incomplete. This is undoubtedly true with regard to the figures available in each country. A detailed discussion of the many sources of error in the statistics of the United States and of foreign countries on this subject will be found in another section, beginning on page 34.

---

[1] The public must be taught that the conduct of labor complicated by a moderate degree of pelvic contraction is quite as serious as a case of appendicitis, and that its proper management requires the highest degree of judgment and skill, while eclampsia or placenta prævia are even more serious.—Williams, J. W. "The midwife problem and medical education in the United States." Trans. Amer. Assn. for Study and Prevention of Infant Mortality, 1911, p. 189.

From that discussion several conclusions may be drawn:

1. Though the figures of the number of deaths from puerperal septicemia and from all other diseases connected with childbirth are certainly incomplete, yet they are reliable as far as they go; they may be accepted as a statement of the minimum number of deaths which have actually occurred as a result of these diseases.

2. All conclusions as to comparative death rates in various years and in various countries can be made only with caution and by bearing in mind the many statistical pitfalls connected with such comparisons.

With a full understanding of the limitations of the figures available, it has seemed worth while to publish the following figures of the deaths in the United States due to childbirth.

## Number of deaths in the United States from childbirth.

In 1913 in the "death-registration area"[1] of the United States 10,010 deaths were reported as due to conditions caused by pregnancy and childbirth. Of these deaths, 4,542 were reported as caused by puerperal septicemia or childbed fever.

Using the death-registration area as a basis, we are justified in estimating that in 1913 in the whole United States 15,376 deaths were due to childbirth, and 6,977 of these were due to childbed fever. As will be shown later, these figures are without doubt a gross underestimate. As it is, they are striking enough—almost 7,000 deaths in one year in this country due to childbed fever, a disease to a large degree easily preventable; and over 8,000 due to the other diseases caused by pregnancy and confinement, most of which are preventable or curable by means well known to science.

## Death rates in the United States from childbirth.

The death rate from all diseases caused by pregnancy and confinement in 1913 in the registration area was 15.8 per 100,000 population (which includes all ages and both sexes). The death rate from puerperal septicemia was 7.2.

These figures, however, mean little to us unless we compare them with the death rates from other preventable diseases. In the same year and area the typhoid rate was 17.9 per 100,000 population; the rate from diphtheria and croup 18.8. The highest death rate from any one disease was that from tuberculosis, 147.6 per 100,000 population. Any such comparison with the rates from diseases to which both sexes and all ages are liable is of course very misleading; but in spite of that fact it is interesting to note that typhoid fever, the disease

---

[1] The death-registration area comprises the States and cities in which the registration of deaths is returned as fairly complete.—U. S. Census. Mortality Statistics, 1911, p. 9. It is estimated that in 1913 the death-registration area included 65.1 per cent of the population of the United States. (See Table I, p. 49.)

against which so great an amount of effort is now directed, has a rate at present but 2 per 100,000 population higher than that from the diseases caused by pregnancy and confinement.

*Death rates per 100,000 women.*—The death rates from childbirth are approximately doubled when worked on the basis of 100,000 women. This will be seen when Tables IV and III (p. 50) are compared. The former gives for the period 1900 to 1910, the annual death rates per 100,000 women in the group of 11 States which were in the death-registration area in 1900, the latter the death rates per 100,000 population in the same group of States for the same period. It is evident that the rates in Table IV for each year are slightly more than twice those in Table III for the same year.

*Death rates per 100,000 women of childbearing age.*—Again, a much higher but a more accurate death rate from these diseases is found when the basis taken is the group which alone is affected by these diseases—women of childbearing age. When the rate is based not upon 100,000 population of both sexes and all ages but upon 100,000 women 15 to 44 years of age, the rate as ordinarily given is multiplied several times.

In 1900,[1] the only year for which the rates can be computed, the death rate in the registration area per 100,000 women 15 to 44 years of age from all diseases of pregnancy and confinement was 50.3; from puerperal infection, 21.6. (See p. 32.) The corresponding rates for the same year per 100,000 population were 13.1 and 5.6. In this year, therefore, the rates are almost quadrupled when based on that group of the population which alone can be affected by these diseases.

Moreover, the death rates as ordinarily given per 100,000 population conceal the fact that the diseases of pregnancy and childbirth are indeed among the most important causes of death of women between 15 and 44 years of age; the actual number of deaths shows this to be the case. In 1913 in the registration area these diseases caused more deaths than any other one cause of death except tuberculosis. In that year there were, among women 15 to 44 years of age, 26,265 deaths from tuberculosis; 9,876 deaths from the diseases of pregnancy and confinement; 6,386 from heart disease; 5,741 from acute nephritis and Bright's disease; 5,065 from cancer; and 4,167 from pneumonia. Other diseases, such as typhoid, appendicitis, and the infectious diseases show far fewer deaths. (See Table V, p. 51.)

*Death rates per 1,000 live births.*—This rate, as will be shown repeatedly throughout the report (see p. 32), gives a far clearer picture of the actual risk of childbirth than do any of the rates so far considered. This rate can be given only for one year, 1910, and only for the provisional birth-registration area for that year. The rate from all diseases caused by pregnancy and confinement is 6.5, from puer-

[1] Census year ending May 31.

peral septicemia, 2.9, and from all other diseases of pregnancy and confinement, 3.6 per 1,000 live births. That is, in this area for every 154 babies born alive one mother lost her life. (See Table VI, p. 52.)

**Is the death rate from childbirth falling?**

Has there been in the last few years any decrease in the death rates from puerperal septicemia and from other diseases caused by pregnancy and confinement? The general opinion of the medical profession and of the laity is that these death rates, and especially the rate from puerperal septicemia, are fast decreasing. The fact that hospital epidemics of puerperal septicemia are now things of the past is thought to be evidence that deaths from this disease are now rare. On the other hand, many obstetricians of wide experience believe that outside of hospitals there has been no great decrease in the death rate from puerperal septicemia.

Dr. Williams,[1] professor of obstetrics, Johns Hopkins University, believes that there has been no great improvement in this country; Dr. Webster,[2] professor of obstetrics, Rush Medical College, University of Chicago, and Dr. Powell[3] hold the same opinion; Dr. De Lee,[4] professor

---

[1] In private practice it is doubtful whether the results are materially better to-day than they were before the introduction of antiseptic methods, for the reason that the doctrines of asepsis have not yet permeated the rank and file of medical men, much less of midwives, to whose care is committed a very large proportion of obstetrical cases. Though, at the same time, it must be admitted that we rarely hear of outbreaks of puerperal infection such as are mentioned in the historical work of Hirsch, who gives the particulars of 216 epidemics occurring between the years 1652 and 1862.

Boehr stated in 1875 that 363,324 women had died from puerperal infection in Prussia during the preceding 60 years, and calculated that every thirtieth married woman eventually perished from it; while Ehlers contended that outside of the well-regulated hospitals the results were equally bad in 1900. Furthermore, Fromme stated, in 1910, that at least 5,000 women succumb each year in Prussia to this preventable malady.

Bacon, in an article based upon the records of the health department of Chicago, showed that for the 40 years prior to 1896 puerperal infection was assigned as the cause of death in 12.75 per cent of the women dying between the ages of 20 and 50 years, varying between 20 per cent in 1873 and 7.3 per cent in 1895. Similar results were reported by Ingerslev, who stated that, even at the present time in Denmark, with the single exception of tuberculosis, puerperal infection is the most frequent cause of death in women during the childbearing period.

The investigations of Boxall, Byers, and Lea show a similar condition in England, where it may be said that outside of the lying-in hospitals this preventable scourge claims as many and perhaps more victims than it did 20 or even 40 years ago.

Moreover, in trying to determine the frequency of puerperal infection, one can not be guided altogether by the mortality statistics, inasmuch as the largest proportion of these cases do not end fatally. On the other hand, anyone who deals much with gynecological patients can not fail to be impressed with the very large proportion whose troubles have originated from febrile affections during the puerperium, which in many instances were clearly due to the neglect of aseptic precautions on the part of the obstetrician or midwife.—Williams, J. W. Obstetrics, 1913, pp. 900, 901.

[2] It is the general impression that there has been a marked diminution in the mortality of puerperal sepsis since the introduction of antiseptics. This is probably true only as regards hospital practice. * * * As regards private practice, it is doubtful if there has been much diminution in mortality, either in Europe or America.—Webster, J. C. A Text-book of Obstetrics, 1903, p. 640.

[3] I am quite sure it is the belief of all who have given attention to this subject, that the mortality from puerperal infection has been diminished little if any in private practice.—Powell, H. H. "Mortality from puerperal infection." Surgery, Gynecology and Obstetrics, 1906, Vol. III, p. 11.

[4] I do not fear to hazard the statement that 8,000 women die annually in the United States from childbed infections. When one considers that the majority of cases of puerperal infection get well, the conclusion is inevitable that the disease is still—in these modern aseptic and antiseptic times—very prevalent.—De Lee, J. B. Principles and Practice of Obstetrics, 1913, p. 870.

of obstetrics, Northwestern University, comments on the great prevalence of puerperal septicemia in spite of our present knowledge of asepsis. Dr. Moran[1] points out the lack of decrease in the figures as given in the census reports, as does also Dr. Davis[2] in a recent volume. Dr. Edgar,[3] professor of obstetrics and clinical midwifery, Cornell University Medical College, on the other hand, believes that there has been a decrease.

We need a definite answer to this question, based on a study of unassailable statistics. Unfortunately the available figures on this subject for this country and foreign countries have many possibilities of error, as will be shown in a later section (see p. 34). The errors have been avoided as far as possible; those which can not be avoided must be considered in reading the following summary. Especially to be remembered is the fact that in recent years great improvement has been made in the registration of deaths from childbirth and childbed fever.

According to the evidence available, these death rates are apparently not decreasing. During the 23 years ending in 1913 in this country no definite decrease in the death rate from the diseases caused by pregnancy and confinement can be demonstrated; nor can any decrease in the death rate from puerperal septicemia be shown.

In the registration area as a whole the death rates have shown no decline in the years between 1890 and 1913. The death rate from all diseases caused by pregnancy and confinement, which was 15.3 in 1890, fell to 13 in 1902, and then with annual fluctuations rose to 16 in 1911; in 1913 the rate was 15.8. The annual average for the period 1901 to 1905 was 14.2; for the period 1906 to 1910, 15.5. (See Table I, p. 49.)

The death rate from all diseases caused by pregnancy and confinement for the group of eight States which have been included in the death-registration area from 1890 to 1913[4] also has shown no decrease during the course of these 23 years. There was a slight fall in the rate for the year 1900 as compared with that for the year 1890, followed by a slight rise. (See Table II, p. 49.) In 1890 the rate was 14.1 per 100,000 population; in 1900, 12.6; in 1913 it was 14.3.

The death rates for a second group of States[4] (those included in the death-registration area since 1900) show between 1900 and 1913 a

[1] Moran, J. F. "The endowment of motherhood," Jour. Amer. Med. Assn., 1915, Vol. LXIV, p. 122.

[2] It is probable that very few physicians realize that with the great progress of preventive medicine and aseptic surgery that there has not been a similar increase in the safety of maternity.—Davis, C. H. Painless Childbirth, Eutocia, and Nitrous Oxid-Oxygen Analgesia, 1916, p. 62.

[3] It is very difficult to estimate the frequency of puerperal infection outside of hospitals * * * but it is undoubtedly much less than it used to be.—Edgar, J. C. The Practice of Obstetrics, 1903, p. 752.

[4] Selected for study because good methods of death registration may be assumed to have become established, and also because comparisons of the rates of such a group of States are not open to the error due to the changing character of the registration area.

64614°—17——3

slight increase, from 12.9 to 14.9, with the high point 15.5 in 1911. (See Table III, p. 50). These rates are more fully discussed on page 38.

The death rates from puerperal septicemia or childbed fever during these years in each group of States have run parallel with those from the whole group of diseases connected with childbirth; they, too, have shown practically no change in 13 years.

It is probable that the improvement in reporting deaths from childbirth may account for the apparent rise in the rates since 1900; it may also perhaps conceal a slight improvement in actual conditions since that time; but it is safe to say that any marked decrease in the actual death rate from childbirth during the last 13 years could not have been masked by this error.

In these years what has been the change in the death rates from other preventable diseases? These death rates tell a very different story from that of the rates from childbirth. They give a bare outline of the remarkable achievements of modern medicine in the prevention of certain diseases.

DIAGRAM I.—DEATH RATES PER 100,000 POPULATION FROM TYPHOID, DIPHTHERIA AND CROUP, AND DISEASES CAUSED BY PREGNANCY AND CONFINEMENT IN THE DEATH-REGISTRATION AREA OF THE UNITED STATES, 1900 TO 1913.

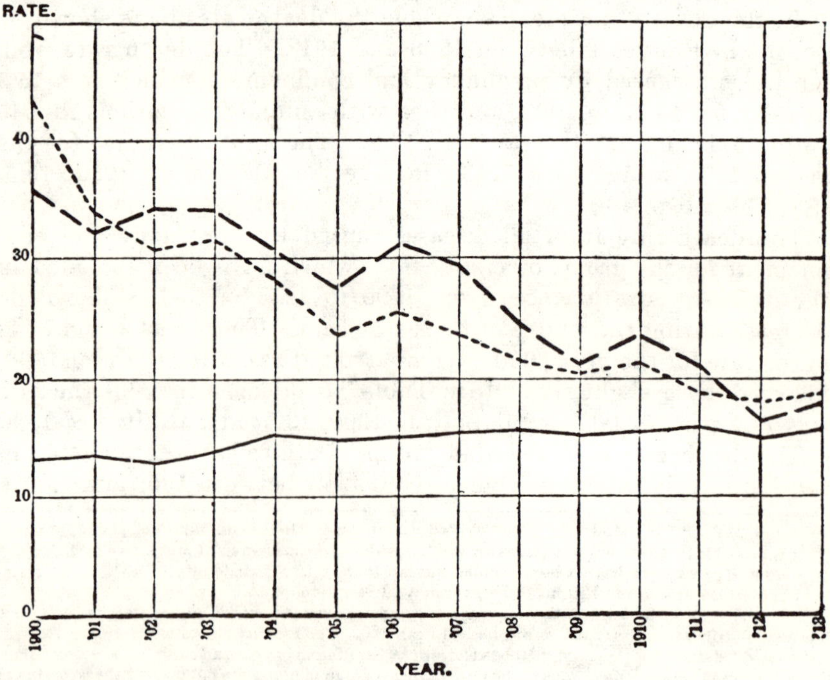


— — — — — TYPHOID.
.................. DIPHTHERIA AND CROUP.
———————— DISEASES OF PREGNANCY AND CONFINEMENT.

DIAGRAM 2.—DEATH RATES PER 100,000 POPULATION FROM TUBERCULOSIS AND PNEUMONIA IN THE DEATH-REGISTRATION AREA OF THE UNITED STATES, 1900 TO 1913.

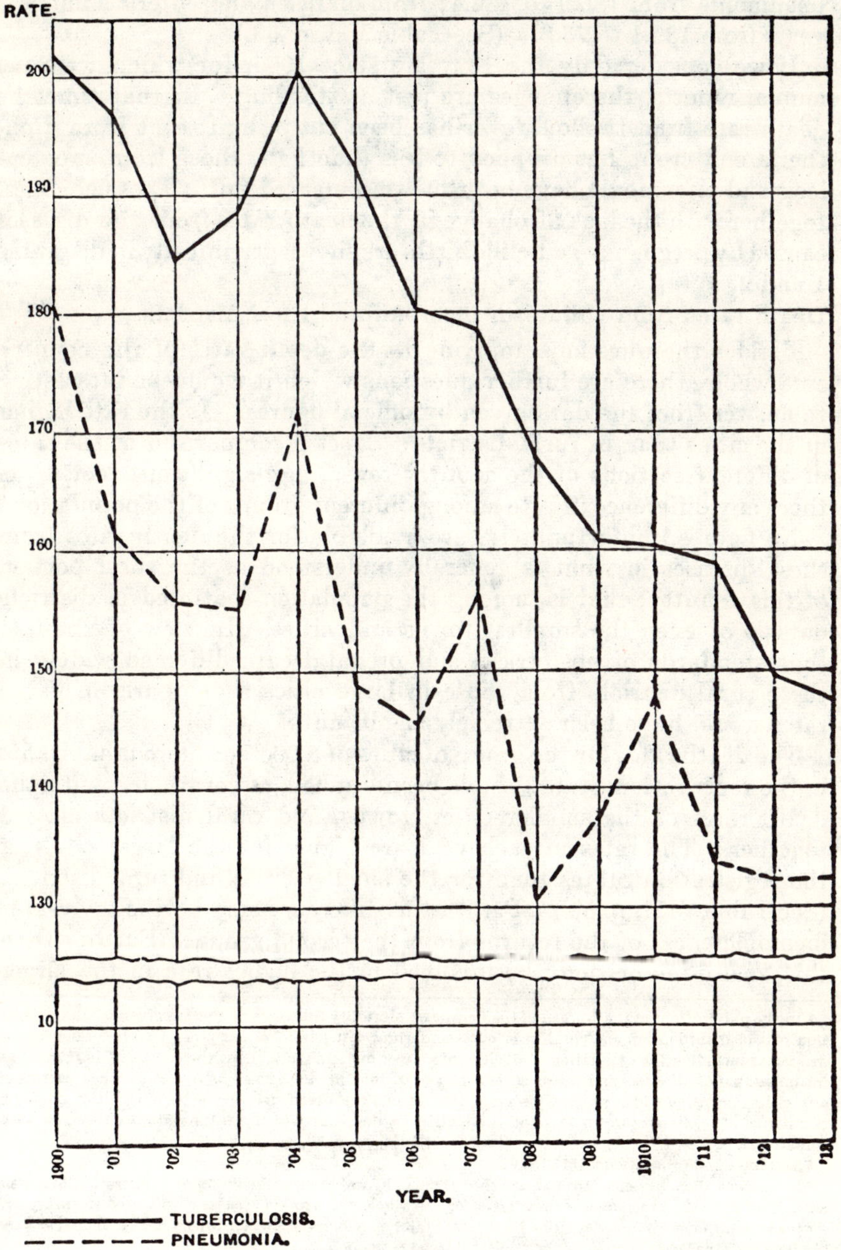

Between 1890 and 1913 the death rate from typhoid fever in the death-registration area fell from 46.3 to 17.9; that from diphtheria and croup from 97.8 to 18.8; from tuberculosis from 252 to 147.6; from pneumonia from 186.9 to 132.4; from diarrhea and enteritis under 2 years from 139.1 to 75.2. (See Table VII, p. 53.)

If we consider only the 13 years since 1900, for which we have annual reports, the changes are just as startling. In that time the death rate from typhoid fever has been cut in half; that from diphtheria and croup has dropped to less than half; those from tuberculosis and pneumonia have both shown a marked fall. These changes, together with the lack of change in the death rates from the diseases caused by pregnancy and childbirth, are shown graphically in diagrams 1 and 2.

**Death rates from childbirth in urban and rural districts.**

Besides the questions applying to the death rates of the country as a whole, there are further questions which it would be interesting to answer from the data given by official figures. Is the rate higher in the cities than in rural districts? Does a comparison of the rates of different sections of the country reveal any significant facts? Is there any difference in rate among different groups of the population?

No figures,[1] unfortunately, are available for the death rates from these diseases in what is generally understood as the rural portion of this country; that is, among the population scattered in districts outside of even the smallest towns and cities. In view of the fact that standards of obstetrical and prenatal care differ so widely in these rural districts from those in large cities a comparison of the rates would have been extremely significant.

The death rates for the group of cities of 8,000 [2] or more inhabitants in the registration States [3] have been studied, as contrasted with the death rates of the smaller cities, towns, and rural districts classed together. The rates in each year are higher for the larger cities of the registration States than for the smaller cities and rural districts. (See Table VIII, p. 53.) Part of this difference may be due to greater incompleteness of the returns from the second group. Further than this, many factors may be involved in the higher rate in the larger

[1] In the publications of the Bureau of the Census on Mortality Statistics figures are given for the population classified into urban and rural or of cities and rural districts. For the years 1900 to 1909 urban is defined as including the population of all cities of 8,000 or more inhabitants at the census of 1900; rural as including that of all cities and towns of less than 8,000 inhabitants, as well as of the districts outside of any cities, towns, or villages. For the years 1910 to 1913 the division is made between cities having a population of 10,000 or more in 1910 and those cities having less than 10,000 inhabitants, together with rural districts.

[2] Ten thousand inhabitants, 1910 to 1913.

[3] It has been thought better to compare the urban and rural rates in the group of registration States in each year rather than to compare these rates for the whole registration area as constituted in each year. As the registration area includes cities in several States of which the smaller towns and rural districts are not included, the latter comparison would seem to be scarcely fair.

cities. While some of the larger cities afford better provision for obstetrical and prenatal care than do the smaller cities and rural districts, this is not true of all; moreover, the larger cities probably show a much higher rate among the less favored than among the more favored groups of their inhabitants. Overcrowding, overwork, low incomes, ignorance of the need for good obstetrical care and how it can be obtained may all play their part in producing this high rate in the larger cities.

The figures do not show a decrease in the death rates from childbirth in the larger cities in recent years. The death rates of the whole group of cities of 8,000 [1] or more inhabitants in the registration States for the years 1900 to 1913 (see Table VIII, p. 53) show no decline. The rate in 1900 was 14.9; in 1913, 17.2.

The rates from childbirth for the same period in a group of 7 large cities have been studied. (See Table IX, p. 54.)

The rates for New York City alone show a definite and steady decline: in 1905 the rate per 100,000 inhabitants was 20.3; in 1913, 14.1.

The rates of Boston, Buffalo, Detroit, Jersey City, and Washington show wide annual fluctuations, but no general tendency to increase or decrease. The rate of Newark, on the other hand, shows an increase.

**Death rates from childbirth in different States.**

The death rates of only 11 States (including the District of Columbia) can be studied through a period of time (1900 to 1913) long enough to justify any conclusions. These States, unfortunately, do not represent any widely different sections of the country, as they include only the New England States, two Middle Atlantic States (New York and New Jersey), the District of Columbia, and two North Central States (Indiana and Michigan). The western and southern sections of the country are unrepresented.

Though the rates for each State vary considerably from year to year, it will be noted that certain States show high average rates; among these are the District of Columbia, Michigan, and Rhode Island, whose rates are 17.6, 17.1, and 16.8, respectively. (See Table X, p. 54.) Other States show comparatively low average rates; for example, New Hampshire (11.2) and Maine (11.8). It seems premature at this time to draw any conclusions as to the cause of these differences in rates in different States. When the rates are available for all sections of the country, a comparison of rates for different large sections presenting similar problems will be very useful.

---

[1] Ten thousand inhabitants, 1910 to 1913.

**Death rates from childbirth of white and colored population.**

No facts brought out in this study are as striking as the difference in rates from childbirth of the white and colored population of the death-registration area. In some cases the rates for the colored population are almost double those for the white. Table XI, page 56, which gives the rates so divided, demonstrates this difference. In 1913 the death rate from all diseases caused by pregnancy and confinement was 15.2 per 100,000 white population and 26.1 per 100,000 colored. In the same year the rate from puerperal septicemia was 6.9 for the white population and 11.5 for the colored. A similar relation is shown by the rates for each year from 1910 to 1913. Although the rates can be given only for four years, and are based on small figures, yet they show differences so marked that they picture without doubt a very great difference in standards of care at childbirth in these two groups. When all the Southern States are included in the death-registration area the magnitude of this problem undoubtedly will be shown by the death rates from childbirth in these States. At present but a small percentage of the colored population of the United States is represented by the figures available.

**Comparison of the average death rates from childbirth in certain foreign countries and in the United States.**

Are the death rates from these diseases in the death-registration area of the United States higher or lower than those in other civilized countries? Have these rates in other countries been falling or rising in the last 13 years, while the rates of this country have been apparently stationary? These questions, like all those of comparative international statistics, are of immense interest, but they involve many difficulties and sources of error. These are discussed on page 41. They should be considered in reading the following summary.

In order to make possible a comparison of the death rates from these causes for 15 foreign countries with those for the United States, an average rate has been computed for the years 1900 to 1910[1] for each of the countries, using the same method as that in use in the United States. When the 16 countries studied are arranged in order, with the one having the lowest rate first, the death-registration area of the United States stands fourteenth on the list. (See Table XII, p. 56.) Only two countries, Switzerland and Spain, have higher rates; many of the countries, however, show rates differing but little from that of the United States. Markedly low rates are those of Sweden (6), Norway (7.8), and Italy (8.9); a strikingly high rate is that of Spain (19.6).

The death rate from childbirth per 1,000 live births is not available for the death-registration area of the United States, but can be given

---

[1] Or for that portion of this period for which figures are available.

only for the small number of States and cities included in the provisional birth-registration area and for one year, 1910. (See p. 31.) This rate, 6.5, is considerably higher than that for 1910 of any of the countries studied. When the average rates for a number of years of the 15 countries are reckoned per 1,000 live births and arranged in order, it will be seen that the same group of countries—Sweden, Italy, and Norway—shows the lowest rates. (See Table XIII, p. 56.) Spain in this table shows the rate which is next to the highest, while Belgium now has the highest rate. For a comparative study of the rates of these countries the rates per 1,000 live births give undoubtedly the clearest picture of the actual conditions.

These rates show a wide variation. While in Sweden but one mother is lost for every 430 babies born alive, in Belgium one mother dies for every 172 babies, and in Spain one for every 175 babies born alive. The rates in Belgium and Spain are two and a half times as high as the rate in Sweden.

Far more significant than a comparison of actual death rates of various countries is a comparison of the changes which have occurred in these death rates in each country in recent years. England and Wales, Ireland, Japan, New Zealand, and Switzerland have shown a decrease in the death rate per 1,000 live births from all diseases caused by pregnancy and confinement; but, in this group, only in England and Wales and in Ireland has the death rate from puerperal septicemia decreased; in the other three countries this rate has remained practically the same, though the total rate has decreased.

In Australia, Belgium, Hungary, Italy, Norway, Prussia, Spain, and Sweden both the rate from childbirth and that from puerperal septicemia remained almost stationary during the periods studied.

The total rate for Scotland shows a definite increase, though the rate from puerperal septicemia has decreased. (See Table XVI, p. 66.)

**Conclusions.**

In the foregoing pages the attempt has been made to draw, from available statistics, answers to certain important and urgent questions relating to the hazards of childbirth in this country and in other countries. It has been shown that a large number of women die year after year in this country from childbed fever, a disease proved over 40 years ago to be almost entirely preventable; and that a still larger number die from other conditions connected with childbirth which are known to be to a large degree preventable or curable. The proportionately small number of women lost from these causes in certain foreign countries demonstrates the needlessness of the greater part of our losses. There is no evidence, moreover, of any great advance made during the last 13 years in this country in the prevention of disease and death due to childbirth, though the same period has been marked by a notable decrease in the death rates of certain other diseases which have been proved preventable.

What is the cause of these conditions in this country? At the root of the matter, apparently, lie two chief causes: First, general ignorance of the dangers connected with childbirth and the need of skilled care and proper hygiene in order to prevent them; second, such difficulties related to the provision of proper obstetrical care as are characteristic of conditions in this country.

A general realization of certain of the fundamental facts related to the bearing of children has only begun; this function has always been looked upon with a mixture of ignorance and fatalism. The hazards to health and life connected with childbirth have been either ignored or accepted as unavoidable accidents. By most people childbirth is regarded as an entirely normal process, and, happily, in the great majority of cases this is true. But the figures given in this report show that it is not true of all. Each year there is a vast number of normal deliveries, and among them the relatively small but absolutely very large number of complicated cases is lost sight of. On the other hand, most people regard such illness and deaths as do occur as unpreventable. Only very gradually and incompletely are women beginning to realize the simple facts that certain accidents and complications occur in a definite percentage of cases of childbirth, but that almost always these may be avoided or cured if women exercise the proper hygiene during pregnancy, secure proper supervision during that time, and have skilled attendance at labor. Like other essentials of hygiene and preventive medicine these principles are at last becoming public property instead of being the exclusive possession of physicians. But in this case progress has been very slow. Knowledge of the need for good care at childbirth is essential; the lack of such knowledge and of a demand for this care has been, probably, the chief factor in producing the present indifference to this phase of preventive medicine.

The husbands of women bearing children do not realize that money paid for skilled service at childbirth is one of the most necessary family expenditures; hence, obstetrics has become one of the worst paid though one of the most taxing branches of medicine. Dr. Williams [1] speaks of the small fees usually paid for maternity care and says that "doctors who are obliged to live from their practice can not reasonably be expected to give much better service than they are paid for." Naturally enough, the lack of interest of physicians in obstetrics is partly due to this fact. No doubt another reason why many able physicians dislike this branch of practice is the fact that they feel strongly the responsibility assumed in the care of

[1] Williams, J. W. "The midwife problem and medical education in the United States." Trans. Amer. Assn. for Study and Prevention of Infant Mortality, 1911, p. 190.

women at childbirth; yet they are frequently called upon to take this responsibility in the face of conditions which they can not control and which threaten the safety of their patients. A conscientious physician does not willingly undertake the conduct of a difficult case of labor outside a hospital and without skilled assistance; but frequently he must do so, either because there is no hospital or trained nurse available, or because the patient and her family are unable or unwilling to pay for the needed help. The physician either must give up the case to an attendant who is less skillful and careful than himself or must take the risk that puerperal septicemia or some other complication may occur. If either follows he has the blame. Altogether a physician has little incentive to specialize and acquire great skill in this branch.

Necessarily the same apparent indifference to the importance of obstetrics is reflected in the courses of many medical colleges. Dr. Williams[1] pointed out in 1911 that in the majority of medical colleges in the United States instruction in this subject was grossly neglected; that graduates from these colleges beginning their practice were totally unprepared to manage any but absolutely normal cases of confinement, and that they were untrained in the practice of the principles of asepsis as applied to this branch. Other papers and discussions in the Transactions of the American Association for Study and Prevention of Infant Mortality have emphasized the same facts. In the five years since the article of Williams was written some improvement in these conditions has undoubtedly taken place, as would be expected in connection with the present remarkable tendency toward the raising of standards of medical education in the United States. However. there is no question that further improvement is greatly needed.

Communities are still to a great extent indifferent to or ignorant of the number of lives of women lost yearly from childbirth; many communities which are proud of their low typhoid or diphtheria rates ignore their high rates from childbed fever. Communities are only beginning to realize that among their chief concerns is the protection of the babies born within their limits, and necessarily also of the mothers of those babies before and at confinement.

The second fundamental cause of the high death rates from childbirth in this country previously spoken of—that is, the difficulty of obtaining adequate care—is seen to depend to a large extent on the first, the general ignorance of need for good care. As women, their husbands, physicians, and communities realize the absolute need of skilled care for the prevention of needless deaths from childbirth, methods for providing such care will be developed. In this development special problems will have to be solved in each type of commu-

[1] Williams, J. W. Supra cit., p. 182.

nity, and in each section of the country—North, South, East, and West. These problems are different from those of foreign countries. While the methods being employed in such countries for reducing the maternal death rate may be suggestive, special methods adapted to the conditions in this country will probably have to be worked out. Of the greatest value, however, as examples, are pieces of work such as that now being carried on in England and other European countries for maternal and infant welfare, that of the New Zealand Society for the Health of Women and Children, the work of the Victorian Order of Nurses of Canada, and of the mayor of the little French town of Villiers-le-duc.[1]

Certain typical problems, characteristic of especial types of communities in this country, may be outlined briefly. In many of the larger cities excellent prenatal and obstetrical care can be obtained by those who can pay considerable sums for it and who realize its importance sufficiently to be willing to do so. In many cities, also, much progress has been made in the provision, through obstetrical clinics and hospitals, of good prenatal and obstetrical care, free or at low cost, for those who otherwise could not afford it. Yet even in a city well supplied with such clinics the number of women reached is relatively small in comparison with the total number of women who bear their children without adequate care during pregnancy and labor. In many large cities, especially those with a large percentage of foreign or of colored population, the untrained midwife is a much-discussed problem. It is well known, moreover, that women of moderate means, who represent a very large proportion of women bearing children, have, in most modern cities, received least benefit from improvements in standards of prenatal and obstetrical care. In working out plans for decreasing the death rate from childbirth in large cities the interests of this group can not be ignored. The problem must be considered as one which must be solved for all classes in a community; it must be realized that it is a problem of the greatest importance to the community as a whole. A very hopeful tendency is the one shown already in some cities, to look upon such service not as a charity but as a concern of the municipality as truly as the protection of its homes from fire and burglary or its milk and water supply from contamination.

In rural districts the problems are essentially different. In many such districts, especially in the North and West, where pioneer conditions still prevail, the question is not one of good or bad obstetrical care but of the inaccessibility of any care at all at this time. Many women bear their children with no attendant other than the hus-

---

[1] Rapport sur un Arreté Municipal pris par M. Morel de Villiers. Bulletin de l'Académie de Médecine. 1904. 3e série, Vol. LI, p. 222. Moore, S. G. "The Milroy lectures on infantile mortality and the relative practical value of measures directed to its prevention." Lecture III, Lancet, 1916. Vol. CXC, p. 943.

band, a relative, or a neighbor. The nearest physician may be many miles away, the nearest hospital much farther. The expense of calling a physician must necessarily be great, and usually is not considered justifiable. These women have of course no care during pregnancy; if complications develop they are unforeseen, and help is not available. As help in household tasks is usually unprocurable, many women must take up their work much sooner than they should. It may be urged that in practice it would be quite impossible for women living under rural conditions to be provided with such skilled supervision during pregnancy and such care at and after confinement as are now considered ideal. It certainly is not true, however, that a feasible community plan could not be worked out, if the interest of the community demanded it. Such a plan would necessarily recognize two main problems: (1) The best practical care of normal cases and (2) the detection of abnormal cases and their care.

A unit plan for a rural county would perhaps include:

1. A rural nursing service, centering at the county seat, with nurses especially equipped to discern the danger signs of pregnancy. The establishment of such a service would undoubtedly be the most economical first step in creating the network of agencies which will assure proper care for both normal and abnormal cases. In the rural counties in the United States which already have established nurses, the growth of this work will be watched with the greatest interest.

2. An accessible county center for maternal and infant welfare at which mothers may obtain simple information as to the proper care of themselves during pregnancy as well as of their babies.

3. A county maternity hospital, or beds in a general hospital, for the proper care of abnormal cases and for the care of normal cases when it is convenient for the women to leave their homes for confinement. Such a hospital necessarily would be accessible to all parts of the county.

4. Skilled attendance at confinement obtainable by each woman in the county.

As examples have been chosen the special problems in large cities and in pioneer rural districts. Other types of communities in this country present some of the same problems or others just as urgent. In each community, large or small, the essential problem is the same—how to bring about a general realization of the need for adequate care for each woman at childbirth, and how to secure such care.

This report attempts to open for lay discussion and medical study the subject of the preventable loss of life caused by childbirth in this country. Greater interest in the subject surely will lead to the development of new and successful methods for the prevention of these needless deaths.

# PART II. DETAILED ANALYSIS OF METHODS AND STATISTICAL DATA.[1]

## DISCUSSION OF CERTAIN TERMS AND METHODS USED IN THIS REPORT.

### International Classification of Causes of Death.

Official mortality statistics are derived from the returns of the causes of the deaths which occur annually. Such a return is made on the death certificate by the attending physician or by some person assumed to be familiar with the facts as regards the cause of death. Before the establishment in 1900 of the International Classification of Diseases and Causes of Death many different methods were used in different countries for the classification of these causes as returned on the certificates. The resultant confusion made difficult or impossible the comparison of the mortality statistics of various countries and led to the proposal of this uniform method of classification, called the "International Classification." Various countries have adopted this system of classification at various times; the United States Bureau of the Census adopted it for use in the calendar year 1900; Great Britain for use in 1911. It is planned to keep this classification up to date through revisions at 10-year intervals. The second revision was made in 1909, and a considerable number of changes were made. Differences in classification between the International List of Causes of Death and the lists in use in countries where the International has not been adopted and between the different revisions of the International List are extremely important, as will be shown, in any comparison of the death rates of various countries and of the same country for a series of years.[2]

In the detailed International List of Causes of Death, second decennial revision, Paris, 1909, the heading "VII—The Puerperal State" includes: (134) Accidents of pregnancy; (135) Puerperal hæmorrhage; (136) Other accidents of labor; (137) Puerperal septichæmia; (138) Puerperal albuminuria and convulsions; (139) Phlegmasia alba dolens, embolus, sudden death; (140) Following childbirth (not otherwise defined); (141) Puerperal diseases of the breast.

The abridged International List of Causes of Death (same revision) makes but two divisions of all the causes of death included in the detailed list under The Puerperal State. These divisions are:

(31) Puerperal septichæmia (puerperal fever, peritonitis), corresponding to number (137) of the detailed list.

---

[1] Part II will be of interest chiefly to students of statistics.

[2] For a discussion of this subject see Bureau de la statistique générale de la France: Statistique Internationale du Mouvement de la Population, 1913, p. 155*.

(32) Other puerperal accidents of pregnancy and labor, corresponding to Nos. (134), (135), (136), (138), (139), (140), and (141) in the detailed list.

In this report in the discussion of the Census figures and the tables, the classification of deaths according to the International List of Causes of Death, second revision, is used. The names for the different groups have been slightly changed, as it was felt that the names used in the International List give a misleading or obscure impression to those unfamiliar with this list.

In giving deaths and death rates the following terms and classification are used:

(a) *Childbirth, or all diseases caused by pregnancy and confinement,* which is the sum of (b) and (c) and corresponds to VII—The Puerperal State of the detailed International List and to the sum of (31) and (32) of the abridged International List.

(b) *Puerperal septicemia, or childbed fever,* which corresponds to (31) Puerperal septichæmia of the abridged International List, and to (137) Puerperal septichæmia of the detailed International List.

(c) *All other diseases caused by pregnancy and confinement,* which corresponds to (32) Other puerperal accidents of pregnancy and labor of the abridged International List, (134) to (136), and (138) to (141) of the detailed International List.

A few words of explanation may be useful with regard to these diseases and complications. In the term "accidents of pregnancy" the word "accident" is not used in its ordinary sense but in the sense of complications due to the pregnant condition. It includes miscarriage, severe hemorrhage during pregnancy, uncontrollable vomiting, and other complications.

"Puerperal hæmorrhage" includes severe hemorrhage at or following labor. It includes placenta prævia.

"Other accidents of labor" includes cases of difficult labor, operative delivery, rupture of the womb, and other complications, except hemorrhage, occurring at the time of labor.

"Puerperal septichæmia" (childbed or milk fever) is an infection coming on after labor or miscarriage.

"Puerperal albuminuria or convulsions," or "eclampsia," is an acute toxemia occurring during pregnancy, or during or after confinement, characterized, in its severest form, by convulsions.

"Phlegmasia alba dolens," often known as "milk leg," is a disease characterized by the swelling of a leg after confinement or miscarriage. The cause is the stoppage of a large vein of the thigh by a blood clot.

"Embolus" means blood clot. Sudden death may result from the carrying of such a blood clot to the heart or lungs.

"Following childbirth" (not otherwise defined) includes among other conditions insanity occurring after pregnancy or labor.

"Puerperal diseases of the breast" include inflammation or infection of the breast during lactation.

**Death-registration area.**

The statistics of causes of death are available only for a certain portion of the United States, included in the so-called "death-registration area." Unlike other civilized countries, the United States has no uniform laws for the registration of births and deaths. Moreover, the efficiency of enforcement of existing laws varies greatly in the different States. The Bureau of the Census in 1880 therefore established a "death-registration area," which comprises "States and cities in which the registration of deaths is returned as fairly complete (at least 90 per cent of the total), and from which transcripts of the deaths recorded under the State laws or municipal ordinances are obtained by the Bureau of the Census."[1] In 1880 this area included but 17 per cent of the total population of the United States. As States and cities have passed better laws and obtained better enforcement they have been added to the registration area; the latter has increased greatly in size, but even in 1913 included only 65.1 per cent of the population of the United States. For the remaining 34.9 per cent of the population of the country we have no reliable statistics. This 34.9 per cent includes the population of the greater number of the Southern States and of many Middle Western and Western States outside of certain registration cities in these States which are included in the area. No statements can be made, therefore, of the number of deaths from any cause in the United States as a whole; only an estimate can be made on the assumption that for any cause of death the same rate prevails in the remainder of the United States as in the death-registration area.

**Provisional birth-registration area.**

The registration of births is still more incomplete in this country than is the registration of deaths. For 1910 the United States Bureau of the Census established a "provisional birth-registration area," including the New England States, Pennsylvania, Michigan, New York City, and Washington, D. C.[2]

**Methods of computing the death rates from all causes connected with pregnancy and confinement.**

(1) *Death rates per 100,000 inhabitants.*—Trask[3] gives the definition, "Death rates may be expressed as the ratio of the total number of deaths, taken as a unit, to the population. For example: 1 in 60. The usual method, however, is to express these rates in terms of the

[1] U. S. Census. Mortality Statistics, 1911, p. 9.
[2] U. S. Census. Mortality Statistics, 1911, p. 25.
[3] Trask, J. W. "Vital statistics." U. S. Public Health Service, Supp. to the Public Health Reports, No. 12, p. 59.

number of deaths per 1,000 population, or in some instances per 10,000 or even 100,000, or 1,000,000." In the publications of the United States Bureau of the Census the death rates of all diseases, including those of the diseases connected with childbirth, are usually expressed in terms of the number of deaths per 100,000 total population. But a death rate computed in this way obviously gives a very misleading impression with regard to a disease to which only one group of the population is liable. In computing the death rate from the diseases connected with childbirth, only women of childbearing age should be considered, or, still better, only women actually bearing children in a given year. All individuals of all ages and both sexes may be exposed each year to a risk of typhoid fever, pneumonia, or tuberculosis; but during the year only the women pregnant or bearing children are exposed to the risk of death from the diseases connected with these functions.

(2) *Death rates per 100,000 women.*—This method of computing rates is somewhat superior to that of computing the deaths per 100,000 total inhabitants. It is used to some extent in foreign reports. These rates have been computed from estimates of female population furnished by the United States Bureau of the Census for the years 1900 to 1910 for the group of 11 States within the death-registration area in 1900. These are given in Table IV, on page 50.

(3) *Death rates per 100,000 women of childbearing age.*[1]—Such a rate, which is a much more accurate one than either of those mentioned above, can be computed for the registration area for only one year, the census year 1900. For that year only has the age and sex distribution of the registration area been published. The number of women 15 to 44 years of age in the registration area in that year was 7,383,154.[2] The number of deaths from childbirth among women 15 to 44 years was 3,712; of these 1,594 were from puerperal septicemia and 2,118 from all other diseases of pregnancy and confinement.[3] The death rates were, therefore, from childbirth or all diseases caused by pregnancy and confinement, 50.3; from puerperal septicemia, 21.6; and from all other diseases of pregnancy and confinement, 28.7.

(4) *Death rates per 1,000 births.*—As shown above, the method of computation of death rates which gives the clearest picture of the hazards of childbirth is that which takes into account only the women giving birth to children in that year. This is the method in use in a large number of foreign countries. The advantages of the method are self-evident.[4] A demonstration of the superiority of

[1] The female population between the ages of 15 and 45 years as determined by census enumeration, or by estimation for intercensal and postcensal years.—Trask, J. W. Supra cit., p. 23.

[2] U. S. Twelfth Census, 1900. Vital Statistics, Part I, p. XLII.

[3] U. S. Twelfth Census, 1900. Vital Statistics, Part II, p. 242.

[4] Each death rate is in terms of registered, i. e., living, births. This is a more accurate measure than a statement per 1,000 of total population or per 1,000 total or married women at childbearing ages.—Newsholme, A. Maternal Mortality in Connection with Childbearing. Grt. Brit. Local Govt. Bd., Supp. to Report of Medical Officer for 1914-15, p. 24.

this method of computation is obtained by a study of the tables giving the death rates from these diseases for foreign countries. In certain countries, as for instance Belgium and Hungary, there has been in recent years an apparent fall in the average death rates as computed per 100,000 population, while the average rates computed per 1,000 live births have remained stationary or risen. This phenomenon is due, evidently, to a decline in the birth rate in these countries during these years, and shows how misleading the rates as given per 100,000 population undoubtedly are in countries with declining birth rates. Whether a fall in the birth rate has occurred in the United States is not known. If it has occurred in the registration area, it would mean that the slight rise in rates per 100,000 population between 1900 and 1913 means a greater rise in rates computed according to the number of births. Such an error might compensate for the opposite error due to the more complete registration of deaths from childbirth in the later years of this period.

In computing the rates per 1,000 births two methods are in use: The computation of the number of deaths per 1,000 total births and that per 1,000 live births. Both methods depend upon an accurate registration of births; the first method is used in those foreign countries in which all births including stillbirths are required to be reported; the second, in those countries where only live births are reported. The first is probably the better method, because by it the whole number of women bearing children in a certain year is considered. But even this rate is not absolutely accurate. While the number of deaths includes those from diseases connected with miscarriage, the whole number of women having miscarriages is not used as a base, but only the number of those bearing stillborn and live children. Miscarriages are not reportable in any country, although a number of miscarriages (as the term is usually defined) probably are reported as stillbirths in certain countries. The fact that women having miscarriages are not considered in the base would lead to a somewhat higher death rate than that which would express absolutely the number of deaths per 1,000 women at risk. On the other hand, in the computation of this rate the fact is not taken into consideration that a certain number of births are multiple; that is, the number of births is larger than the number of women bearing children. Still another objection to the use of this rate, especially in the comparison of the rates of different countries, is the fact that the definition of stillbirth varies greatly according to the laws of different countries;[1] that is, in one country many cases may be reported as stillbirths which in another country, having a different

[1] Royal Statistical Society. "Report of special committee on infantile mortality." Journal of the Royal Statistical Society, 1913, Vol. LXXVI, p. 27.

64614°—17——5

interpretation of this term, might not be reported at all, as they would be classed as miscarriages.

The second method, in which the number of deaths per 1,000 live births is considered, is that used by foreign countries in which the registration of stillbirths is not required. England and Wales, Ireland, Scotland, and New Zealand are among this number.

The variation in different countries with regard to the definition of stillbirth causes a difficulty in the use of this method. In three of the countries studied—France, Belgium, and Spain—the term stillbirth includes infants alive at birth but dying before the registration of birth, i. e., within one to three days of birth. Because of these various difficulties, death rates for the foreign countries have been, wherever possible, computed by both methods.

On account of the lack of accurate birth registration neither method has been used in computing rates for the United States. Only for States and cities in the provisional birth-registration area, and for one year, 1910, can the death rates per 1,000 live births be given. These are shown in Table VI, page 52.

## SOURCES OF ERROR IN THE STUDY OF DEATH RATES FROM CHILDBIRTH.

In all mortality statistics, and especially in those with which we are especially concerned in this bulletin, there are two general sources of inaccuracy in the figures: First, the figures for each year may be inaccurate, or may give an incomplete picture of actual conditions because of many different factors, such as incompleteness or inaccuracy of the figures, inappropriate methods of classification or computation, etc. Second, the figures for different years may not be comparable simply because of the great improvements that are made each year in methods of registration, computation, and classification. With the object in view of giving each year as accurate and clear a picture of the actual conditions as possible, tremendous advance in methods has been made yearly in this country and in other countries. This very advance, however, brings with it many difficulties in comparing the figures for the years before such improvements were instituted with those of the years after that time. Each year the figures give us more accurate information of the actual number of deaths and of the death rates; yet each year the comparison of the figures for that year with those in the past is fraught with more danger of error. In general, therefore, the study of the actual number of deaths and the death rates for the last years for which figures are obtainable is more valuable than any comparison of rates for different years. All these sources of error will now be discussed in detail.

**Inaccuracy of returns.**

As all mortality statistics depend upon the returns of the cause of death as given by the physician or other person on the death certificates, their value depends on the degree of accuracy of diagnosis shown by these returns. As Hoffman[1] has pointed out, the returns for countries in which a medical certificate of the cause of death is not required must be of very small value. He states, however, that "For most of the civilized countries this requirement is met to a reasonably satisfactory degree."

The objection has frequently been raised, however, that there is a large percentage of error even in the returns made by physicians due to mistakes in diagnosis, such errors being more numerous in the case of certain diseases than of others. This matter has been considered by the United States Bureau of the Census.[2] Hoffman[3] defends the general validity of the death returns. He admits that there is serious risk of error in the "Careless or superficial use of the data of mortality statistics, irrespective of the diseases dealt with: for, as pointed out by Longstaff, * * * 'there are numerous fallacies to which the classification of deaths according to their alleged causes is liable,' and he enumerates particularly * * * the more or less varying proportions of indefinite causes, the deliberate falsification of returns for personal or family reasons, and the effect of the progress of medical science, improved diagnosis, etc." Hoffman, however, concludes: "All of these reasons notwithstanding, the conclusion appears to be incontrovertible that on the whole the present system of death registration is entitled to confidence and the results approximately represent the true state of the nation's health."

With regard to the diseases in question, however, inaccuracy of the returns undoubtedly constitutes a special source of error in the figures for all countries. The statistics of deaths due to puerperal septicemia (childbed fever or infection at the time of miscarriage or childbirth) are without question very incomplete. Many deaths due to this disease are reported, for obvious reasons, as due to some other condition or to some general condition, such as septicemia, pyemia, and the like. This fault in all statistics on the subject has been commented on very frequently both in this country and in foreign countries.[4]

---

[1] Hoffman, F. L. The Mortality from Cancer Throughout the World, 1915, p. 2.

[2] U. S. Census. Mortality Statistics, 1912, p. 24.

[3] Hoffman, F. L. Supra cit., p. 3.

[4] (a) It is very difficult to make accurate statements as to the frequency of puerperal infection, especially when it occurs outside of hospital practice. Concerning this condition the vital statistics of the health officers of the various American cities are of no value, inasmuch as the vast majority of deaths from this disease are returned as being due to malaria, typhoid fever, pneumonia, or other causes.—Williams, J. W. Obstetrics, 1913, p. 900. (b) It is very difficult to estimate the frequency of puerperal infection outside of hospitals, since many deaths are reported as due to typhoid, malaria, pneumonia, etc.—Edgar, J. C. The Practice of Obstetrics, 1903, p. 772. (c) It is not unlikely, furthermore, that in a considerable number of deaths due to childbearing the fact that they are associated with childbearing escapes certification.

It follows, however, that almost never is a case reported as due to infection at confinement when it is really due to some other cause; in other words, the figures though undoubtedly incomplete are reliable as far as they go; they are a statement of the minimum number of cases which have occurred. As Newsholme remarks,[1] many cases of puerperal septicemia probably are reported as due to other conditions associated with childbirth; so that the total figures for all diseases associated with this condition should always be noted, although it may be the figures for puerperal septicemia in which our immediate interest lies.

Many deaths due to other complications of pregnancy and confinement are also undoubtedly reported under other headings. This is especially true of cases of puerperal albuminuria and convulsions, which are reported as due to acute nephritis or simply to convulsions; and of hemorrhage or phlebitis following miscarriage or labor, reported without reference to their connection with childbirth.

**Limited area and short period of time represented by figures.**

In the United States the limited area of the country (the death-registration area) for which any figures are available is an element of weakness in the statistics. Though this area and its population are absolutely very large, they can not be considered as representative of the entire country. Any estimate based on the figures for the registration area is open to criticism on account of differences in age and sex distribution in different parts of the country.

In the United States the short period for which any figures are available lessens greatly the value of a study such as this. In foreign countries comparisons of the death rates for a long series of years may be made, even though errors due to lack of comparability of the figures may occur. In this country information is available

---

Deaths from puerperal fever are likely also to be understated; and the desirability is confirmed of basing inferences as to excessive mortality from childbearing on all the conditions concerned in this mortality, and not merely on the death returns for puerperal fever.—Newsholme, A. Supra cit., pp. 26, 30. (*d*) It may be objected that owing to faulty registration and deficient death certification the returns are not reliable. That this objection may have some weight in estimating the amount of mortality, especially as regards puerperal fever (in which for obvious reasons the death returns are avowedly defective), I fully admit; but, as this communication seeks to compare the mortality of one year with that of another and of one part of the kingdom with that of another, and as the sources of error apply to each, the result can not be materially affected. In estimating the true amount of mortality, however, a mental correction should certainly be made for this obvious source of error.—Boxall, R. "The mortality of childbirth," Lancet, 1893, Vol. II, p. 10. (*e*) Warren, S. P. "The prevalence of puerperal septicemia in private practice at the present time, contrasted with that of a generation ago." Amer. Jour. of Obstetrics, 1905, Vol. LI, p. 301.

[1] But the above extreme local variations in the proportion between deaths from puerperal fever and from other dangers of childbearing suggest that in death certification there may be local variations in the extent to which deaths from puerperal fever are returned under the heading of other conditions associated with childbearing. * * * On the whole, it is likely that in comparing counties and county boroughs with each other, the safest plan is to utilize only the death rates from the two sets of conditions taken together.—Newsholme, A. Supra cit., p. 26.

only for the census years 1880, 1890, and 1900 and for the calendar years from 1900 to 1913, inclusive. Moreover, the area covered by the reports previous to 1890 was so small that any comparison between years prior to 1890 and years subsequent to that date has seemed unwise.

**Methods of computation.**

In the United States the computation of the death rates from the diseases in question by a method (computation per 100,000 total population) giving but an inaccurate picture of the facts is necessarily a source of error in the study. This method also makes difficult a comparison of the death rates with those of foreign countries.

**Sources of error in comparisons of death rates of different years.**

There are many special sources of error involved in the comparison of death rates of the registration area of the United States from these causes in different years.

First. Differences in the constitution of the death-registration area cause one of the most important difficulties in comparison. As before stated, the death-registration area is not an unchanging entity, but has been added to almost yearly as registration has improved in various States and cities. This constant increase constitutes a serious source of error in comparing the death rates for this area for different years. Within the course of the years studied, States or cities having a particularly high or low rate from the disease in question may have been added to the registration area.[1] This difficulty is so serious that in making comparisons of the death rates in the registration area of the United States from a certain disease through a series of years the publications of the United States Bureau of the Census always point out the influence which the inclusion of a certain State may have had upon the rate of the disease in question for the registration area.

The same method may be applied, for example, to a comparison of the death rates from childbirth in the registration area for the years 1909 and 1910. In 1909 the rate for the registration area was 15.3; in 1910, 15.7. In 1910, however, four States—Minnesota, Montana, Utah, and North Carolina [2]—were added to the registration area and one State—South Dakota—was dropped. In that year the death rate from childbirth in Minnesota was 11.9 per 100,000 inhabitants, in Montana 16.4, in Utah 18.4, and in the municipalities of North Carolina 30.7. That in South Dakota in 1909 was 21.7 for the urban and 12.9 for the rural portions of the State. Evidently the exact determination of the effect which the inclusion or exclusion of any one of these States exerted upon the death rate of the registration area is a complicated matter.

---

[1] U. S. Census. Mortality Statistics, 1909, p. 9.

[2] Municipalities of 1,000 or more inhabitants in 1900.

It was thought wise, therefore, in this study to make, in addition to a comparison of the death rates from childbirth in the registration area for 1890 and from 1900 to 1913, a comparison of the death rates shown (1) for the same series of years by the group of States which have been registration States since 1890, and (2) for the years 1900 to 1913 by the group of States which have been registration States since 1900. Obviously these two comparisons contain no error due to changes in the groups of States compared from year to year.

The group of eight States which have been registration States since 1890 includes all the New England States except Maine, also New York, New Jersey, and the District of Columbia. (See Table II, p. 49.) For this group of States no permanent decrease has occurred in the death rate from childbirth per 100,000 population in the 23 years studied. There was a decrease in the rate between 1890 and 1900, followed by a rise, and then by slightly fluctuating rates. The rates for 1890[1] and 1913, however, are almost identical—14.1 and 14.3 per 100,000 inhabitants.

The rates for the second group of 11 States show no decline but rather an increase in the 13 years from 1900 to 1913. These States have been registration States since 1900 and include, besides the 8 above mentioned, Maine, Michigan, and Indiana. The death rate from childbirth in 1900[2] was 13.4; in 1913, 14.9; with fluctuations between 12.7 and 15.5.

The fact that the death rates from childbirth show no decrease in the registration area from 1890 to 1913 (see Table I, p. 49) is therefore corroborated by the two comparisons just made. The rates for this area also show fluctuations from year to year, but are nearly identical for 1890 and 1913, i. e., 15.3 and 15.8.

This possible source of error in the comparison of the rates in the registration area for different years, therefore, is shown to be of practical unimportance.

A comparison of the three Tables I, II, and III brings out several interesting facts. Tables I and II both show a decline in the rates between 1890 and 1900; this fall is followed by a corresponding rise and fluctuating rates. The rates for the group of 8 States shown in Table II are almost uniformly slightly lower for each year than are those of the death-registration area shown in Table I.

Second. The most important source of error in the comparisons of the death rates of various years is due to the improvements which have been made yearly in the accuracy of the returns of the cause of death. In each State, newly admitted to the registration area, improvements are made continually in the completeness and accuracy of the death returns. In addition one special improvement has been made in the returns in the registration area.

---

[1] Census year ending May 31.

[2] Calendar year

It has already been pointed out with regard to the diseases under consideration that deaths due to puerperal septicemia and to other complications of pregnancy and confinement are frequently reported as due to such indefinite causes as septicemia, pyemia, hemorrhage, phlebitis, convulsions, etc. In several foreign countries the attempt has been made for some years to render the records more complete by making inquiries as to cases of death of women of childbearing age where the cause of death is an indefinite one of this character. To each physician making such a report for a woman of childbearing age a confidential inquiry is sent, asking whether or not the cause of death had any relation to childbirth or miscarriage. Boxall[1] states that this has been done in England since 1881 and has resulted in an increase of about 12 per cent in the number of cases reported as due to puerperal septicemia. In this country since about 1906[2] the State registrars of vital statistics have cooperated with the United States Bureau of the Census in making their reports more complete through this practice.

For several years[2] the Census Bureau has made an inquiry in many cases where the cause of death of a woman of childbearing age has been returned to it as septicemia, pyemia, or peritonitis, and additional cases of puerperal septicemia have been added in this way. That bureau is unable, however, to estimate the percentage of cases which have thus been added. In a test[3] in which a number of letters of inquiry were sent to physicians returning deaths as due to meningitis, paralysis, convulsions, pneumonia, and peritonitis, 102 cases returned as peritonitis were thus investigated. Eight cases were changed to puerperal septicemia following the answer to these inquiries. The following statement is made: "If the percentages of change resulting from this investigation, which, though limited, may prove to be fairly representative, be applied to the numbers of deaths compiled from the various causes for the registration area for 1911, * * * some of the definite causes would be increased as follows: * * * Puerperal septicemia from 4,376 to 4,560, or 4.2 per cent."[3]

Without doubt, therefore, the records in this country since 1906, and especially since 1912, are more complete than those for previous years.[4]

Obviously greater accuracy of the returns leads to an apparent rise in rate, even when the true death rate is stationary or declining slightly. It is impossible to estimate how great has been the influence

---

[1] Boxall, R. "Mortality in childbed, both in hospital and in general practice," Jour. of Obstetrics and Gynæcology of the British Empire, 1905. Vol. VII, p. 322; Newsholme, A. Supra cit., p. 25.

[2] Statement by Chief Statistician for Vital Statistics, U. S. Bureau of the Census.

[3] U. S. Census. Mortality Statistics, 1911, pp. 37, 38.

[4] Similar improvements in the records for other causes of death have been made in recent years through the method of making similar inquiries with regard to deaths reported as due to such indefinite causes as simple meningitis, paralysis without specified cause, etc. See U. S. Census. Mortality Statistics, 1912, pp. 23, 24, and Dublin, L. I., and Kopf, E. W. "An experiment in the compilation of mortality statistics," Quart. Public. of the Amer. Stat. Assn., 1913. Vol. XIII, p. 639.

of this factor upon the death rates of childbirth and of puerperal septicemia since 1900. As an index the changes in the death rates for the death-registration area from the indefinite causes, "purulent infection and septicemia," "simple peritonitis," "convulsions," and "hemorrhage, other diseases of the circulatory system," between 1900 and 1913 should be studied.

It is significant that the average death rate from purulent infection and septicemia, which in 1901–1905 was 6.1 per 100,000 population, fell in 1906–1910 to 3.8 and then decreased steadily, being 2.8 in 1913.[1] In the same way the death rate from simple peritonitis, which was 10.8 in 1901–1905, fell to 6.1 in 1906–1910 and 2.7 in 1913.[1] The other causes mentioned have shown a decline which is much less marked.

As these death rates represent those of the entire population, not those of women of childbearing age, their decline can be ascribed only in part to the fact that a number of cases formerly returned as due to these causes are now ascribed to puerperal septicemia and other diseases caused by pregnancy and confinement. It is plain, however, that this factor has been a very important one in determining their decrease.

In general, then, it may be stated that recent improvements in death certification must be borne in mind in making comparisons of the death rates from childbirth since 1900; that these improvements probably account for the apparent rise in the death rate between 1900 and 1913, and may, indeed, conceal a slight actual decrease in the rates during those years. It is not, however, probable that any substantial decrease in rate has been concealed in this way.

The comparisons made in Tables II and III of rates for the group of 8 States which have been in the registration area since 1890 and for that of 11 States which have been in this area since 1900 are probably less subject to this source of error than is a comparison of rates for the registration area. In the States in which registration has been good for a number of years improvements made in the returns for the more recent years will not be so marked a factor.

Third. A third source of error in the comparison of death rates for various years in this country results from the changes in classification of causes of death which have been made. In the United States the International List of Causes of Death was adopted for use in the calendar year 1900. A different classification was in use before that time. The group of diseases included in the older classification under "Affections connected with pregnancy" are included under the title "The puerperal state," Division VII of the detailed International List (see p. 29), corresponding to the terms "Child-

[1] U. S. Census. Mortality Statistics, 1913, pp. 53, 54.

birth" or "All diseases caused by pregnancy and confinement" as used in this bulletin. Therefore these large groups can be compared for the census years 1890 and 1900 and the calendar years 1900 to 1913. The title puerperal septicemia of the older classification does not correspond, however, to that of "puerperal septichæmia" of the International Classification. Nevertheless, it has been thought best to print the figures for puerperal septicemia for the census years 1890 and 1900 with the warning that these figures are not exactly comparable with the figures for this disease for the calendar years 1900 to 1913. At the second revision of the International Classification, in force for the registration area January 1, 1910, several changes were made in the classification of the group of diseases with which we are concerned, i. e., "The puerperal state." These changes do not affect the whole group, but only the subgroups, especially No. 137, "Puerperal septichæmia." Three causes of deaths included under this heading under the first revision were removed and included under other headings; these are: Puerperal toxemia, included now under 138; puerperal phlebitis, changed to a separate heading, 139; and retention of the placenta, now included under 135. No other groups previously not included were added to "Puerperal septichæmia" in that year. These changes would naturally cause a decrease in the number of deaths ascribed to puerperal septicemia and a corresponding decrease in the death rate for this disease, with an increase in the rate of those included under "Other diseases caused by pregnancy and confinement." This must be remembered in comparing the rates for years succeeding 1910 with those preceding it, both in the United States and in all other countries studied. How far this change in the death rate for puerperal septicemia compensates in the United States for the opposite error due to the more complete returns for this disease brought about by the inquiries sent by the Bureau of the Census it would be impossible to say.

**Sources of error in a study of foreign statistics.**

It may be claimed that a comparison of the vital statistics of various foreign countries involves a certain risk of error due to differences in the methods of registration employed in the various countries and in the degrees of accuracy of the returns. For instance, the comparatively low death rate of a certain country may be explained as being due to the incompleteness of the returns in that country. Beyond this source of error, which can not be avoided, two other especial sources appear to exist in the comparison of the death rates from the diseases caused by childbirth. The first one is that already treated at some length, i. e., the development of errors due to the different methods used by different countries in computing the rates. This source of error has been avoided by reckoning the rates uniformly for each country in the group considered according to two different methods, i. e., per 100,000 total population and per 1,000 live births. While neither method of computation is an ideal one, it has been necessary to use them as they alone give a basis of comparison of the rates of all the countries considered.

A second source of error has also been alluded to; it is the lack of uniformity in methods of classification of the causes of death. Many of the countries under consideration have not used the International Classification at all, or only for a portion of the period studied. As the best means available for avoiding this difficulty, the figures for each country have been used as published in the Statistique Internationale du Mouvement de la Population d'après les Registres d'Etat Civil, prepared by the Ministère du Travail, Bureau de la Statistique Générale of France. In this publication figures for countries not using the International Classification have been rearranged to conform as nearly as possible to the divisions of the International List. Figures, however, are available from this source only up to the year 1910; for the years following, figures have been obtained from the latest available original reports of each country. For those countries not using the International Classification the figures have been rearranged in the same way to conform to it as nearly as possible.[1]

Slight differences in methods of classification will probably not affect the death rates to any great extent, nor will they often affect the number of deaths, and consequently the death rates, of the whole group of diseases—"The puerperal state," or "All diseases caused by pregnancy and confinement." Only the proportion of deaths to be ascribed to either of the two subgroups "puerperal septicemia" and "other diseases caused by pregnancy and confinement," will be affected. A rearrangement of the deaths within the group, ascribing a larger number of deaths to puerperal septicemia will bring, of course, a decrease in those reported as due to "other diseases caused by pregnancy and confinement." For this reason, therefore, the total number of deaths for the large group and the death rate for this group are more important than those of the subgroups. (See p. 36.) An exception to the statement in regard to the differences in method of classification must be made for the figures of England and Wales. Previous to 1911, the year in which the International Classification was adopted, a certain group of deaths almost universally included under the large group "The puerperal state" or "All diseases caused by pregnancy and confinement" was not included in the English and Welsh figures, i. e., deaths due to puerperal nephritis and albuminuria. Consequently in these earlier years the reports of deaths

[1] On pages 57 to 59 will be found especial notes as to difficulties encountered in the reclassification of the figures of various countries.

ascribed to childbirth or all diseases caused by pregnancy and confinement are incomplete and the death rates from this group of causes are lower than would have been the case had the International Classification been used. This fact must be remembered in making comparisons between England and Wales and other countries. The amount of the error, which is not a very large one, can be estimated by noting the number of deaths annually reported from this cause for the years 1911 to 1914. (See p. 58; also Table XV, p. 60.) Whether or not there is the same incompleteness in the figures of other countries could not be learned from the reports.

In general, foreign statistics have been used in this report as giving a rough estimate of actual conditions. Unfortunately more exact information is not in existence. It has not been considered wise, in view of the possibilities of error in the material, to use any method of analysis which assumes a higher degree of accuracy than can be attributed to all the existing figures.

## FOREIGN STATISTICS.

**Comparison of the average death rates from childbirth in certain foreign countries and in the United States.**

1. *Average death rates per 100,000 population.*—In order to obtain a basis for comparison with the rates for the death-registration area of the United States the average rates for 15 foreign countries have been reckoned according to the number of deaths per 100,000 population. These rates are given in Table XII, on page 56, in which the countries are arranged in order, the one having the lowest rate being first. Many of the countries show rates differing but very little from that of the United States. The rates for 9 of the 16 countries vary between 12.4 and 15.2, while that of the registration area is 14.9. Other facts brought out by this table are mentioned on page 22.

2. *Average death rates per 1,000 live births.*—It has been realized that the average death rate from these diseases as above computed gives a very misleading idea of the actual death rate on the basis of the number of women bearing children. Differences in the age and sex composition of the population of the countries studied, and, above all, differences in the birth rate, obviously lead to great error. Unfortunately the rate per 1,000 births can not be given for the death-registration area of the United States, though it can be given for one year (1910) for the provisional birth-registration area. This rate is 6.5 per 1,000 live births. The comparison of such a rate, for a limited area of a country reckoned only for one year, with average rates of other countries reckoned for a series of years, is of course unfair. Still it is a noteworthy fact that the rate for this small area of the United States is considerably higher than that for any country in the group considered.

Table XIII, page 56, gives the average death rates reckoned per 1,000 live births for the 15 foreign countries already studied arranged in order, the one having the lowest rate being first. The order here shows a considerable variation from that in the previous table. However, the same group of countries shows the lowest rates computed according to either method of computation; these are Sweden, Italy, and Norway. Similarly, the highest rates in both tables are shown by a second group of countries—Belgium, Spain, Switzerland, Australia, and Scotland. The rates for Ireland form an exception. The rate for that country, reckoned per 100,000 inhabitants, is only moderately high; reckoned per 1,000 live births, however, it is one of the higher rates.

3. *Percentage of deaths caused by puerperal septicemia.*—Another interesting feature of the foreign figures is the great variation shown among the different countries in the percentage of the total deaths from childbirth which are ascribed to puerperal septicemia. Table XIV gives these figures for each country for as large a part of the period 1900 to 1910 as figures are available. As pointed out frequently throughout this report, on account of the inaccurate returns from puerperal septicemia the total rate from childbirth is a more reliable one than is the rate from puerperal septicemia; therefore, sweeping conclusions can not be based on these comparisons. Otherwise these figures would be extremely significant, as the deaths from puerperal septicemia are the most easily preventable of all the deaths from childbirth. In the larger number (11) of the 15 foreign countries studied the deaths from puerperal septicemia constitute from 30 to 50 per cent of the total number of deaths from childbirth. In the registration area of the United States they represent 44 per cent. Norway, 51.2 per cent, and Spain, 62.8 per cent, show the only two percentages higher than 50; New Zealand, 25.2 per cent, and Hungary, 26.7 per cent, show markedly low percentages.

**Comparison of the changes in the death rates from childbirth in certain foreign countries for the years 1900 to 1913.**

Far more valuable than a comparison of average rates of foreign countries is a study of the rates of each country for a series of years in order to discover whether they are decreasing or increasing and to compare such changes in the various countries. While it may be dangerous on account of different methods of registration and classification to compare the rates of different countries, no such source of error is attached to the comparison of rates in the same country for a number of years. The period 1900 to 1913 (or the latest year for which figures are available) is a very short one for a study of a change in death rates. It would have been far more interesting to study the death rates for a long series of years in each country, choosing a period beginning before the introduction of methods of asepsis. But such a study for the complete list of countries considered was not thought advisable, because of the difficulties caused by variations in classification of causes of death in the earlier years.

In order to study the rates for any increase or decrease occurring during the last 13 years, the rates per 1,000 [1] live births will be used rather than those per 100,000 population. In several countries—Belgium, Hungary, Italy, Norway, Prussia, and Spain—the rate from childbirth per 100,000 population apparently has fallen during the period, while the rate per 1,000 live births has remained almost the same, or has risen. The cause of this inconsistency, as explained on page 33, is the fact that in these countries the birth rate or the proportionate number of births to the number of inhabitants has decreased.

Average death rates for the foreign countries studied are given for periods of from 3 to 5 years in Table XVI. Differences in averages from period to period are more significant than differences in rates from year to year, and they indicate more accurately and readily whether death rates in a given country are increasing or decreasing.

In preparing Table XVI it would have been more satisfactory to base averages on identical five-year periods for all countries, but since the periods for which the information was available varied so widely in different countries, this procedure was impracticable, and the complete periods were divided into as nearly uniform subperiods as possible.

The countries will be considered in different groups.

*Countries showing a decrease in the death rates from all diseases caused by pregnancy and confinement.*—England and Wales show a fall in the total death rate from these diseases and also a fall in the death rate from puerperal septicemia in the years between 1900 and 1914.[2] The total death rate per 1,000 live births fell from 4.4 in 1900–1904 to 3.7 in 1910–1914. The death rate from puerperal septicemia per 1,000 live births was 1.9 in 1900–1904, and 1.4 in 1910–1914. The still greater apparent drop in the rates per 100,000 inhabitants will be noted. This decrease in the rates from these diseases in England and Wales since 1900 is especially important because the lack of decrease for a long period of time before 1900 has been the subject of considerable discussion.

Boxall [3] in 1893 and 1905 published two reports which aroused medical interest. Based on studies of the figures published by the

---

[1] The rate per 1,000 live births will be found in column 8 of Table XV, p. 60.

[2] In studying the figures after 1910, only the figures given as 1911 (a) and 1912 (a), etc., must be compared with the figures of years before 1910, for the reasons explained on p. 58.

[3] Boxall, R. "The mortality of childbirth," Lancet, 1893, Vol. II, p. 9; "Mortality in childbed, both in hospital and in general practice." Jour. of Obstetrics and Gynæcology of the British Empire, 1905, Vol. VII, p. 315.

registrar general, these reports comment on the lack of decrease in the total mortality from childbirth and from puerperal septicemia in the period since the introduction of methods of antisepsis.

Sir Arthur Newsholme, medical officer of the Local Government Board of England, published last year a most interesting report on maternal mortality in connection with childbearing in England and Wales.[1] The report in question will no doubt be the inspiration of studies of this subject in many countries, just as it has been of the present report on conditions in the United States. He finds that from 1874 to 1893 there was no decline in the rates from puerperal septicemia, or from other conditions associated with childbirth, but that since 1895 there has been a marked decline in the rate from puerperal septicemia and a decline in the total rate from childbirth. There has been, however, little change in the death rate from conditions other than puerperal septicemia caused by childbirth. He writes: "Even so far as puerperal fever is concerned, notwithstanding the improvement already secured, it must be regarded as highly unsatisfactory that in 1914 for every 644 infants born 1 mother lost her life from puerperal infection, either present before the birth of the infant, or more often acquired during or soon after its birth. A large portion of this mortality, with its still greater amount of associated sickness, could at once be prevented were adequate antenatal care and skilled attendance under satisfactory conditions at and after birth made available."[1]

The interest in this subject in England is reflected in several acts which have been passed in recent years with the object of securing better antenatal and confinement care for all women at childbirth. These are the midwives act, 1902; the notification of births act, 1907; the notification of births (extension) act, 1915, the maternity benefits under the national insurance act, and the voting of grants by Parliament in aid of work done by local authorities and voluntary agencies to promote maternal and child welfare work.

The rates for Ireland show a decrease in the death rate from childbirth. In 1902 to 1906 the rate was 5.8; in 1911 to 1914 it was 5.2. There was also a slight decrease in the rate from puerperal septicemia.

Japan shows also a fall in the rate from childbirth from 4.2 in 1901–1904 to 3.6 in 1909–1912. The death rate from puerperal septicemia, however, has increased slightly.

The rates for New Zealand and Switzerland have also shown a decline in the periods studied.

*Countries showing almost stationary rates from the diseases caused by pregnancy and confinement.*—This group includes all the remaining countries considered except Scotland. In several of these countries

[1] Newsholme, A. Maternal Mortality in Connection with Childbearing. Grt. Brit. Local Govt. Bd., Supp. to Report of Medical Officer for 1914-15, pp. 22, 23.

there has been a slight fall or rise in the rates between the first and last period, amounting in each case to less than 0.5 of 1 per 1,000 live births.

In Prussia no demonstrable fall has occurred in the rate per 1,000 live births from all diseases caused by pregnancy and confinement, nor in that from puerperal septicemia. The total rate in 1903 to 1906 was 3.2; in 1907 to 1910 it was 3.1.

The almost stationary rates for Australia, Belgium, Hungary, Italy, Norway, Spain, and Sweden will also be noted in the tables.

In all of these countries numerous physicians have called attention to the stationary or rising death rates from childbirth and from childbed fever. A large medical literature has grown up on this subject. Von Herff[1] comments on the figures published by Krohme, showing for Prussia an increasing death rate from puerperal septicemia in the years 1901 to 1904. He attributes it to the laxity of physicians in carrying out antiseptic methods and to the unnecessarily frequent use of forceps and to other obstetrical operations. Buess[2] and Winter[3] are among those who have written more recently on the question of these death rates in Switzerland, East Prussia, and other European countries.

*Countries showing a rise in rates.*—The total mortality rate from diseases of childbirth for Scotland has shown a definite increase from 5.1 per 1,000 live births in 1901–1905 to 5.8 in 1911–1914. This increase, however, has not been due apparently to an increase in the rate from puerperal septicemia; in fact, this rate has shown a fall.

---

[1] Von Herff, O. "Wie ist der zunehmenden Kindbettfiebersterblichkeit zu steuern? Minderung der Operationen. Besserung der Desinfektion in der Hauspraxis." Münchener Medizinische Wochenschrift, 1907, Vol. LIV, p. 1017.

[2] Buess. Zeitschrift für Geburtshülfe und Gynäkologie, 1915, Vol. LXXVII, p. 735.

[3] Winter. "Die Bekämpfung des Kindbettfiebers in Ostpreussen." Deutsche Medizinische Wochenschrift, 1908, Vol. XXXIV, p. 2244.

# PART III. GENERAL TABLES.

TABLE I.—*Population, deaths, and death rates per 100,000 population in the death-registration area from diseases caused by pregnancy and confinement, 1890 and 1900 to 1913.*

| Year.[1] | Population of death-registration area. | | Deaths from diseases caused by pregnancy and confinement. | | | | | |
|---|---|---|---|---|---|---|---|---|
| | | | Number. | | | Rate per 100,000 population. | | |
| | Total. | Per cent of population of United States. | Total. | Puerperal septicemia. | All other. | Total. | Puerperal septicemia. | All other. |
| 1890[2] | 19,659,440 | 31.4 | 3,011 | [3] 1,383 | 1,628 | 15.3 | [3] 7.0 | 8.3 |
| 1900[2] | 28,807,269 | 37.9 | 3,772 | [3] 1,619 | 2,153 | 13.1 | [3] 5.6 | 7.5 |
| 1900 | 30,765,618 | 40.5 | 4,106 | 1,769 | 2,337 | 13.3 | 5.7 | 7.6 |
| 1901 | 31,370,952 | 40.3 | 4,294 | 1,882 | 2,412 | 13.7 | 6.0 | 7.7 |
| 1902 | 32,029,815 | 40.4 | 4,164 | 1,813 | 2,351 | 13.0 | 5.7 | 7.3 |
| 1903 | 32,701,083 | 40.4 | 4,569 | 1,992 | 2,577 | 14.0 | 6.1 | 7.9 |
| 1904 | 33,345,163 | 40.4 | 5,109 | 2,291 | 2,818 | 15.3 | 6.9 | 8.5 |
| 1905 | 34,052,201 | 40.4 | 5,077 | 2,309 | 2,768 | 14.9 | 6.8 | 8.1 |
| 1906 | 41,983,419 | 48.9 | 6,341 | 2,622 | 3,719 | 15.1 | 6.2 | 8.9 |
| 1907 | 43,016,990 | 49.2 | 6,719 | 2,908 | 3,811 | 15.6 | 6.8 | 8.9 |
| 1908 | 46,789,913 | 52.5 | 7,344 | 3,271 | 4,073 | 15.7 | 7.0 | 8.7 |
| 1909 | 50,870,518 | 56.1 | 7,791 | 3,427 | 4,364 | 15.3 | 6.7 | 8.6 |
| 1910 | 53,843,896 | 58.3 | 8,455 | 3,892 | 4,563 | 15.7 | 7.2 | 8.5 |
| 1911 | 59,275,977 | 63.1 | 9,456 | 4,376 | 5,080 | 16.0 | 7.4 | 8.6 |
| 1912 | 60,427,247 | 63.2 | 9,035 | 3,905 | 5,130 | 15.0 | 6.5 | 8.5 |
| 1913 | 63,298,718 | 65.1 | 10,010 | 4,542 | 5,468 | 15.8 | 7.2 | 8.6 |
| Annual average: | | | | | | | | |
| 1901 to 1905 | 32,699,843 | .......... | 4,643 | 2,057 | 2,586 | 14.2 | 6.3 | 7.9 |
| 1906 to 1910 | 47,300,947 | .......... | 7,330 | 3,224 | 4,106 | 15.5 | 6.8 | 8.7 |

[1] Calendar year, unless otherwise specified.
[2] Census year ending May 31.
[3] Figures for puerperal septicemia for the census years 1890 and 1900 not comparable with those for later years. See p. 41.

TABLE II.—*Deaths and death rates per 100,000 population in the 8 States within the death-registration area in 1890*[1] *from diseases caused by pregnancy and confinement, 1890 and 1900 to 1913.*

| Year.[2] | Deaths from diseases caused by pregnancy and confinement. | | | | | |
|---|---|---|---|---|---|---|
| | Number. | | | Rate per 100,000 population. | | |
| | Total. | Puerperal septicemia. | All other. | Total. | Puerperal septicemia. | All other. |
| 1890[3] | 1,655 | [4] 698 | 957 | 14.1 | [4] 6.0 | 8.2 |
| 1900[3] | 1,806 | [4] 791 | 1,015 | 12.6 | [4] 5.5 | 7.1 |
| 1900 | 1,905 | 798 | 1,107 | 13.3 | 3.0 | 7.7 |
| 1901 | 1,903 | 747 | 1,156 | 13.0 | 5.1 | 7.9 |
| 1902 | 1,842 | 762 | 1,080 | 12.4 | 5.1 | 7.2 |
| 1903 | 1,998 | 801 | 1,197 | 13.1 | 5.3 | 7.9 |
| 1904 | 2,305 | 996 | 1,309 | 14.9 | 6.4 | 8.4 |
| 1905 | 2,434 | 1,033 | 1,401 | 15.4 | 6.5 | 8.9 |
| 1906 | 2,434 | 989 | 1,445 | 15.0 | 6.1 | 8.9 |
| 1907 | 2,595 | 1,086 | 1,509 | 15.6 | 6.5 | 9.1 |
| 1908 | 2,450 | 1,050 | 1,400 | 14.4 | 6.2 | 8.2 |
| 1909 | 2,537 | 1,034 | 1,503 | 14.5 | 5.9 | 8.6 |
| 1910 | 2,608 | 1,145 | 1,463 | 14.6 | 6.4 | 8.2 |
| 1911 | 2,722 | 1,179 | 1,543 | 14.9 | 6.4 | 8.4 |
| 1912 | 2,574 | 1,049 | 1,525 | 13.9 | 5.6 | 8.2 |
| 1913 | 2,707 | 1,140 | 1,567 | 14.3 | 6.0 | 8.3 |

[1] Excluding Delaware.
[2] Calendar year, unless otherwise specified.
[3] Census year ending May 31.
[4] Figures for puerperal septicemia for the census years 1890 and 1900 not comparable with those for later years. See p. 41.

TABLE III.—*Deaths and death rates per 100,000 population in the 11 States within the death-registration area in 1900 from diseases caused by pregnancy and confinement, 1900 to 1913.*

| Year.[1] | Deaths from diseases caused by pregnancy and confinement. | | | | | |
|---|---|---|---|---|---|---|
| | Number. | | | Rate per 100,000 population. | | |
| | Total. | Puerperal septicemia. | All other. | Total. | Puerperal septicemia. | All other. |
| 1900[2] | 2,568 | [3] 1,150 | 1,418 | 12.9 | [3] 5.8 | 7.1 |
| 1900 | 2,682 | 1,155 | 1.527 | 13.4 | 5.8 | 7.6 |
| 1901 | 2,704 | 1,124 | 1,580 | 13.3 | 5.5 | 7.8 |
| 1902 | 2,626 | 1,092 | 1,534 | 12.7 | 5.3 | 7.4 |
| 1903 | 2,778 | 1,153 | 1,625 | 13.2 | 5.5 | 7.7 |
| 1904 | 3,216 | 1,403 | 1,813 | 15.1 | 6.6 | 8.5 |
| 1905 | 3,219 | 1,401 | 1,818 | 14.8 | 6.4 | 8.4 |
| 1906 | 3,229 | 1,302 | 1,927 | 14.5 | 5.9 | 8.7 |
| 1907 | 3.448 | 1,476 | 1,972 | 15.2 | 6.5 | 8.7 |
| 1908 | 3,343 | 1,431 | 1,912 | 14.4 | 6.2 | 8.2 |
| 1909 | 3,422 | 1,453 | 1,969 | 14.5 | 6.1 | 8.3 |
| 1910 | 3,641 | 1,624 | 2,017 | 15.1 | 6.7 | 8.4 |
| 1911 | 3,806 | 1,748 | 2,058 | 15.5 | 7.1 | 8.4 |
| 1912 | 3.527 | 1,488 | 2,039 | 14.1 | 6.0 | 8.2 |
| 1913 | 3,789 | 1,661 | 2,128 | 14.9 | 6.5 | 8.4 |

[1] Calendar year, unless otherwise specified.
[2] Census year ending May 31.
[3] Figures for puerperal septicemia for the census year 1900 not comparable with those for later years. See p. 41.

TABLE IV.—*Death rates per 100,000 female population in the 11 States within the death-registration area in 1900 from diseases caused by pregnancy and confinement, 1900 to 1910.*

| Year. | Death rate per 100,000 female population from diseases caused by pregnancy and confinement. | | | Year. | Death rate per 100,000 female population from diseases caused by pregnancy and confinement. | | |
|---|---|---|---|---|---|---|---|
| | Total. | Puerperal septicemia. | All other. | | Total. | Puerperal septicemia. | All other. |
| 1900 | 26.9 | 11.6 | 15.3 | 1906 | 29.2 | 11.8 | 17.5 |
| 1901 | 26.7 | 11.1 | 15.6 | 1907 | 30.6 | 13.1 | 17.5 |
| 1902 | 25.5 | 10.6 | 14.9 | 1908 | 29.1 | 12.4 | 16.6 |
| 1903 | 26.6 | 11.0 | 15.5 | 1909 | 29.2 | 12.4 | 16.8 |
| 1904 | 30.3 | 13.2 | 17.1 | 1910 | 30.4 | 13.6 | 16.9 |
| 1905 | 29.8 | 13.0 | 16.8 | | | | |

TABLE V.—*Number of deaths of women from 15 to 44 years of age in the death-registration area from each cause and class of causes included in the abridged International List of Causes of Death (revision of 1909),*[1] *1913.*

[Computed from figures in Mortality Statistics, 1913, pp. 338 to 349, in which causes of death are given according to the detailed International List of Causes of Death.]

| Abridged International List No. | Cause of death. | Number of deaths. |
|---|---|---|
| 13, 14, 15 | Tuberculosis of the lungs, tuberculous meningitis, other forms of tuberculosis | 26,265 |
| 31, 32 | Puerperal septicemia (puerperal fever, peritonitis) and other puerperal accidents of pregnancy and labor | 9,876 |
| 19 | Organic diseases of the heart | 6,386 |
| 29 | Acute nephritis and Bright's disease | 5,741 |
| 16 | Cancer and other malignant tumors | 5,065 |
| 22 | Pneumonia | 4,167 |
| 35 | Violent deaths (suicide excepted) | 3,262 |
| 1 | Typhoid fever | 2,706 |
| 30 | Noncancerous tumors and other diseases of the female genital organs | 2,669 |
| 26 | Appendicitis and typhlitis | 1,620 |
| 36 | Suicide | 1,562 |
| 23 | Other diseases of the respiratory system (tuberculosis excepted) | 1,458 |
| 18 | Cerebral hemorrhage and softening | 1,398 |
| 24 | Diseases of the stomach (cancer excepted) | 940 |
| 27 | Hernia, intestinal obstruction | 854 |
| 28 | Cirrhosis of the liver | 598 |
| 9 | Influenza | 489 |
| 17 | Simple meningitis | 484 |
| 8 | Diphtheria and croup | 330 |
| 12 | Other epidemic diseases | 312 |
| 6 | Scarlet fever | 307 |
| 5 | Measles | 304 |
| 3 | Malaria | 250 |
| 21 | Chronic bronchitis | 184 |
| 20 | Acute bronchitis | 90 |
| 33 | Congenital debility and malformations | 24 |
| 11 | Cholera nostras | 18 |
| 4 | Smallpox | 16 |
| 7 | Whooping cough | 9 |
| 2 | Typhus fever | 2 |
| 10 | Asiatic cholera | ........ |
| 37 | Other diseases | 11,688 |
| 38 | Unknown or ill-defined diseases | 458 |

[1] Except No. 25, diarrhea and enteritis (under 2 years), and No. 34, senility.

TABLE VI.—*Population, live births, deaths, and death rates per 100,000 population and per 1,000 live births from diseases caused by pregnancy and confinement, by States and principal cities in the provisional birth-registration area,*[1] *1910.*

| State and city. | Population July 1, 1910 (estimated). | Live births, 1910. | Deaths from diseases caused by pregnancy and confinement. | | | | | | | | |
|---|---|---|---|---|---|---|---|---|---|---|---|
| | | | Total. | | | Puerperal septicemia. | | | All other. | | |
| | | | Number. | Rate. | | Number. | Rate. | | Number. | Rate. | |
| | | | | Per 100,000 population. | Per 1,000 live births. | | Per 100,000 population. | Per 1,000 live births. | | Per 100,000 population. | Per 1,000 live births. |
| Provisional birth-registration area | 22,222,401 | 502,390 | 3,652 | 16.4 | 6.5 | 1,612 | 7.3 | 2.9 | 2,040 | 9.2 | 3.6 |
| Connecticut | 1,119,109 | 27,291 | 148 | 13.2 | 5.4 | 65 | 5.8 | 2.4 | 83 | 7.4 | 3.0 |
| Maine | 713,382 | 15,578 | 110 | 14.8 | 7.1 | 46 | 6.2 | 3.0 | 64 | 8.6 | 4.1 |
| Massachusetts | 3,381,657 | 86,766 | 412 | 12.2 | 4.7 | 166 | 4.9 | 1.9 | 216 | 7.3 | 2.8 |
| Michigan | 2,820,108 | 63,566 | 474 | 16.8 | 7.5 | 196 | 7.0 | 3.1 | 278 | 9.9 | 4.4 |
| New Hampshire | 430,972 | 9,385 | 52 | 12.1 | 5.5 | 18 | 4.2 | 1.9 | 34 | 7.9 | 3.6 |
| Pennsylvania | 7,693,866 | 202,613 | 1,441 | 18.7 | 7.1 | 656 | 8.5 | 3.2 | 785 | 10.2 | 3.9 |
| Rhode Island | 545,282 | 13,439 | 82 | 15.0 | 6.1 | 27 | 5.0 | 2.0 | 55 | 10.1 | 4.1 |
| Vermont | 356,216 | 7,351 | 61 | 17.1 | 8.3 | 22 | 6.2 | 3.0 | 39 | 10.9 | 5.3 |
| New York City | 4,799,639 | 129,355 | 802 | 16.7 | 6.2 | 376 | 7.8 | 2.9 | 426 | 8.9 | 3.3 |
| Washington, D. C | 332,173 | 7,016 | 70 | 21.1 | 10.0 | 40 | 12.0 | 5.7 | 30 | 9.0 | 4.3 |
| Principal cities in foregoing States | 4,182,418 | 109,755 | 744 | 17.8 | 6.8 | 357 | 8.5 | 3.3 | 387 | 9.3 | 3.5 |
| Bridgeport | 102,709 | 2,976 | 15 | 14.6 | 5.0 | 6 | 5.8 | 2.0 | 9 | 8.8 | 3.0 |
| New Haven | 134,145 | 3,772 | 19 | 14.2 | 5.0 | 10 | 7.5 | 2.7 | 9 | 6.7 | 2.4 |
| Boston | 673,744 | 17,758 | 94 | 14.0 | 5.3 | 38 | 5.6 | 2.1 | 56 | 8.3 | 3.2 |
| Fall River | 119,864 | 4,591 | 15 | 12.5 | 3.3 | 6 | 5.0 | 1.3 | 9 | 7.5 | 2.0 |
| Lowell | 106,761 | 2,631 | 8 | 7.5 | 3.0 | 1 | .9 | .4 | 7 | 6.6 | 2.7 |
| Worcester | 146,736 | 3,921 | 20 | 13.6 | 5.1 | 12 | 8.2 | 3.1 | 8 | 5.5 | 2.0 |
| Detroit | 470,118 | 11,960 | 97 | 20.6 | 8.1 | 48 | 10.2 | 4.0 | 49 | 10.4 | 4.1 |
| Grand Rapids | 113,168 | 2,693 | 20 | 17.7 | 7.4 | 5 | 4.4 | 1.9 | 15 | 13.3 | 5.6 |
| Philadelphia | 1,551,395 | 38,667 | 290 | 18.7 | 7.5 | 142 | 9.1 | 3.7 | 148 | 9.5 | 3.8 |
| Pittsburgh | 535,384 | 15,059 | 120 | 22.4 | 8.0 | 71 | 13.3 | 4.7 | 49 | 9.2 | 3.3 |
| Providence | 225,424 | 5,727 | 46 | 20.4 | 8.0 | 18 | 8.0 | 3.1 | 28 | 12.4 | 4.9 |

[1] As established by United States Bureau of the Census. See Mortality Statistics, 1911.

TABLE VII.—*Death rates per 100,000 population in the death-registration area from certain important causes of death, 1890 and 1900 to 1913.*

| Year.[1] | Death rate per 100,000 population from— | | | | | | | | | | |
|---|---|---|---|---|---|---|---|---|---|---|---|
| | Typhoid fever. | Diphtheria and croup. | Measles. | Whooping cough. | Scarlet fever. | Tuberculosis (all forms). | Pneumonia (all forms). | Diarrhea and enteritis (under 2 yrs.). | Diseases caused by pregnancy and confinement. | | |
| | | | | | | | | | Total. | Puerperal septicemia. | All other. |
| 1890 [2] | 46.3 | 97.8 | 13.5 | 15.8 | 13.6 | 252.0 | 186.9 | 139.1 | 15.3 | [3] 7.0 | 8.3 |
| 1900 [2] | 33.8 | 45.2 | 13.2 | 12.7 | 11.6 | 190.9 | 192.0 | 97.5 | 13.1 | [3] 5.6 | 7.5 |
| 1900 | 35.9 | 43.3 | 12.5 | 12.1 | 10.2 | 201.9 | 180.5 | 108.8 | 13.3 | 5.7 | 7.6 |
| 1901 | 32.3 | 34.0 | 7.3 | 9.7 | 13.1 | 196.9 | 161.4 | 90.9 | 13.7 | 6.0 | 7.7 |
| 1902 | 34.3 | 30.8 | 9.5 | 12.0 | 12.6 | 184.5 | 155.7 | 84.0 | 13.0 | 5.7 | 7.3 |
| 1903 | 34.1 | 31.7 | 9.8 | 15.8 | 12.2 | 188.5 | 155.1 | 81.6 | 14.0 | 6.1 | 7.9 |
| 1904 | 31.7 | 28.3 | 11.0 | 6.5 | 10.8 | 200.7 | 171.4 | 90.9 | 15.3 | 6.9 | 8.5 |
| 1905 | 27.8 | 23.6 | 7.5 | 10.6 | 6.7 | 192.3 | 148.8 | 97.0 | 14.9 | 6.8 | 8.1 |
| 1906 | 31.3 | 25.7 | 12.1 | 15.1 | 7.7 | 180.2 | 145.5 | 101.4 | 15.1 | 6.2 | 8.9 |
| 1907 | 29.5 | 23.6 | 10.0 | 11.3 | 10.0 | 178.5 | 156.5 | 96.6 | 15.6 | 6.8 | 8.9 |
| 1908 | 24.3 | 21.5 | 9.9 | 10.6 | 11.9 | 167.6 | 130.9 | 95.2 | 15.7 | 7.0 | 8.7 |
| 1909 | 21.1 | 20.4 | 9.6 | 9.6 | 11.4 | 160.8 | 137.6 | 87.8 | 15.3 | 6.7 | 8.6 |
| 1910 | 23.5 | 21.4 | 12.3 | 11.4 | 11.6 | 160.3 | 147.7 | 100.8 | 15.7 | 7.2 | 8.5 |
| 1911 | 21.0 | 18.9 | 10.0 | 11.3 | 8.8 | 158.9 | 133.7 | 77.4 | 16.0 | 7.4 | 8.6 |
| 1912 | 16.5 | 18.2 | 7.0 | 9.3 | 6.7 | 149.5 | 132.3 | 70.3 | 15.0 | 6.5 | 8.5 |
| 1913 | 17.9 | 18.8 | 12.8 | 10.0 | 8.7 | 147.6 | 132.4 | 75.2 | 15.8 | 7.2 | 8.6 |

[1] Calendar year, unless otherwise specified.
[2] Census year ending May 31.
[3] Figures for puerperal septicemia for the census years 1890 and 1900 not comparable with those for later years. See p. 41.

TABLE VIII.—*Deaths and death rates per 100,000 population in cities of at least 8,000 [1] population and in smaller cities and rural districts in the death-registration States from diseases caused by pregnancy and confinement, 1900 to 1913.*

| Year. | Deaths from diseases caused by pregnancy and confinement. | | | | | | | | | | | |
|---|---|---|---|---|---|---|---|---|---|---|---|---|
| | Number. | | | | | | Rate per 100,000 population. | | | | | |
| | Total. | | Puerperal septicemia. | | All other. | | Total. | | Puerperal septicemia. | | All other. | |
| | Cities of at least 8,000 population. | Cities of less than 8,000 population and rural districts. | Cities of at least 8,000 population. | Cities of less than 8,000 population and rural districts. | Cities of at least 8,000 population. | Cities of less than 8,000 population and rural districts. | Cities of at least 8,000 population. | Cities of less than 8,000 population and rural districts. | Cities of at least 8,000 population. | Cities of less than 8,000 population and rural districts. | Cities of at least 8,000 population. | Cities of less than 8,000 population and rural districts. |
| 1900 | 1,595 | 1,087 | 713 | 442 | 882 | 645 | 14.9 | 11.7 | 6.7 | 4.8 | 8.3 | 6.9 |
| 1901 | 1,607 | 1,097 | 661 | 463 | 946 | 634 | 14.4 | 12.0 | 5.9 | 5.1 | 8.5 | 7.0 |
| 1902 | 1,575 | 1,051 | 710 | 382 | 865 | 669 | 13.7 | 11.5 | 6.2 | 4.2 | 7.5 | 7.3 |
| 1903 | 1,659 | 1,119 | 715 | 438 | 944 | 681 | 14.1 | 12.1 | 6.1 | 4.7 | 8.0 | 7.4 |
| 1904 | 1,968 | 1,248 | 892 | 511 | 1,076 | 737 | 16.4 | 13.4 | 7.4 | 5.5 | 8.9 | 7.9 |
| 1905 | 2,069 | 1,150 | 937 | 464 | 1,132 | 686 | 16.8 | 12.3 | 7.6 | 5.0 | 9.1 | 7.3 |
| 1906 | 3,060 | 2,063 | 1,308 | 761 | 1,752 | 1,302 | 16.8 | 13.2 | 7.2 | 4.9 | 9.6 | 8.3 |
| 1907 | 3,245 | 2,145 | 1,427 | 821 | 1,818 | 1,324 | 17.3 | 13.5 | 7.6 | 5.2 | 9.7 | 8.3 |
| 1908 | 3,384 | 2,654 | 1,532 | 1,085 | 1,852 | 1,569 | 16.6 | 14.5 | 7.5 | 5.9 | 9.1 | 8.6 |
| 1909 | 3,734 | 2,936 | 1,678 | 1,212 | 2,056 | 1,724 | 16.2 | 13.8 | 7.3 | 5.7 | 8.9 | 8.1 |
| 1910 | 4,271 | 3,123 | 2,029 | 1,305 | 2,242 | 1,818 | 17.0 | 13.8 | 8.1 | 5.8 | 8.9 | 8.0 |
| 1911 | 4,543 | 3,926 | 2,202 | 1,678 | 2,341 | 2,248 | 16.5 | 14.6 | 8.0 | 6.2 | 8.5 | 8.4 |
| 1912 | 4,463 | 3,551 | 1,997 | 1,417 | 2,466 | 2,134 | 15.9 | 13.1 | 7.1 | 5.2 | 8.8 | 7.9 |
| 1913 | 5,031 | 4,013 | 2,353 | 1,717 | 2,678 | 2,296 | 17.2 | 13.8 | 8.0 | 5.9 | 9.2 | 7.9 |

[1] For the years 1900 to 1909, inclusive, basis of division was 8,000 according to the census of 1900; for the years 1910 to 1913, inclusive, basis of division was 10,000 according to the census of 1910.

TABLE IX.—*Death rates per 100,000 population in cities that had at least 200,000 population in 1900, and were within the death-registration States of 1900, from diseases caused by pregnancy and confinement, 1900 to 1913.*

| Year. | Boston. | Buffalo. | Detroit. | Jersey City. | New York. | Newark. | Washington. |
|---|---|---|---|---|---|---|---|
| 1900 | 18.5 | 9.1 | 24.7 | 15.9 | 19.3 | 12.6 | 15.4 |
| 1901 | 13.4 | 15.3 | 19.5 | 16.0 | 17.7 | 14.8 | 23.6 |
| 1902 | 14.7 | 12.5 | 15.7 | 16.4 | 16.4 | 16.8 | 15.2 |
| 1903 | 17.4 | 18.1 | 15.0 | 12.0 | 15.7 | 9.7 | 18.0 |
| 1904 | 15.8 | 16.0 | 16.3 | 17.3 | 19.0 | 14.6 | 17.6 |
| 1905 | 14.1 | 12.9 | 16.7 | 17.6 | 20.3 | 16.3 | 17.7 |
| 1906 | 15.0 | 20.4 | 15.7 | 18.4 | 18.3 | 18.1 | 17.0 |
| 1907 | 15.9 | 19.8 | 17.1 | 11.6 | 18.9 | 16.9 | 16.8 |
| 1908 | 12.1 | 16.1 | 18.5 | 24.2 | 17.1 | 20.0 | 17.7 |
| 1909 | 20.7 | 13.4 | 14.6 | 15.6 | 16.3 | 19.7 | 17.1 |
| 1910 | 14.0 | 12.5 | 20.6 | 17.1 | 16.7 | 18.0 | 21.1 |
| 1911 | 19.4 | 10.2 | 21.6 | 21.8 | 15.8 | 19.8 | 16.9 |
| 1912 | 17.9 | 13.0 | 17.7 | 18.1 | 14.8 | 20.6 | 14.0 |
| 1913 | 20.6 | 13.9 | 26.5 | 18.1 | 14.1 | 23.2 | 18.1 |

TABLE X.—*Death rates per 100,000 population in the 11 States within the death-registration area in 1900 from diseases caused by pregnancy and confinement, 1900 to 1913.*

| Year. | Death rate per 100,000 population from diseases caused by pregnancy and confinement. | | | | | | | | | | | |
|---|---|---|---|---|---|---|---|---|---|---|---|---|
| | Connecticut. | | | District of Columbia. | | | Indiana. | | | Maine. | | |
| | Total. | Puerperal septicemia. | All other. | Total. | Puerperal septicemia. | All other. | Total. | Puerperal septicemia. | All other. | Total. | Puerperal septicemia. | All other. |
| 1900 | 13.0 | 5.7 | 7.3 | 15.4 | 5.4 | 10.0 | 10.4 | 4.8 | 5.6 | 9.4 | 3.0 | 6.3 |
| 1901 | 11.9 | 4.4 | 7.5 | 23.6 | 10.5 | 13.0 | 10.2 | 5.0 | 5.2 | 11.0 | 4.1 | 6.9 |
| 1902 | 13.4 | 5.0 | 8.4 | 15.2 | 5.9 | 9.3 | 9.0 | 3.8 | 5.2 | 15.2 | 6.1 | 9.1 |
| 1903 | 13.2 | 4.4 | 8.7 | 18.0 | 9.2 | 8.8 | 10.5 | 5.4 | 5.1 | 13.1 | 3.9 | 9.2 |
| 1904 | 13.2 | 4.8 | 8.4 | 17.6 | 8.0 | 9.7 | 12.3 | 5.8 | 6.4 | 12.7 | 5.3 | 7.4 |
| 1905 | 15.0 | 5.7 | 9.3 | 17.7 | 6.2 | 11.5 | 12.3 | 6.5 | 5.7 | 11.7 | 5.1 | 6.5 |
| 1906 | 13.6 | 5.4 | 8.2 | 17.0 | 7.7 | 9.3 | 11.2 | 4.8 | 6.3 | 10.1 | 2.3 | 7.7 |
| 1907 | 13.4 | 6.4 | 7.0 | 16.8 | 7.3 | 9.5 | 13.3 | 7.1 | 6.3 | 10.8 | 4.3 | 6.6 |
| 1908 | 11.7 | 4.3 | 7.4 | 17.7 | 4.7 | 13.1 | 13.2 | 6.1 | 7.0 | 11.2 | 4.1 | 7.1 |
| 1909 | 13.1 | 4.1 | 9.0 | 17.1 | 7.6 | 9.5 | 14.5 | 7.2 | 7.3 | 10.6 | 4.6 | 6.0 |
| 1910 | 13.2 | 5.8 | 7.4 | 21.1 | 12.0 | 9.0 | 16.6 | 8.8 | 7.8 | 14.8 | 6.2 | 8.6 |
| 1911 | 11.3 | 5.0 | 6.3 | 16.9 | 7.4 | 9.5 | 17.7 | 10.9 | 6.8 | 13.4 | 3.9 | 9.5 |
| 1912 | 15.2 | 5.3 | 9.9 | 14.0 | 4.4 | 9.6 | 16.5 | 8.7 | 7.8 | 10.1 | 2.8 | 7.3 |
| 1913 | 12.1 | 4.7 | 7.4 | 18.1 | 6.9 | 11.2 | 15.1 | 8.0 | 7.2 | 11.3 | 3.7 | 7.7 |
| Annual average, 1900 to 1913 | 13.1 | 5.1 | 8.0 | 17.6 | 7.4 | 10.2 | 13.1 | 6.7 | 6.4 | 11.8 | 4.2 | 7.6 |

TABLE X.—*Death rates per 100,000 population in the 11 States within the death-registration area in 1900 from diseases caused by pregnancy and confinement, 1900 to 1913*—Continued.

| Year. | Death rate per 100,000 population from diseases caused by pregnancy and confinement—Continued. | | | | | | | | | | | |
|---|---|---|---|---|---|---|---|---|---|---|---|---|
| | Massachusetts. | | | Michigan. | | | New Hampshire. | | | New Jersey. | | |
| | Total. | Puerperal septicemia. | All other. | Total. | Puerperal septicemia. | All other. | Total. | Puerperal septicemia. | All other. | Total. | Puerperal septicemia. | All other. |
| 1900 | 11.1 | 3.7 | 7.4 | 18.5 | 8.8 | 9.7 | 8.0 | 2.4 | 5.6 | 12.8 | 4.9 | 7.9 |
| 1901 | 9.4 | 3.2 | 6.2 | 19.0 | 9.1 | 9.9 | 7.0 | 3.1 | 3.9 | 9.9 | 3.8 | 6.1 |
| 1902 | 9.5 | 3.1 | 6.4 | 18.1 | 7.7 | 10.4 | 6.7 | 2.6 | 4.1 | 11.0 | 4.8 | 6.2 |
| 1903 | 11.7 | 4.0 | 7.7 | 16.7 | 7.4 | 9.3 | 10.5 | 3.8 | 6.7 | 11.5 | 4.6 | 6.9 |
| 1904 | 13.3 | 4.5 | 8.8 | 19.8 | 8.6 | 11.2 | 9.1 | 3.3 | 5.7 | 12.7 | 6.3 | 6.4 |
| 1905 | 11.9 | 4.0 | 7.9 | 14.8 | 6.2 | 8.6 | 12.6 | 3.3 | 9.3 | 13.3 | 6.2 | 7.0 |
| 1906 | 12.5 | 3.9 | 8.5 | 16.3 | 6.4 | 9.9 | 14.9 | 5.0 | 9.9 | 14.6 | 6.2 | 8.3 |
| 1907 | 12.8 | 4.3 | 8.4 | 15.7 | 6.4 | 9.3 | 10.6 | 3.1 | 7.5 | 13.1 | 5.2 | 7.8 |
| 1908 | 11.0 | 4.0 | 6.9 | 16.9 | 6.9 | 10.0 | 10.1 | 2.3 | 7.7 | 14.5 | 7.1 | 7.5 |
| 1909 | 14.6 | 5.1 | 9.4 | 15.0 | 6.9 | 8.2 | 13.1 | 4.4 | 8.6 | 12.7 | 5.7 | 7.0 |
| 1910 | 12.2 | 4.9 | 7.3 | 16.8 | 7.0 | 9.9 | 12.1 | 4.2 | 7.9 | 15.5 | 7.5 | 8.1 |
| 1911 | 14.8 | 6.1 | 8.7 | 17.5 | 8.5 | 9.0 | 13.6 | 4.2 | 9.5 | 16.1 | 7.7 | 8.4 |
| 1912 | 13.1 | 5.3 | 7.8 | 14.7 | 6.2 | 8.5 | 15.2 | 5.1 | 10.1 | 15.2 | 6.1 | 9.2 |
| 1913 | 14.4 | 5.3 | 9.1 | 19.7 | 9.3 | 10.4 | 13.5 | 4.1 | 9.4 | 16.2 | 7.8 | 8.4 |
| Annual average, 1900 to 1913 | 12.4 | 4.4 | 7.9 | 17.1 | 7.5 | 9.6 | 11.2 | 3.7 | 7.6 | 13.7 | 6.1 | 7.6 |

| Year. | New York. | | | Rhode Island. | | | Vermont. | | |
|---|---|---|---|---|---|---|---|---|---|
| | Total. | Puerperal septicemia. | All other. | Total. | Puerperal septicemia. | All other. | Total. | Puerperal septicemia. | All other. |
| 1900 | 14.1 | 6.5 | 7.6 | 20.8 | 8.4 | 12.4 | 13.4 | 4.9 | 8.4 |
| 1901 | 15.1 | 6.2 | 8.9 | 18.9 | 6.8 | 12.1 | 9.6 | 2.9 | 6.7 |
| 1902 | 13.7 | 6.0 | 7.7 | 15.8 | 7.1 | 8.7 | 11.3 | 3.8 | 7.5 |
| 1903 | 14.0 | 6.0 | 8.0 | 13.5 | 5.9 | 7.6 | 14.7 | 3.5 | 11.2 |
| 1904 | 16.0 | 7.3 | 8.7 | 20.6 | 10.6 | 10.0 | 16.9 | 5.4 | 11.5 |
| 1905 | 16.9 | 7.8 | 9.1 | 20.8 | 8.9 | 11.8 | 18.9 | 4.3 | 14.6 |
| 1906 | 15.9 | 7.0 | 9.0 | 17.8 | 6.9 | 10.9 | 15.9 | 4.0 | 12.0 |
| 1907 | 17.1 | 7.7 | 9.4 | 19.5 | 8.1 | 11.4 | 27.0 | 7.1 | 19.9 |
| 1908 | 15.7 | 7.2 | 8.5 | 16.7 | 6.0 | 10.8 | 18.9 | 6.2 | 12.7 |
| 1909 | 14.9 | 6.3 | 8.7 | 15.4 | 7.3 | 8.1 | 18.9 | 9.0 | 9.9 |
| 1910 | 15.1 | 6.7 | 8.4 | 15.0 | 5.0 | 10.1 | 17.1 | 6.2 | 10.9 |
| 1911 | 15.0 | 6.6 | 8.4 | 15.9 | 5.2 | 10.8 | 13.7 | 4.5 | 9.2 |
| 1912 | 13.5 | 6.0 | 7.6 | 14.1 | 5.1 | 9.0 | 13.7 | 2.2 | 11.4 |
| 1913 | 14.0 | 6.2 | 7.8 | 12.6 | 4.0 | 8.6 | 15.3 | 4.7 | 10.6 |
| Annual average, 1900 to 1913 | 15.1 | 6.7 | 8.4 | 16.8 | 6.7 | 10.1 | 16.1 | 4.9 | 11.2 |

TABLE XI.—*Deaths and death rates per 100,000 population in the death-registration area from diseases caused by pregnancy and confinement, by color of decedent, 1910 to 1913.*

| Year. | Deaths from diseases caused by pregnancy and confinement. | | | | | | | | | | | |
|---|---|---|---|---|---|---|---|---|---|---|---|---|
| | Number. | | | | | | Rate per 100,000 population. | | | | | |
| | Total. | | Puerperal septicemia. | | All other. | | Total. | | Puerperal septicemia. | | All other. | |
| | White. | Colored. | White. | Colored. | White. | Colored. | White. | Colored. | White. | Colored. | White. | Colored. |
| 1910...... | 7,902 | 553 | 3,609 | 283 | 4,293 | 270 | 15.3 | 25.6 | 7.0 | 13.1 | 8.3 | 12.5 |
| 1911...... | 8,783 | 673 | 4,038 | 338 | 4,745 | 335 | 15.5 | 26.8 | 7.1 | 13.5 | 8.4 | 13.3 |
| 1912...... | 8,365 | 670 | 3,580 | 325 | 4,785 | 345 | 14.5 | 26.0 | 6.2 | 12.6 | 8.3 | 13.4 |
| 1913...... | 9,167 | 843 | 4,170 | 372 | 4,997 | 471 | 15.2 | 26.1 | 6.9 | 11.5 | 8.3 | 14.6 |

TABLE XII.—*Average death rates per 100,000 population in certain countries from diseases caused by pregnancy and confinement, 1900 to 1910.*

| Country. | Death rate per 100,000 population from diseases caused by pregnancy and confinement. | | | Country. | Death rate per 100,000 population from diseases caused by pregnancy and confinement. | | |
|---|---|---|---|---|---|---|---|
| | Total. | Puerperal septicemia. | All other. | | Total. | Puerperal septicemia. | All other. |
| Sweden [1] | 6.0 | 2.4 | 3.5 | Japan [1] | 13.3 | 4.5 | 8.8 |
| Norway | 8.1 | 4.1 | 3.9 | Australia [5] | 14.1 | 4.7 | 9.4 |
| Italy | 8.9 | 3.3 | 5.7 | Belgium [3] | 14.8 | 5.8 | 9.0 |
| France [2] | 10.3 | 4.8 | 5.5 | Scotland [1] | 14.8 | 5.5 | 9.4 |
| Prussia [3] | 10.4 | 4.7 | 5.8 | United States [6] | 14.9 | 6.5 | 8.3 |
| England and Wales | 11.1 | 4.7 | 6.5 | Switzerland | 15.2 | 6.4 | 8.8 |
| New Zealand | 12.4 | 3.1 | 9.3 | Spain [1] | 19.6 | 12.3 | 7.3 |
| Ireland [4] | 12.9 | 4.5 | 8.4 | Austria | (7) | 6.6 | (7) |
| Hungary | 13.3 | 3.6 | 9.8 | | | | |

[1] Rates based on figures for 1901 to 1910.
[2] Rates based on figures for 1906 to 1910.
[3] Rates based on figures for 1903 to 1910.
[4] Rates based on figures for 1902 to 1910.
[5] Rates based on figures for 1907 to 1910.
[6] Rates based on figures for death-registration area which increased from year to year; in 1900 it comprised 40.5 per cent of the total population of the United States and in 1910, 58.3 per cent.
[7] Figures not available.

TABLE XIII.—*Average death rates per 1,000 live births in certain foreign countries from diseases caused by pregnancy and confinement, 1900 to 1910.*

| Country. | Death rate per 1,000 live births from diseases caused by pregnancy and confinement. | | | Country. | Death rate per 1,000 live births from diseases caused by pregnancy and confinement. | | |
|---|---|---|---|---|---|---|---|
| | Total. | Puerperal septicemia. | All other. | | Total. | Puerperal septicemia. | All other. |
| Sweden [1] | 2.3 | 0.9 | 1.4 | France [3] | 5.2 | 2.4 | 2.8 |
| Italy | 2.7 | 1.0 | 1.7 | Scotland [1] | 5.2 | 1.9 | 3.3 |
| Norway | 2.9 | 1.5 | 1.4 | Australia [4] | 5.3 | 1.8 | 3.5 |
| Prussia [2] | 3.2 | 1.4 | 1.8 | Ireland [5] | 5.5 | 1.9 | 3.6 |
| Hungary | 3.6 | 1.0 | 2.6 | Switzerland | 5.6 | 2.4 | 3.3 |
| England and Wales | 4.1 | 1.7 | 2.4 | Spain [1] | 5.7 | 3.6 | 2.1 |
| Japan [1] | 4.1 | 1.4 | 2.7 | Belgium [2] | 5.8 | 2.3 | 3.5 |
| New Zealand | 4.6 | 1.2 | 3.5 | Austria | (6) | 1.9 | (6) |

[1] Rates based on figures for 1901 to 1910.
[2] Rates based on figures for 1903 to 1910.
[3] Rates based on figures for 1906 to 1910.
[4] Rates based on figures for 1907 to 1910.
[5] Rates based on figures for 1902 to 1910.
[6] Figures not available.

TABLE XIV.—*Deaths in certain countries from diseases caused by pregnancy and confinement and number and per cent of such deaths from puerperal septicemia, 1900 to 1910.*

| Country. | Deaths from diseases caused by pregnancy and confinement. | | | Country. | Deaths from diseases caused by pregnancy and confinement. | | |
|---|---|---|---|---|---|---|---|
| | Total. | Puerperal septicemia. | | | Total. | Puerperal septicemia. | |
| | | Number. | Per cent. | | | Number. | Per cent. |
| Sweden[1] | 3,179 | 1,294 | 40.7 | Hungary | 29,273 | 7,824 | 26.7 |
| Norway | 2,032 | 1,041 | 51.2 | Japan[1] | 63,908 | 21,494 | 33.6 |
| Italy | 32,651 | 11,901 | 36.4 | Australia[5] | 2,388 | 800 | 33.5 |
| France[2] | 20,217 | 9,424 | 46.6 | Belgium[3] | 8,588 | 3,392 | 39.5 |
| Prussia[3] | 31,680 | 14,151 | 44.7 | Scotland[1] | 6,839 | 2,522 | 36.9 |
| England and Wales | 41,691 | 17,433 | 41.8 | United States[6] | 63,969 | 28,176 | 44.0 |
| New Zealand | 1,190 | 300 | 25.2 | Switzerland | 5,897 | 2,485 | 42.1 |
| Ireland[4] | 5,109 | 1,792 | 35.1 | Spain[1] | 37,504 | 23,557 | 62.8 |

[1] Figures for 1901 to 1910.
[2] Figures for 1906 to 1910.
[3] Figures for 1903 to 1910.
[4] Figures for 1902 to 1910.
[5] Figures for 1907 to 1910.
[6] Figures for death-registration area which increased from year to year; in 1900 it comprised 40.5 per cent of the total population of the United States and in 1910, 58.3 per cent.

## COMMENT ON SOURCES OF STATISTICS FOR FOREIGN COUNTRIES.

The following paragraphs present, by countries, the sources of the figures subsequent to 1910 in Table XV for foreign countries and also notes on certain of these figures which call for comment or explanation. Unless otherwise specified the figures for all countries for the years 1900 to 1910, inclusive, are taken from the Statistique Internationale du Mouvement de la Population d'après les Registres de l'Etat Civil, of the Bureau de la statistique générale de la France. The figures for 1900 come from the volume published in 1907; those for 1901 to 1910 from that published in 1913.

These foreign sources were used only for the figures in columns 1, 3, 4, 9, and 13, from which the figures in columns 2, 5, 6, 7, 8, 10, 11, 12, 14, 15, and 16 were computed. Blank spaces indicate that statistics were not available. Similarly, where a table begins with data for a year subsequent to 1900, it indicates that the figures for the earlier years were not available, unless otherwise noted.

*Australia* (p. 60).—Bureau of census and statistics. Population and vital statistics. Bulletins 29 and 30. 1911–1912.

*Austria* (p. 60).—Statistisches Centralcommission. Österreichisches statistisches Handbuch für die im Reichsrathe vertretenen Königreiche und Länder. Nebst einem Anhange für die gemeinsamen Angelegenheiten der österreichischungarischen Monarchie. Hrsg. von der statistischen Centralcommission. XXXI Jahrgang. 1911.

The statistics for Austria give the deaths from puerperal septicemia only. The figures for deaths from other diseases of pregnancy and confinement were not available.

The population for 1911 could not be secured from official publications, and was therefore estimated. In making this estimate, one-tenth of the increase from 1900 to 1910 was added to the figure for 1910.

*Belgium* (p. 60).—Ministère de l'intérieur et de l'instruction publique. Annuaire statistique de la Belgique. 1912–13.

The population is that estimated as of December 31 of each year.

Belgium classifies stillbirths as "mort-nés et autres enfants présentés sans vie."

*England and Wales* (p. 61).—74th–77th annual reports of the registrar general of births, deaths, and marriages in England and Wales, 1911 to 1914.

Several points should be noted in the figures for England and Wales.

I. The registrar general's reports, prior to 1911, grouped deaths from diseases of pregnancy and confinement into the two large groups "puerperal septic diseases" and "diseases of pregnancy and childbirth (not septic)," and included phlegmasia alba dolens in puerperal septic diseases. For the years 1900 to 1910 the figures used are those given by the Statistique Internationale. The deaths from phlegmasia alba dolens have apparently been subtracted from puerperal septic diseases and have been added to the other group, thus making the classification conform more nearly to the international nomenclature. Therefore, while the figures for "deaths from all diseases caused by pregnancy and confinement" will agree with the official English figures, those for the two other groups, prior to 1911, will not.

II. As the registrar general's report for 1914 gives a table of deaths for the years 1900 to 1914 according to the detailed list of causes of death in use prior to 1911, this table has been used as the source for the figures for England and Wales after 1910, so that the statistics after 1910 can be compared with those of earlier years.

The number of deaths from puerperal septicemia for the years after 1910 is slightly lower when the deaths are classified according to the International Classification than when they are classified according to the older method, as given in table for England and Wales. The deaths from other diseases of pregnancy and confinement are, of course, correspondingly higher. This difference can be seen from the following:

*Number of deaths from puerperal septicemia.*

| Year. | According to the International Classification. | According to the classification in use prior to 1911. |
|---|---|---|
| 1911 | 1,262 | 1,267 |
| 1912 | 1,216 | 1,223 |
| 1913 | 1,108 | 1,119 |
| 1914 | 1,365 | 1,372 |

III. The International Classification was not used in England until 1911, and deaths from puerperal nephritis and albuminuria were not distinguished as puerperal until after 1910. For England and Wales, therefore, the figures are presented for 1911 to 1914, inclusive, in two ways: (*a*) According to use in England prior to 1911, excluding deaths from puerperal nephritis and albuminuria; and (*b*) including deaths from puerperal nephritis and albuminuria.

The number of these deaths was as follows:

*Deaths from puerperal nephritis and albuminuria.*

| Year: | |
|---|---|
| 1911 | 177 |
| 1912 | 174 |
| 1913 | 221 |
| 1914 | 198 |

*Hungary* (p. 61).—Statisztikai hivatal. Magyar statisztikai evkönyv. 1911.

The figures given for Hungary include those for Fiume and Croatia-Slavonia.

*Ireland* (p. 62).—51st detailed annual report of the registrar general of marriages, births, and deaths in Ireland in 1914.

I. The registrar general's reports for Ireland, up through 1914, classify deaths from diseases of pregnancy and confinement into two large groups—puerperal septic diseases and diseases of pregnancy and childbirth (not septic), and include phlegmasia alba dolens in puerperal septic diseases. This was the method used in England and Wales prior to 1911. See note on England and Wales.

In the figures for Ireland, given by the Statistique Internationale, apparently no correction has been made as in the case of England and Wales, but in the table here given the figures have been corrected to make them comparable with those for England and Wales and for other countries. To make this correction the deaths from phlegmasia alba dolens were subtracted from deaths from puerperal septic diseases and added to the other group. Thus while the figures for "deaths from all diseases of pregnancy and confinement" will agree with the official Irish figures and with those given in the Statistique Internationale, those for the other two groups will not.

II. The figures for 1900 and for 1901 are not given because in those years the registrar general's reports did not include under puerperal septic diseases either pyemia or septicemia.

*Italy* (p. 62).—Direzione generale della statistica. Statistica delle cause di morte. 1911–1913.

Movimento de la popolazione. 1913.

Only columns 1, 3, and 4 for 1900 to 1910 were taken from the Statistique Internationale. The above original Italian sources were used, as in the Statistique Internationale the deaths from "other diseases of pregnancy and confinement" and the deaths from "noncancerous tumors and other diseases of the female genital organs" were added together, for several years. (The figures here given were probably not available when the Statistique Internationale was published.)

*Japan* (p. 63).—Bureau de la statistique générale. Mouvement de la population de l'empire du Japon for 1911 and 1912.

The population is that estimated as of December 31 of each year.

*New Zealand* (p. 63).—Registrar general's office. Statistics of the Dominion of New Zealand. 1911–1914.

*Norway* (p. 63).—Statistiske centralbureau. Statistisk aarbok for kongeriget norge. 1914.

The population for 1911 and 1912 is that estimated as of December 31.

*Scotland* (p. 64).—57th–60th annual reports of the registrar general for Scotland. 1911–1914.

The registrar general's reports for Scotland prior to 1911, like those of England and Wales and Ireland, included phlegmasia alba dolens under puerperal septic diseases. As in the case of Ireland, the figures given by the Statistique Internationale have apparently not been corrected. However, in the table here given the figures have been corrected by the method described above in the comment on the statistics for Ireland.

*Sweden* (p. 65).—Statistiska centralbyrån. Statistisk årsbok för Sverige. 1915.

The population is that estimated as of December 31 of each year.

*Switzerland* (p. 65).—Statistisches Bureau. Statistisches Jahrbuch der Schweiz. 1914.

TABLE XV.—*Population, births, deaths, and death rates per 100,000 population, per 1,000 births, and per 1,000 live births from diseases caused by pregnancy and confinement in certain foreign countries for specified years.*

| Country and year. | Population July 1 each year (estimated). | Births. | | | Deaths from diseases caused by pregnancy and confinement. | | | | | | | | | | | |
|---|---|---|---|---|---|---|---|---|---|---|---|---|---|---|---|---|
| | | | | | Total. | | | | Puerperal septicemia. | | | | All other. | | | |
| | | | | | | Rate. | | | | Rate. | | | | Rate. | | |
| | | Total. | Live births. | Still-births. | Number. | Per 100,000 population. | Per 1,000 births. | Per 1,000 live births. | Number. | Per 100,000 population. | Per 1,000 births. | Per 1,000 live births. | Number. | Per 100,000 population. | Per 1,000 births. | Per 1,000 live births. |
| | 1 | 2 | 3 | 4 | 5 | 6 | 7 | 8 | 9 | 10 | 11 | 12 | 13 | 14 | 15 | 16 |
| **Australia:** | | | | | | | | | | | | | | | | |
| 1907 | 4,124,000 | ..... | 110,347 | ..... | 614 | 14.9 | ..... | 5.6 | 179 | 4.3 | ..... | 1.6 | 435 | 10.5 | ..... | 3.9 |
| 1908 | 4,194,000 | ..... | 111,515 | ..... | 606 | 14.4 | ..... | 5.4 | 202 | 4.8 | ..... | 1.8 | 404 | 9.6 | ..... | 3.6 |
| 1909 | 4,275,000 | ..... | 114,071 | ..... | 577 | 13.5 | ..... | 5.1 | 201 | 4.7 | ..... | 1.8 | 376 | 8.8 | ..... | 3.3 |
| 1910 | 4,370,000 | ..... | 116,801 | ..... | 591 | 13.5 | ..... | 5.1 | 218 | 5.0 | ..... | 1.9 | 373 | 8.5 | ..... | 3.2 |
| 1911 | 4,490,000 | ..... | 122,193 | ..... | 615 | 13.7 | ..... | 5.0 | 209 | 4.7 | ..... | 1.7 | 406 | 9.0 | ..... | 3.3 |
| 1912 | 4,645,000 | ..... | 133,088 | ..... | 644 | 13.9 | ..... | 4.8 | 231 | 5.0 | ..... | 1.7 | 413 | 8.9 | ..... | 3.1 |
| **Austria:** | | | | | | | | | | | | | | | | |
| 1900 | 25,976,000 | 995,537 | 967,939 | 27,598 | ..... | ..... | ..... | ..... | 1,952 | 7.5 | 2.0 | 2.0 | ..... | ..... | ..... | ..... |
| 1901 | 26,279,000 | 988,985 | 961,501 | 27,484 | ..... | ..... | ..... | ..... | 1,944 | 7.4 | 2.0 | 2.0 | ..... | ..... | ..... | ..... |
| 1902 | 26,535,000 | 1,010,843 | 984,240 | 26,603 | ..... | ..... | ..... | ..... | 1,922 | 7.2 | 1.9 | 2.0 | ..... | ..... | ..... | ..... |
| 1903 | 26,780,000 | 969,960 | 943,053 | 26,007 | ..... | ..... | ..... | ..... | 1,780 | 6.6 | 1.8 | 1.9 | ..... | ..... | ..... | ..... |
| 1904 | 27,021,000 | 987,425 | 961,430 | 25,995 | ..... | ..... | ..... | ..... | 1,911 | 7.1 | 1.9 | 2.0 | ..... | ..... | ..... | ..... |
| 1905 | 27,229,000 | 945,978 | 921,764 | 24,214 | ..... | ..... | ..... | ..... | 1,622 | 6.0 | 1.7 | 1.8 | ..... | ..... | ..... | ..... |
| 1906 | 27,448,000 | 987,166 | 961,258 | 25,908 | ..... | ..... | ..... | ..... | 1,692 | 6.2 | 1.7 | 1.8 | ..... | ..... | ..... | ..... |
| 1907 | 27,706,000 | 966,911 | 942,160 | 24,742 | ..... | ..... | ..... | ..... | 1,609 | 5.8 | 1.7 | 1.7 | ..... | ..... | ..... | ..... |
| 1908 | 27,950,000 | 965,593 | 941,375 | 24,218 | ..... | ..... | ..... | ..... | 1,822 | 6.5 | 1.9 | 1.9 | ..... | ..... | ..... | ..... |
| 1909 | 28,186,000 | 965,096 | 941,239 | 23,857 | ..... | ..... | ..... | ..... | 1,734 | 6.2 | 1.8 | 1.8 | ..... | ..... | ..... | ..... |
| 1910 | 28,427,000 | 946,820 | 923,545 | 23,275 | ..... | ..... | ..... | ..... | 1,770 | 6.2 | 1.9 | 1.9 | ..... | ..... | ..... | ..... |
| 1911 | 28,672,000 | 920,945 | 898,702 | 22,243 | ..... | ..... | ..... | ..... | 1,712 | 6.0 | 1.9 | 1.9 | ..... | ..... | ..... | ..... |
| **Belgium:** | | | | | | | | | | | | | | | | |
| 1900 | 6,694,000 | 202,790 | 193,789 | 9,001 | 1,016 | 15.6 | 5.2 | 5.4 | ..... | ..... | ..... | ..... | ..... | ..... | ..... | ..... |
| 1901 | 6,800,000 | 209,340 | 200,077 | 9,263 | 1,055 | 15.5 | 5.0 | 5.3 | ..... | ..... | ..... | ..... | ..... | ..... | ..... | ..... |
| 1902 | 6,896,000 | 204,846 | 195,871 | 8,975 | 1,080 | 15.7 | 5.3 | 5.5 | ..... | ..... | ..... | ..... | ..... | ..... | ..... | ..... |
| 1903 | 6,985,000 | 200,870 | 192,301 | 8,569 | 1,205 | 17.3 | 6.0 | 6.3 | 432 | 6.2 | 2.2 | 2.2 | 773 | 11.1 | 3.8 | 4.0 |
| 1904 | 7,075,000 | 200,333 | 191,721 | 8,612 | 1,179 | 16.7 | 5.9 | 6.1 | 445 | 6.3 | 2.2 | 2.3 | 734 | 10.4 | 3.7 | 3.8 |

| | | | | | | | | | | | | | | | | |
|---|---|---|---|---|---|---|---|---|---|---|---|---|---|---|---|---|
| 1905 | 7,161,000 | 196,029 | 187,437 | 8,592 | 995 | 13.9 | 5.1 | 5.3 | 389 | 5.4 | 2.0 | 2.1 | 606 | 8.5 | 3.1 | 3.2 |
| 1906 | 7,239,000 | 191,775 | 186,271 | 8,501 | 1,029 | 11.2 | 5.3 | 5.5 | 403 | 5.6 | 2.1 | 2.2 | 626 | 8.6 | 3.2 | 3.4 |
| 1907 | 7,318,000 | 193,419 | 185,138 | 8,311 | 1,053 | 11.4 | 5.4 | 5.7 | 407 | 5.6 | 2.1 | 2.2 | 646 | 8.8 | 3.3 | 3.5 |
| 1908 | 7,386,000 | 192,397 | 183,834 | 8,563 | 1,121 | 15.2 | 5.8 | 6.1 | 466 | 6.3 | 2.4 | 2.5 | 655 | 8.9 | 3.4 | 3.6 |
| 1909 | 7,452,000 | 184,70[illegible] | 176,431 | 8,269 | 1,039 | 13.9 | 5.6 | 5.9 | 439 | 5.9 | 2.4 | 2.5 | 600 | 8.1 | 3.2 | 3.4 |
| 1910 | 7,421,000 | 184,42[illegible] | 176,413 | 8,008 | 967 | 13.0 | 5.2 | 5.5 | 411 | 5.5 | 2.2 | 2.3 | 556 | 7.5 | 3.0 | 3.2 |
| 1911 | 7,490,000 | 179,35[illegible] | 171,802 | 7,557 | 1,024 | 13.7 | 5.7 | 6.0 | 398 | 5.3 | 2.2 | 2.3 | 626 | 8.4 | 3.5 | 3.6 |
| 1912 | 7,571,000 | 178,97[illegible] | 171,187 | 7,789 | 1,122 | 14.8 | 6.3 | 6.6 | 476 | 6.3 | 2.7 | 2.8 | 646 | 8.5 | 3.6 | 3.8 |
| **England and Wales:** | | | | | | | | | | | | | | | | |
| 1900 | 32,249,000 | ... | 927,062 | ... | 4,455 | 13.8 | ... | 4.8 | 1,941 | 6.0 | ... | 2.1 | 2,514 | 7.8 | ... | 2.7 |
| 1901 | 32,612,000 | ... | 929,807 | ... | 4,394 | 13.5 | ... | 4.7 | 2,005 | 6.1 | ... | 2.2 | 2,389 | 7.3 | ... | 2.6 |
| 1902 | 32,951,000 | ... | 940,509 | ... | 4,205 | 12.8 | ... | 4.5 | 1,908 | 5.8 | ... | 2.0 | 2,297 | 7.0 | ... | 2.4 |
| 1903 | 33,293,000 | ... | 948,271 | ... | 3,857 | 11.6 | ... | 4.1 | 1,581 | 4.7 | ... | 1.7 | 2,276 | 6.8 | ... | 2.4 |
| 1904 | 33,639,000 | ... | 945,389 | ... | 3,667 | 10.9 | ... | 3.9 | 1,560 | 4.6 | ... | 1.7 | 2,107 | 6.3 | ... | 2.2 |
| 1905 | 33,989,000 | ... | 929,293 | ... | 3,905 | 11.5 | ... | 4.2 | 1,631 | 4.8 | ... | 1.8 | 2,274 | 6.7 | ... | 2.4 |
| 1906 | 34,342,000 | ... | 935,081 | ... | 3,757 | 10.9 | ... | 4.0 | 1,538 | 4.5 | ... | 1.6 | 2,219 | 6.5 | ... | 2.4 |
| 1907 | 34,699,000 | ... | 918,042 | ... | 3,520 | 10.1 | ... | 3.8 | 1,381 | 4.0 | ... | 1.5 | 2,139 | 6.2 | ... | 2.3 |
| 1908 | 35,059,000 | ... | 940,383 | ... | 3,361 | 9.6 | ... | 3.6 | 1,312 | 3.7 | ... | 1.4 | 2,049 | 5.8 | ... | 2.2 |
| 1909 | 35,424,000 | ... | 914,472 | ... | 3,379 | 9.5 | ... | 3.7 | 1,357 | 3.8 | ... | 1.5 | 2,022 | 5.7 | ... | 2.2 |
| 1910 | 35,792,000 | ... | 896,962 | ... | 3,191 | 8.9 | ... | 3.6 | 1,219 | 3.4 | ... | 1.4 | 1,972 | 5.5 | ... | 2.2 |
| 1911a[1] | 36,190,000 | ... | 881,138 | ... | 3,236 | 8.9 | ... | 3.7 | 1,267 | 3.5 | ... | 1.4 | 1,969 | 5.4 | ... | 2.2 |
| 1911b | ... | ... | ... | ... | 3,413 | 9.4 | ... | 3.9 | ... | ... | ... | ... | 2,146 | 5.9 | ... | 2.4 |
| 1912a | 36,382,000 | ... | 872,737 | ... | 3,299 | 9.1 | ... | 3.8 | 1,223 | 3.4 | ... | 1.4 | 2,076 | 5.7 | ... | 2.4 |
| 1912b | ... | ... | ... | ... | 3,473 | 9.5 | ... | 4.0 | ... | ... | ... | ... | 2,250 | 6.2 | ... | 2.6 |
| 1913a | 36,606,000 | ... | 881,890 | ... | 3,271 | 8.9 | ... | 3.7 | 1,119 | 3.1 | ... | 1.3 | 2,152 | 5.9 | ... | 2.4 |
| 1913b | ... | ... | ... | ... | 3,492 | 9.5 | ... | 4.0 | ... | ... | ... | ... | 2,373 | 6.5 | ... | 2.7 |
| 1914a | 36,961,000 | ... | 879,096 | ... | 3,469 | 9.4 | ... | 3.9 | 1,372 | 3.7 | ... | 1.6 | 2,097 | 5.7 | ... | 2.4 |
| 1914b | ... | ... | ... | ... | 3,667 | 9.9 | ... | 4.2 | ... | ... | ... | ... | 2,285 | 6.2 | ... | 2.6 |
| **France:** | | | | | | | | | | | | | | | | |
| 1906 | 39,282,000 | 84[illegible],173 | 806,847 | 37,326 | 4,067 | 10.4 | 4.8 | 5.0 | 1,873 | 4.8 | 2.2 | 2.3 | 2,194 | 5.6 | 2.6 | 2.7 |
| 1907 | 39,279,000 | 80[illegible],446 | 772,681 | 36,765 | 4,499 | 11.5 | 5.6 | 5.8 | 2,117 | 5.4 | 2.6 | 2.7 | 2,382 | 6.1 | 2.9 | 3.1 |
| 1908 | 39,368,000 | 82[illegible],714 | 792,178 | 37,536 | 3,982 | 10.1 | 4.8 | 5.0 | 1,855 | 4.7 | 2.2 | 2.3 | 2,127 | 5.4 | 2.6 | 2.7 |
| 1909 | 39,421,000 | 8[illegible]5,641 | 769,565 | 36,076 | 4,097 | 10.4 | 5.1 | 5.3 | 1,900 | 4.8 | 2.4 | 2.5 | 2,197 | 5.6 | 2.7 | 2.9 |
| 1910 | 39,528,000 | 8[illegible]0,399 | 774,390 | 36,009 | 3,572 | 9.0 | 4.4 | 4.6 | 1,679 | 4.2 | 2.1 | 2.2 | 1,893 | 4.8 | 2.3 | 2.4 |
| **Hungary:** | | | | | | | | | | | | | | | | |
| 1900 | 19,144,000 | 7[illegible]8,673 | 752,718 | 15,955 | 2,606 | 13.6 | 3.4 | 3.5 | 636 | 3.3 | .8 | .8 | 1,970 | 10.3 | 2.6 | 2.6 |
| 1901 | 19,342,000 | 7[illegible]7,224 | 731,721 | 15,503 | 2,789 | 14.4 | 3.7 | 3.8 | 687 | 3.6 | .9 | .9 | 2,102 | 10.9 | 2.8 | 2.9 |
| 1902 | 19,513,000 | 7[illegible]5,641 | 759,739 | 15,902 | 2,665 | 13.7 | 3.4 | 3.5 | 622 | 3.2 | .8 | .8 | 2,043 | 10.5 | 2.6 | 2.7 |
| 1903 | 19,669,000 | [illegible]40,405 | 725,239 | 15,166 | 2,562 | 13.0 | 3.5 | 3.5 | 571 | 2.9 | .8 | .8 | 1,991 | 10.1 | 2.7 | 2.7 |
| 1904 | 19,832,000 | [illegible]55,526 | 740,799 | 14,727 | 2,678 | 13.5 | 3.5 | 3.6 | 654 | 3.3 | .9 | .9 | 2,024 | 10.2 | 2.7 | 2.7 |
| 1905 | 19,969,000 | [illegible]34,335 | 720,532 | 13,803 | 2,694 | 13.5 | 3.7 | 3.7 | 689 | 3.5 | .9 | 1.0 | 2,005 | 10.0 | 2.7 | 2.8 |
| 1906 | 20,099,000 | [illegible]48,060 | 733,953 | 14,107 | 2,490 | 12.4 | 3.3 | 3.4 | 602 | 3.0 | .8 | .8 | 1,888 | 9.4 | 2.5 | 2.6 |
| 1907 | 20,200,000 | [illegible]55,653 | 740,867 | 14,786 | 2,552 | 12.6 | 3.4 | 3.4 | 720 | 3.6 | 1.0 | 1.0 | 1,832 | 9.0 | 2.4 | 2.5 |

[1] See explanatory note on p. 58.

TABLE XV. *Population, births, deaths, and death rates per 100,000 population, per 1,000 births, and per 1,000 live births from diseases caused by pregnancy and confinement in certain foreign countries for specified years*—Continued.

| Country and year. | Population July 1 each year (estimated). | Births. Total. | Births. Live births. | Births. Still-births. | Deaths, Total. Number. | Total, Rate per 100,000 population. | Total, Rate per 1,000 births. | Total, Rate per 1,000 live births. | Puerperal septicemia. Number. | Puerperal septicemia, Rate per 100,000 population. | Puerperal septicemia, Rate per 1,000 births. | Puerperal septicemia, Rate per 1,000 live births. | All other. Number. | All other, Rate per 100,000 population. | All other, Rate per 1,000 births. | All other, Rate per 1,000 live births. |
|---|---|---|---|---|---|---|---|---|---|---|---|---|---|---|---|---|
| | 1 | 2 | 3 | 4 | 5 | 6 | 7 | 8 | 9 | 10 | 11 | 12 | 13 | 14 | 15 | 16 |
| Hungary—Continued. | | | | | | | | | | | | | | | | |
| 1908 | 20,426,000 | 771,126 | 755,888 | 15,238 | 2,892 | 14.2 | 3.8 | 3.8 | 880 | 4.4 | 1.2 | 1.2 | 2,003 | 9.8 | 2.6 | 2.6 |
| 1909 | 20,606,000 | 792,354 | 776,395 | 15,959 | 2,839 | 13.8 | 3.6 | 3.7 | 961 | 4.7 | 1.2 | 1.2 | 1,878 | 9.1 | 2.4 | 2.4 |
| 1910 | 20,793,000 | 758,566 | 742,899 | 15,667 | 2,506 | 12.1 | 3.3 | 3.4 | 793 | 3.8 | 1.0 | 1.1 | 1,713 | 8.2 | 2.3 | 2.3 |
| 1911 | 20,958,000 | 747,916 | 732,767 | 15,149 | 2,443 | 11.7 | 3.3 | 3.3 | 869 | 4.1 | 1.2 | 1.2 | 1,574 | 7.5 | 2.1 | 2.1 |
| Ireland: | | | | | | | | | | | | | | | | |
| 1902 | 4,434,000 | ........ | 101,863 | ........ | 635 | 14.3 | ........ | 6.2 | 214 | 4.8 | ........ | 2.1 | 421 | 9.5 | ........ | 4.1 |
| 1903 | 4,416,000 | ........ | 101,831 | ........ | 573 | 13.0 | ........ | 5.6 | 222 | 5.0 | ........ | 2.2 | 351 | 7.9 | ........ | 3.4 |
| 1904 | 4,405,000 | ........ | 103,811 | ........ | 583 | 13.2 | ........ | 5.6 | 206 | 4.7 | ........ | 2.0 | 377 | 8.6 | ........ | 3.6 |
| 1905 | 4,396,000 | ........ | 102,832 | ........ | 573 | 13.0 | ........ | 5.6 | 217 | 4.9 | ........ | 2.1 | 356 | 8.1 | ........ | 3.5 |
| 1906 | 4,393,000 | ........ | 103,536 | ........ | 607 | 13.8 | ........ | 5.9 | 218 | 5.0 | ........ | 2.1 | 389 | 8.9 | ........ | 3.8 |
| 1907 | 4,383,000 | ........ | 101,742 | ........ | 505 | 11.5 | ........ | 5.0 | 152 | 3.5 | ........ | 1.5 | 353 | 8.1 | ........ | 3.5 |
| 1908 | 4,379,000 | ........ | 102,039 | ........ | 530 | 12.1 | ........ | 5.2 | 178 | 4.1 | ........ | 1.7 | 352 | 8.0 | ........ | 3.4 |
| 1909 | 4,380,000 | ........ | 102,759 | ........ | 561 | 12.8 | ........ | 5.5 | 207 | 4.7 | ........ | 2.0 | 354 | 8.1 | ........ | 3.4 |
| 1910 | 4,378,000 | ........ | 101,963 | ........ | 542 | 12.4 | ........ | 5.3 | 178 | 4.1 | ........ | 1.7 | 364 | 8.3 | ........ | 3.6 |
| 1911 | 4,384,000 | ........ | 101,758 | ........ | 514 | 11.7 | ........ | 5.1 | 165 | 3.8 | ........ | 1.6 | 349 | 8.0 | ........ | 3.4 |
| 1912 | 4,385,000 | ........ | 101,035 | ........ | 549 | 12.5 | ........ | 5.4 | 187 | 4.3 | ........ | 1.9 | 362 | 8.3 | ........ | 3.6 |
| 1913 | 4,379,000 | ........ | 100,094 | ........ | 527 | 12.0 | ........ | 5.3 | 163 | 3.7 | ........ | 1.6 | 364 | 8.3 | ........ | 3.6 |
| 1914 | 4,381,000 | ........ | 98,806 | ........ | 497 | 11.3 | ........ | 5.0 | 182 | 4.2 | ........ | 1.8 | 315 | 7.2 | ........ | 3.2 |
| Italy: | | | | | | | | | | | | | | | | |
| 1900 | 32,346,000 | 1,113,055 | 1,067,376 | 45,679 | 3,034 | 9.4 | 2.7 | 2.8 | 1,033 | 3.2 | .9 | 1.0 | 2,001 | 6.2 | 1.8 | 1.9 |
| 1901 | 32,533,000 | 1,104,017 | 1,057,763 | 46,254 | 2,767 | 8.5 | 2.5 | 2.6 | 994 | 3.1 | .9 | .9 | 1,773 | 5.4 | 1.6 | 1.7 |
| 1902 | 32,700,000 | 1,141,749 | 1,093,074 | 48,675 | 2,807 | 8.6 | 2.5 | 2.6 | 1,037 | 3.2 | .9 | .9 | 1,770 | 5.4 | 1.6 | 1.6 |
| 1903 | 32,840,000 | 1,088,797 | 1,042,090 | 46,707 | 2,771 | 8.4 | 2.5 | 2.7 | 1,112 | 3.4 | 1.0 | 1.1 | 1,659 | 5.1 | 1.5 | 1.6 |
| 1904 | 33,016,000 | 1,134,552 | 1,085,431 | 49,121 | 2,981 | 9.0 | 2.6 | 2.7 | 1,082 | 3.3 | 1.0 | 1.0 | 1,899 | 5.8 | 1.7 | 1.7 |

| | | | | | | | | | | | | | | | | |
|---|---|---|---|---|---|---|---|---|---|---|---|---|---|---|---|---|
| 1905 | 33,103,000 | 1,133,970 | 1,084,518 | 40,461 | 3,198 | 9.6 | 2.8 | 2.9 | 977 | 2.9 | .9 | .9 | 2,221 | 6.7 | 2.0 | 2.0 |
| 1906 | 33,325,000 | 1,119,131 | 1,070,978 | 48,153 | 2,701 | 8.4 | 2.5 | 2.6 | 1,021 | 3.1 | .9 | 1.0 | 1,770 | 5.3 | 1.6 | 1.7 |
| 1907 | 33,515,000 | 1,110,756 | 1,062,333 | 48,023 | 3,074 | 9.2 | 2.8 | 2.9 | 1,147 | 3.4 | 1.0 | 1.1 | 1,927 | 5.7 | 1.7 | 1.8 |
| 1908 | 33,827,000 | 1,190,278 | 1,138,813 | 51,465 | 3,315 | 9.8 | 2.8 | 2.9 | 1,245 | 3.7 | 1.0 | 1.1 | 2,070 | 6.1 | 1.7 | 1.8 |
| 1909 | 34,077,000 | 1,166,121 | 1,115,831 | 50,290 | 3,127 | 9.2 | 2.7 | 2.8 | 1,242 | 3.6 | 1.1 | 1.1 | 1,885 | 5.5 | 1.6 | 1.7 |
| 1910 | 34,377,000 | 1,194,747 | 1,144,410 | 50,337 | 2,786 | 8.1 | 2.3 | 2.4 | 1,011 | 2.9 | .8 | .9 | 1,775 | 5.2 | 1.5 | 1.6 |
| 1911 | 34,689,000 | 1,141,036 | 1,093,545 | 47,491 | 2,612 | 7.5 | 2.3 | 2.4 | 920 | 2.7 | .8 | .8 | 1,683 | 4.9 | 1.5 | 1.5 |
| 1912 | 35,020,000 | 1,181,553 | 1,133,985 | 47,568 | 2,743 | 7.8 | 2.3 | 2.4 | 899 | 2.6 | .8 | .8 | 1,814 | 5.3 | 1.6 | 1.6 |
| 1913 | 35,418,000 | 1,169,353 | 1,122,482 | 46,871 | 2,811 | 7.9 | 2.4 | 2.5 | 1,037 | 2.9 | .9 | .9 | 1,774 | 5.0 | 1.5 | 1.6 |
| **Japan:** | | | | | | | | | | | | | | | | |
| 1901 | 45,437,000 | 1,657,080 | 1,501,591 | 155,489 | 6,671 | 14.7 | 4.0 | 4.4 | 1,885 | 4.1 | 1.1 | 1.3 | 4,786 | 10.5 | 2.9 | 3.2 |
| 1902 | 46,022,000 | 1,668,543 | 1,510,835 | 157,708 | 6,556 | 14.2 | 3.9 | 4.3 | 1,983 | 4.3 | 1.2 | 1.3 | 4,573 | 9.9 | 2.7 | 3.0 |
| 1903 | 46,733,000 | 1,643,736 | 1,489,816 | 153,920 | 6,071 | 13.0 | 3.7 | 4.1 | 2,028 | 4.3 | 1.2 | 1.4 | 4,043 | 8.7 | 2.5 | 2.7 |
| 1904 | 47,220,000 | 1,587,429 | 1,440,371 | 147,058 | 5,742 | 12.2 | 3.6 | 4.0 | 1,810 | 3.8 | 1.1 | 1.3 | 3,932 | 8.3 | 2.5 | 2.7 |
| 1905 | 47,678,000 | 1,594,862 | 1,452,770 | 142,092 | 6,185 | 13.0 | 3.9 | 4.3 | 1,878 | 3.9 | 1.2 | 1.3 | 4,307 | 9.0 | 2.7 | 3.0 |
| 1906 | 48,165,000 | 1,544,026 | 1,394,295 | 149,731 | 6,237 | 12.9 | 4.0 | 4.5 | 1,915 | 4.0 | 1.2 | 1.4 | 4,322 | 9.0 | 2.8 | 3.1 |
| 1907 | 48,820,000 | 1,773,286 | 1,614,472 | 158,814 | 6,728 | 13.8 | 3.8 | 4.2 | 2,294 | 4.7 | 1.3 | 1.4 | 4,434 | 9.1 | 2.5 | 2.7 |
| 1908 | 49,589,000 | 1,825,491 | 1,662,815 | 162,676 | 7,091 | 14.3 | 3.9 | 4.3 | 2,570 | 5.2 | 1.4 | 1.5 | 4,521 | 9.1 | 2.5 | 2.7 |
| 1909 | 50,254,000 | 1,855,426 | 1,693,850 | 161,576 | 6,399 | 12.7 | 3.4 | 3.8 | 2,575 | 5.1 | 1.4 | 1.5 | 3,824 | 7.6 | 2.1 | 2.3 |
| 1910 | 50,903,000 | 1,870,249 | 1,712,857 | 157,392 | 6,228 | 12.2 | 3.3 | 3.6 | 2,556 | 5.0 | 1.4 | 1.5 | 3,672 | 7.2 | 2.0 | 2.1 |
| 1911[1] | 51,435,000 | 1,903,122 | 1,747,803 | 155,319 | 6,192 | 12.0 | 3.3 | 3.5 | 2,512 | 4.9 | 1.3 | 1.4 | 3,680 | 7.2 | 1.9 | 2.1 |
| 1912[1] | 52,107,000 | 1,885,219 | 1,737,674 | 147,545 | 5,770 | 11.1 | 3.1 | 3.3 | 2,357 | 4.5 | 1.3 | 1.4 | 3,413 | 6.5 | 1.8 | 2.0 |
| **New Zealand:** | | | | | | | | | | | | | | | | |
| 1900 | 764,000 | ........ | 19,546 | ........ | 75 | 9.8 | ........ | 3.8 | 24 | 3.1 | ........ | 1.2 | 51 | 6.7 | ........ | 2.6 |
| 1901 | 778,000 | ........ | 20,491 | ........ | 90 | 11.6 | ........ | 4.4 | 20 | 2.6 | ........ | 1.0 | 70 | 9.0 | ........ | 3.4 |
| 1902 | 798,000 | ........ | 20,655 | ........ | 110 | 13.8 | ........ | 5.3 | 25 | 3.1 | ........ | 1.2 | 85 | 10.7 | ........ | 4.1 |
| 1903 | 820,000 | ........ | 21,829 | ........ | 128 | 15.6 | ........ | 5.9 | 28 | 3.4 | ........ | 1.3 | 100 | 12.2 | ........ | 4.6 |
| 1904 | 845,000 | ........ | 22,766 | ........ | 106 | 12.5 | ........ | 4.7 | 21 | 2.5 | ........ | .9 | 85 | 10.1 | ........ | 3.7 |
| 1905 | 870,000 | ........ | 23,682 | ........ | 100 | 11.5 | ........ | 4.2 | 21 | 2.4 | ........ | .9 | 79 | 9.1 | ........ | 3.3 |
| 1906 | 896,000 | ........ | 24,252 | ........ | 94 | 10.5 | ........ | 3.9 | 18 | 2.0 | ........ | .7 | 76 | 8.5 | ........ | 3.1 |
| 1907 | 919,000 | ........ | 25,094 | ........ | 116 | 12.6 | ........ | 4.6 | 29 | 3.2 | ........ | 1.2 | 87 | 9.5 | ........ | 3.5 |
| 1908 | 945,000 | ........ | 25,940 | ........ | 119 | 12.6 | ........ | 4.6 | 46 | 4.9 | ........ | 1.8 | 73 | 7.7 | ........ | 2.8 |
| 1909 | 972,000 | ........ | 26,524 | ........ | 135 | 13.9 | ........ | 5.1 | 33 | 3.4 | ........ | 1.2 | 102 | 10.5 | ........ | 3.8 |
| 1910 | 993,000 | ........ | 25,984 | ........ | 117 | 11.8 | ........ | 4.5 | 35 | 3.5 | ........ | 1.3 | 82 | 8.3 | ........ | 3.2 |
| 1911 | 1,015,000 | ........ | 26,354 | ........ | 114 | 11.2 | ........ | 4.3 | 27 | 2.7 | ........ | 1.0 | 87 | 8.6 | ........ | 3.3 |
| 1912 | 1,039,000 | ........ | 27,508 | ........ | 100 | 9.6 | ........ | 3.6 | 19 | 1.8 | ........ | .7 | 81 | 7.8 | ........ | 2.9 |
| 1913 | 1,069,000 | ........ | 27,935 | ........ | 100 | 9.4 | ........ | 3.6 | 29 | 2.7 | ........ | 1.0 | 71 | 6.6 | ........ | 2.5 |
| 1914 | 1,090,000 | ........ | 28,338 | ........ | 118 | 10.8 | ........ | 4.2 | 35 | 3.2 | ........ | 1.2 | 83 | 7.6 | ........ | 2.9 |
| **Norway:** | | | | | | | | | | | | | | | | |
| 1900 | 2,200,000 | 67,765 | 66,149 | 1,616 | 184 | 8.4 | 2.7 | 2.8 | 111 | 5.0 | 1.6 | 1.7 | 73 | 3.3 | 1.1 | 1.1 |
| 1901 | 2,235,000 | 67,935 | 66,207 | 1,728 | 219 | 9.8 | 3.2 | 3.3 | 101 | 4.5 | 1.5 | 1.5 | 118 | 5.3 | 1.7 | 1.8 |
| 1902 | 2,255,000 | 66,854 | 65,262 | 1,592 | 207 | 9.2 | 3.1 | 3.2 | 109 | 4.8 | 1.6 | 1.7 | 98 | 4.3 | 1.5 | 1.5 |
| 1903 | 2,265,000 | 66,797 | 65,155 | 1,642 | 205 | 9.1 | 3.1 | 3.1 | 113 | 5.0 | 1.7 | 1.7 | 92 | 4.1 | 1.4 | 1.4 |
| 1904 | 2,274,000 | 65,533 | 63,955 | 1,578 | 199 | 8.8 | 3.0 | 3.1 | 106 | 4.7 | 1.6 | 1.7 | 93 | 4.1 | 1.4 | 1.5 |

[1] Figures for Dec. 31.

TABLE XV.—*Population, births, deaths, and death rates per 100,000 population, per 1,000 births, and per 1,000 live births from diseases caused by pregnancy and confinement in certain foreign countries for specified years*—Continued.

| Country and year. | Population July 1 each year (estimated). | Births. | | | Deaths from diseases caused by pregnancy and confinement. | | | | | | | | | | | |
|---|---|---|---|---|---|---|---|---|---|---|---|---|---|---|---|---|
| | | | | | Total. | | | | Puerperal septicemia. | | | | All other. | | | |
| | | | | | | Rate. | | | | Rate. | | | | Rate. | | |
| | | Total. | Live births. | Still-births. | Number. | Per 100,000 population. | Per 1,000 births. | Per 1,000 live births. | Number. | Per 100,000 population. | Per 1,000 births. | Per 1,000 live births. | Number. | Per 100,000 population. | Per 1,000 births. | Per 1,000 live births. |
| | 1 | 2 | 3 | 4 | 5 | 6 | 7 | 8 | 9 | 10 | 11 | 12 | 13 | 14 | 15 | 16 |
| **Norway—Continued.** | | | | | | | | | | | | | | | | |
| 1905 | 2,284,000 | 64,158 | 62,698 | 1,460 | 163 | 7.1 | 2.5 | 2.6 | 75 | 3.3 | 1.2 | 1.2 | 88 | 3.9 | 1.4 | 1.4 |
| 1906 | 2,294,000 | 62,743 | 61,316 | 1,427 | 152 | 6.6 | 2.4 | 2.5 | 78 | 3.4 | 1.2 | 1.3 | 74 | 3.2 | 1.2 | 1.2 |
| 1907 | 2,303,000 | 62,151 | 60,722 | 1,429 | 168 | 7.3 | 2.7 | 2.8 | 92 | 4.0 | 1.5 | 1.5 | 76 | 3.3 | 1.2 | 1.3 |
| 1908 | 2,318,000 | 62,286 | 60,866 | 1,420 | 183 | 7.9 | 2.9 | 3.0 | 98 | 4.2 | 1.6 | 1.6 | 85 | 3.7 | 1.4 | 1.4 |
| 1909 | 2,338,000 | 62,846 | 61,407 | 1,439 | 187 | 8.0 | 3.0 | 3.0 | 81 | 3.5 | 1.3 | 1.3 | 106 | 4.5 | 1.7 | 1.7 |
| 1910 | 2,353,000 | 62,890 | 61,461 | 1,429 | 165 | 7.0 | 2.6 | 2.7 | 77 | 3.3 | 1.2 | 1.3 | 88 | 3.7 | 1.4 | 1.4 |
| 1911 | 2,415,000 | 62,867 | 61,468 | 1,399 | ........ | ........ | ........ | ........ | 87 | 3.6 | 1.4 | 1.4 | ........ | ........ | ........ | ........ |
| 1912 | 2,439,000 | 62,581 | 61,151 | 1,430 | ........ | ........ | ........ | ........ | 90 | 3.7 | 1.4 | 1.5 | ........ | ........ | ........ | ........ |
| **Prussia:** | | | | | | | | | | | | | | | | |
| 1900 | 34,254,000 | 1,275,712 | 1,235,719 | 39,993 | 4,074 | 11.9 | 3.2 | 3.3 | ........ | ........ | ........ | ........ | ........ | ........ | ........ | ........ |
| 1901 | 34,802,000 | 1,301,092 | 1,260,379 | 40,713 | 3,992 | 11.5 | 3.1 | 3.2 | ........ | ........ | ........ | ........ | ........ | ........ | ........ | ........ |
| 1902 | 35,366,000 | 1,295,914 | 1,255,686 | 40,228 | 4,080 | 11.5 | 3.1 | 3.2 | ........ | ........ | ........ | ........ | ........ | ........ | ........ | ........ |
| 1903 | 35,930,000 | 1,274,666 | 1,235,213 | 39,453 | 4,120 | 11.5 | 3.2 | 3.3 | 1,986 | 5.5 | 1.6 | 1.6 | 2,134 | 5.9 | 1.7 | 1.7 |
| 1904 | 36,494,000 | 1,304,697 | 1,264,534 | 40,163 | 4,395 | 12.0 | 3.4 | 3.5 | 2,103 | 5.8 | 1.6 | 1.7 | 2,292 | 6.3 | 1.8 | 1.8 |
| 1905 | 37,058,000 | 1,279,992 | 1,241,620 | 38,372 | 3,963 | 10.7 | 3.1 | 3.2 | 1,789 | 4.8 | 1.4 | 1.4 | 2,174 | 5.9 | 1.7 | 1.8 |
| 1906 | 37,628,000 | 1,308,912 | 1,269,611 | 39,301 | 3,722 | 9.9 | 2.8 | 2.9 | 1,456 | 3.9 | 1.1 | 1.1 | 2,266 | 6.0 | 1.7 | 1.8 |
| 1907 | 38,203,000 | 1,298,291 | 1,259,636 | 38,655 | 3,771 | 9.9 | 2.9 | 3.0 | 1,529 | 4.0 | 1.2 | 1.2 | 2,242 | 5.9 | 1.7 | 1.8 |
| 1908 | 38,777,000 | 1,308,283 | 1,269,399 | 38,884 | 3,899 | 10.1 | 3.0 | 3.1 | 1,744 | 4.5 | 1.3 | 1.4 | 2,155 | 5.6 | 1.6 | 1.7 |
| 1909 | 39,352,000 | 1,287,030 | 1,249,040 | 37,990 | 3,913 | 9.9 | 3.0 | 3.1 | 1,772 | 4.5 | 1.4 | 1.4 | 2,141 | 5.4 | 1.7 | 1.7 |
| 1910 | 39,926,000 | 1,256,613 | 1,219,447 | 37,166 | 3,897 | 9.8 | 3.1 | 3.2 | 1,772 | 4.4 | 1.4 | 1.5 | 2,125 | 5.3 | 1.7 | 1.7 |
| **Scotland:** | | | | | | | | | | | | | | | | |
| 1901 | 4,479,000 | ........ | 132,192 | ........ | 627 | 14.0 | ........ | 4.7 | 280 | 6.3 | ........ | 2.1 | 347 | 7.7 | ........ | 2.6 |
| 1902 | 4,507,000 | ........ | 132,267 | ........ | 682 | 15.1 | ........ | 5.2 | 307 | 6.8 | ........ | 2.3 | 375 | 8.3 | ........ | 2.8 |
| 1903 | 4,535,000 | ........ | 133,525 | ........ | 709 | 15.6 | ........ | 5.3 | 291 | 6.4 | ........ | 2.2 | 418 | 9.2 | ........ | 3.1 |
| 1904 | 4,564,000 | ........ | 132,603 | ........ | 615 | 13.5 | ........ | 4.6 | 241 | 5.3 | ........ | 1.8 | 374 | 8.2 | ........ | 2.8 |
| 1905 | 4,592,000 | ........ | 131,410 | ........ | 718 | 15.6 | ........ | 5.5 | 248 | 5.4 | ........ | 1.9 | 470 | 10.2 | ........ | 3.6 |
| 1906 | 4,621,000 | ........ | 132,005 | ........ | 717 | 15.5 | ........ | 5.4 | 263 | 5.7 | ........ | 2.0 | 454 | 9.8 | ........ | 3.4 |
| 1907 | 4,650,000 | ........ | 128,840 | ........ | 686 | 14.8 | ........ | 5.3 | 228 | 4.9 | ........ | 1.8 | 458 | 9.8 | ........ | 3.6 |

| | | | | | | | | | | | | | | | | |
|---|---|---|---|---|---|---|---|---|---|---|---|---|---|---|---|---|
| 1908 | 4,679,000 | ........ | 131,362 | ........ | 676 | 14.4 | ........ | 5.1 | 231 | 4.9 | ........ | 1.8 | 445 | 9.5 | ........ | 3.4 |
| 1909 | 4,708,000 | ........ | 128,669 | ........ | 699 | 14.8 | ........ | 5.4 | 212 | 4.5 | ........ | 1.6 | 487 | 10.3 | ........ | 3.8 |
| 1910 | 4,737,000 | ........ | 124,059 | ........ | 710 | 15.0 | ........ | 5.7 | 221 | 4.7 | ........ | 1.8 | 489 | 10.3 | ........ | 3.9 |
| 1911 | 4,751,000 | ........ | 121,850 | ........ | 699 | 14.7 | ........ | 5.7 | 173 | 3.6 | ........ | 1.4 | 526 | 11.1 | ........ | 4.3 |
| 1912 | 4,741,000 | ........ | 122,790 | ........ | 675 | 14.2 | ........ | 5.5 | 193 | 4.1 | ........ | 1.6 | 482 | 10.2 | ........ | 3.9 |
| 1913 | 4,728,000 | ........ | 120,516 | ........ | 708 | 15.0 | ........ | 5.9 | 160 | 3.4 | ........ | 1.3 | 548 | 11.6 | ........ | 4.5 |
| 1914 | 4,747,000 | ........ | 123,934 | ........ | 746 | 15.7 | ........ | 6.0 | 229 | 4.8 | ........ | 1.8 | 517 | 10.9 | ........ | 4.2 |
| **Spain:** | | | | | | | | | | | | | | | | |
| 1901 | 18,657,000 | 666,2[illegible]2 | 650,649 | 15,603 | 3,674 | 19.7 | 5.5 | 5.6 | 2,178 | 11.7 | 3.3 | 3.3 | 1,496 | 8.0 | 2.2 | 2.3 |
| 1902 | 18,755,000 | 683,1[illegible]3 | 666,687 | 16,466 | 3,494 | 18.6 | 5.1 | 5.2 | 2,116 | 11.3 | 3.1 | 3.2 | 1,378 | 7.3 | 2.0 | 2.1 |
| 1903 | 18,853,000 | 703,5[illegible]8 | 685,265 | 18,303 | 3,771 | 20.0 | 5.4 | 5.5 | 2,362 | 12.5 | 3.4 | 3.4 | 1,409 | 7.5 | 2.0 | 2.1 |
| 1904 | 18,951,000 | 667,125 | 649,878 | 17,247 | 3,885 | 20.5 | 5.8 | 6.0 | 2,465 | 13.0 | 3.7 | 3.8 | 1,420 | 7.5 | 2.1 | 2.2 |
| 1905 | 19,049,000 | 688,058 | 670,651 | 17,407 | 4,115 | 21.6 | 6.0 | 6.1 | 2,715 | 14.3 | 3.9 | 4.0 | 1,400 | 7.3 | 2.0 | 2.1 |
| 1906 | 19,147,000 | 666,874 | 650,385 | 16,489 | 3,860 | 20.2 | 5.8 | 5.9 | 2,469 | 12.9 | 3.7 | 3.8 | 1,391 | 7.3 | 2.1 | 2.1 |
| 1907 | 19,245,000 | 661,981 | 646,374 | 15,607 | 3,930 | 20.4 | 5.9 | 6.1 | 2,549 | 13.2 | 3.9 | 3.9 | 1,381 | 7.2 | 2.1 | 2.1 |
| 1908 | 19,343,000 | 674,125 | 657,701 | 16,424 | 3,725 | 19.3 | 5.5 | 5.7 | 2,316 | 12.0 | 3.4 | 3.5 | 1,409 | 7.3. | 2.1 | 2.1 |
| 1909 | 19,442,000 | 666,551 | 650,415 | 16,136 | 3,613 | 18.7 | 5.5 | 5.6 | 2,280 | 11.7 | 3.4 | 3.5 | 1,363 | 7.0 | 2.0 | 2.1 |
| 1910 | 19,540,000 | 662,934 | 646,787 | 16,147 | 3,407 | 17.4 | 5.1 | 5.3 | 2,107 | 10.8 | 3.2 | 3.3 | 1,300 | 6.7 | 2.0 | 2.0 |
| **Sweden:** | | | | | | | | | | | | | | | | |
| 1900 | 5,117,000 | 141,717 | 138,139 | 3,578 | ........ | ........ | ........ | ........ | 121 | 2.4 | .9 | .9 | ........ | ........ | ........ | ........ |
| 1901 | 5,156,000 | 142,998 | 139,370 | 3,628 | 315 | 6.1 | 2.2 | 2.3 | 152 | 2.9 | 1.1 | 1.1 | 163 | 3.2 | 1.1 | 1.2 |
| 1902 | 5,187,000 | 140,879 | 137,364 | 3,515 | 306 | 5.9 | 2.2 | 2.2 | 146 | 2.8 | 1.0 | 1.1 | 160 | 3.1 | 1.1 | 1.2 |
| 1903 | 5,210,000 | 137,334 | 133,896 | 3,438 | 305 | 5.9 | 2.2 | 2.3 | 128 | 2.5 | .9 | 1.0 | 177 | 3.4 | 1.3 | 1.3 |
| 1904 | 5,241,000 | 138,484 | 134,952 | 3,532 | 288 | 5.5 | 2.1 | 2.1 | 126 | 2.4 | .9 | .9 | 162 | 3.1 | 1.2 | 1.2 |
| 1905 | 5,278,000 | 138,827 | 135,409 | 3,418 | 333 | 6.3 | 2.4 | 2.5 | 169 | 3.2 | 1.2 | 1.2 | 164 | 3.1 | 1.2 | 1.2 |
| 1906 | 5,316,000 | 140,069 | 136,620 | 3,449 | 325 | 6.1 | 2.3 | 2.4 | 124 | 2.3 | .9 | .9 | 201 | 3.8 | 1.4 | 1.5 |
| 1907 | 5,357,000 | 140,330 | 136,793 | 3,537 | 318 | 5.9 | 2.3 | 2.3 | 110 | 2.1 | .8 | .8 | 208 | 3.9 | 1.5 | 1.5 |
| 1908 | 5,404,000 | 142,309 | 138,874 | 3,435 | 295 | 5.5 | 2.1 | 2.1 | 107 | 2.0 | .8 | .8 | 188 | 3.5 | 1.3 | 1.4 |
| 1909 | 5,453,000 | 142,987 | 139,505 | 3,482 | 349 | 6.4 | 2.4 | 2.5 | 113 | 2.1 | .8 | .8 | 236 | 4.3 | 1.7 | 1.7 |
| 1910 | 5,499,000 | 138,976 | 135,625 | 3,351 | 345 | 6.3 | 2.5 | 2.5 | 119 | 2.2 | .9 | .9 | 226 | 4.1 | 1.6 | 1.7 |
| 1911 | 5,562,000 | 136,335 | 132,977 | 3,358 | 354 | 6.4 | 2.6 | 2.7 | 136 | 2.4 | 1.0 | 1.0 | 218 | 3.9 | 1.6 | 1.6 |
| **Switzerland:** | | | | | | | | | | | | | | | | |
| 1900 | 3,302,000 | 97,695 | 94,316 | 3,379 | 523 | 15.8 | 5.4 | 5.5 | 193 | 5.8 | 2.0 | 2.0 | 330 | 10.0 | 3.4 | 3.5 |
| 1901 | 3,341,000 | 100,635 | 97,028 | 3,607 | 586 | 17.5 | 5.8 | 6.0 | 250 | 7.5 | 2.5 | 2.6 | 336 | 10.1 | 3.3 | 3.5 |
| 1902 | 3,385,000 | 99,993 | 96,481 | 3,512 | 500 | 14.8 | 5.0 | 5.2 | 196 | 5.8 | 2.0 | 2.0 | 304 | 9.0 | 3.0 | 3.2 |
| 1903 | 3,429,000 | 97,119 | 93,824 | 3,295 | 554 | 16.2 | 5.7 | 5.9 | 237 | 6.9 | 2.4 | 2.5 | 317 | 9.2 | 3.3 | 3.4 |
| 1904 | 3,472,000 | 98,300 | 94,867 | 3,433 | 590 | 17.0 | 6.0 | 6.2 | 257 | 7.4 | 2.6 | 2.7 | 333 | 9.6 | 3.4 | 3.5 |
| 1905 | 3,516,000 | 98,057 | 94,653 | 3,404 | 551 | 15.7 | 5.6 | 5.8 | 253 | 7.2 | 2.6 | 2.7 | 298 | 8.5 | 3.0 | 3.1 |
| 1906 | 3,560,000 | 98,971 | 95,595 | 3,376 | 495 | 13.9 | 5.0 | 5.2 | 191 | 5.4 | 1.9 | 2.0 | 304 | 8.5 | 3.1 | 3.2 |
| 1907 | 3,604,000 | 97,696 | 94,508 | 3,188 | 553 | 15.3 | 5.7 | 5.9 | 261 | 7.2 | 2.7 | 2.8 | 292 | 8.1 | 3.0 | 3.1 |
| 1908 | 3,647,000 | 99,468 | 96,245 | 3,223 | 554 | 15.2 | 5.6 | 5.8 | 227 | 6.2 | 2.3 | 2.4 | 327 | 9.0 | 3.3 | 3.4 |
| 1909 | 3,691,000 | 97,296 | 94,112 | 3,184 | 544 | 14.7 | 5.6 | 5.8 | 238 | 6.4 | 2.4 | 2.5 | 306 | 8.3 | 3.1 | 3.3 |
| 1910 | 3,735,000 | 96,669 | 93,514 | 3,155 | 417 | 12.0 | 4.6 | 4.8 | 182 | 4.9 | 1.9 | 1.9 | 265 | 7.1 | 2.7 | 2.8 |
| 1911 | 3,781,000 | 94,185 | 91,320 | 2,865 | 501 | 13.3 | 5.3 | 5.5 | 245 | 6.5 | 2.6 | 2.7 | 256 | 6.8 | 2.7 | 2.8 |
| 1912 | 3,831,000 | 95,171 | 92,196 | 2,975 | 484 | 12.6 | 5.1 | 5.2 | 218 | 5.7 | 2.3 | 2.4 | 266 | 6.9 | 2.8 | 2.9 |

TABLE XVI.—*Average death rates per 100,000 population and per 1,000 live births from diseases caused by pregnancy and confinement in certain foreign countries for specified periods of years.*

| Country and specified period of years. | Death rate from diseases caused by pregnancy and confinement. | | | | | |
|---|---|---|---|---|---|---|
| | Total. | | Puerperal septicemia. | | All other. | |
| | Per 100,000 population. | Per 1,000 live births. | Per 100,000 population. | Per 1,000 live births. | Per 100,000 population. | Per 1,000 live births. |
| **Australia:** | | | | | | |
| Whole period | 14.0 | 5.2 | 4.8 | 1.8 | 9.2 | 3.4 |
| 1907–1909 | 14.3 | 5.3 | 4.6 | 1.7 | 9.6 | 3.6 |
| 1910–1912 | 13.7 | 5.0 | 4.9 | 1.8 | 8.8 | 3.2 |
| **Austria:** | | | | | | |
| Whole period | | | 6.5 | 1.9 | | |
| 1900–1903 | | | 7.2 | 2.0 | | |
| 1904–1907 | | | 6.2 | 1.8 | | |
| 1908–1911 | | | 6.2 | 1.9 | | |
| **Belgium:** | | | | | | |
| Whole period | 14.7 | 5.9 | 5.8 | 2.3 | 8.8 | 3.5 |
| 1903–1907 | 15.3 | 5.8 | 5.8 | 2.2 | 9.5 | 3.6 |
| 1908–1912 | 14.1 | 6.0 | 5.9 | 2.5 | 8.3 | 3.5 |
| **England and Wales:** | | | | | | |
| Whole period | 10.6 | 4.0 | 4.3 | 1.6 | 6.3 | 2.4 |
| 1900–1904 | 12.5 | 4.4 | 5.5 | 1.9 | 7.0 | 2.5 |
| 1905–1909 | 10.3 | 3.9 | 4.2 | 1.6 | 6.2 | 2.3 |
| 1910–1914a [1] | 9.1 | 3.7 | 3.4 | 1.4 | 5.6 | 2.3 |
| **France:** | | | | | | |
| Whole period | 10.3 | 5.2 | 4.8 | 2.4 | 5.5 | 2.8 |
| 1906–1910 | 10.3 | 5.2 | 4.8 | 2.4 | 5.5 | 2.8 |
| **Hungary:** | | | | | | |
| Whole period | 13.2 | 3.6 | 3.6 | 1.0 | 9.6 | 2.6 |
| 1900–1903 | 13.7 | 3.6 | 3.2 | .8 | 10.4 | 2.7 |
| 1904–1907 | 13.0 | 3.5 | 3.3 | .9 | 9.7 | 2.6 |
| 1908–1911 | 12.9 | 3.6 | 4.2 | 1.2 | 8.7 | 2.4 |
| **Ireland:** | | | | | | |
| Whole period | 12.6 | 5.4 | 4.4 | 1.9 | 8.2 | 3.6 |
| 1902–1906 | 13.5 | 5.8 | 4.9 | 2.1 | 8.6 | 3.7 |
| 1907–1910 | 12.2 | 5.2 | 4.1 | 1.8 | 8.1 | 3.5 |
| 1911–1914 | 11.9 | 5.2 | 4.0 | 1.7 | 7.9 | 3.5 |
| **Italy:** | | | | | | |
| Whole period | 8.7 | 2.7 | 3.1 | 1.0 | 5.5 | 1.7 |
| 1900–1904 | 8.8 | 2.7 | 3.2 | 1.0 | 5.6 | 1.7 |
| 1905–1909 | 9.2 | 2.8 | 3.4 | 1.0 | 5.9 | 1.8 |
| 1910–1913 | 7.9 | 2.4 | 2.8 | .9 | 5.1 | 1.6 |
| **Japan:** | | | | | | |
| Whole period | 13.0 | 4.0 | 4.5 | 1.4 | 8.5 | 2.6 |
| 1901–1904 | 13.5 | 4.2 | 4.2 | 1.3 | 9.3 | 2.9 |
| 1905–1908 | 13.5 | 4.3 | 4.5 | 1.4 | 9.1 | 2.9 |
| 1909–1912 | 12.0 | 3.6 | 4.9 | 1.5 | 7.1 | 2.1 |
| **New Zealand:** | | | | | | |
| Whole period | 11.7 | 4.4 | 3.0 | 1.1 | 8.8 | 3.3 |
| 1900–1904 | 12.7 | 4.8 | 2.9 | 1.1 | 9.8 | 3.7 |
| 1905–1909 | 12.3 | 4.5 | 3.2 | 1.2 | 9.1 | 3.3 |
| 1910–1914 | 10.5 | 4.0 | 2.8 | 1.1 | 7.8 | 3.0 |
| **Norway:** | | | | | | |
| Whole period | 8.1 | 2.9 | 4.1 | 1.5 | 3.9 | 1.4 |
| 1900–1903 | 9.1 | 3.1 | 4.8 | 1.7 | 4.3 | 1.4 |
| 1904–1907 | 7.4 | 2.7 | 3.8 | 1.4 | 3.6 | 1.3 |
| 1908–1910 | 7.6 | 2.9 | 3.7 | 1.4 | 4.0 | 1.5 |
| **Prussia:** | | | | | | |
| Whole period | 10.4 | 3.2 | 4.7 | 1.4 | 5.8 | 1.8 |
| 1903–1906 | 11.0 | 3.2 | 5.0 | 1.5 | 6.0 | 1.8 |
| 1907–1910 | 9.9 | 3.1 | 4.4 | 1.4 | 5.5 | 1.7 |
| **Scotland:** | | | | | | |
| Whole period | 14.9 | 5.4 | 5.0 | 1.8 | 9.8 | 3.6 |
| 1901–1905 | 14.8 | 5.1 | 6.0 | 2.1 | 8.7 | 3.0 |
| 1906–1910 | 14.9 | 5.4 | 4.9 | 1.8 | 10.0 | 3.6 |
| 1911–1914 | 14.9 | 5.8 | 4.0 | 1.5 | 10.9 | 4.2 |
| **Spain:** | | | | | | |
| Whole period | 19.6 | 5.7 | 12.3 | 3.6 | 7.3 | 2.1 |
| 1901–1905 | 20.1 | 5.7 | 12.6 | 3.6 | 7.5 | 2.1 |
| 1906–1910 | 19.2 | 5.7 | 12.1 | 3.6 | 7.1 | 2.1 |
| **Sweden:** | | | | | | |
| Whole period | 6.0 | 2.4 | 2.4 | 1.0 | 3.6 | 1.4 |
| 1901–1904 | 5.8 | 2.2 | 2.7 | 1.0 | 3.2 | 1.2 |
| 1905–1908 | 6.0 | 2.3 | 2.4 | .9 | 3.6 | 1.4 |
| 1909–1911 | 6.3 | 2.6 | 2.2 | .9 | 4.1 | 1.7 |
| **Switzerland:** | | | | | | |
| Whole period | 14.9 | 5.6 | 6.4 | 2.4 | 8.5 | 3.2 |
| 1900–1904 | 16.3 | 5.8 | 6.7 | 2.4 | 9.6 | 3.4 |
| 1905–1908 | 15.0 | 5.7 | 6.5 | 2.4 | 8.5 | 3.2 |
| 1909–1912 | 13.1 | 5.3 | 5.9 | 2.4 | 7.3 | 2.9 |

[1] See explanatory note on p. 58.

U. S. DEPARTMENT OF LABOR
JAMES J. DAVIS, Secretary
CHILDREN'S BUREAU
GRACE ABBOTT, Chief

# THE NUTRITION AND CARE OF CHILDREN IN A MOUNTAIN COUNTY OF KENTUCKY

By

LYDIA ROBERTS

Bureau Publication No. 110

WASHINGTON
GOVERNMENT PRINTING OFFICE
1922

# CONTENTS.

## ILLUSTRATIONS.



## CHARTS.

## LETTER OF TRANSMITTAL.

June 14, 1922.

Sir: There is transmitted herewith a report on the Nutrition and Care of Children in a Mountain County of Kentucky, by Lydia Roberts. The physical examinations were made by Dr. Frances Sage Bradley, assisted by E. Ida McCune, and Ethel M. Springer assisted in the direction of the field work. The visiting of the homes was done by Ella Ross and Alta Nelson. The investigation was planned by Miss Roberts, and the report written by her.

Respectfully submitted.

Grace Abbott, *Chief.*

Hon. James J. Davis,
*Secretary of Labor.*

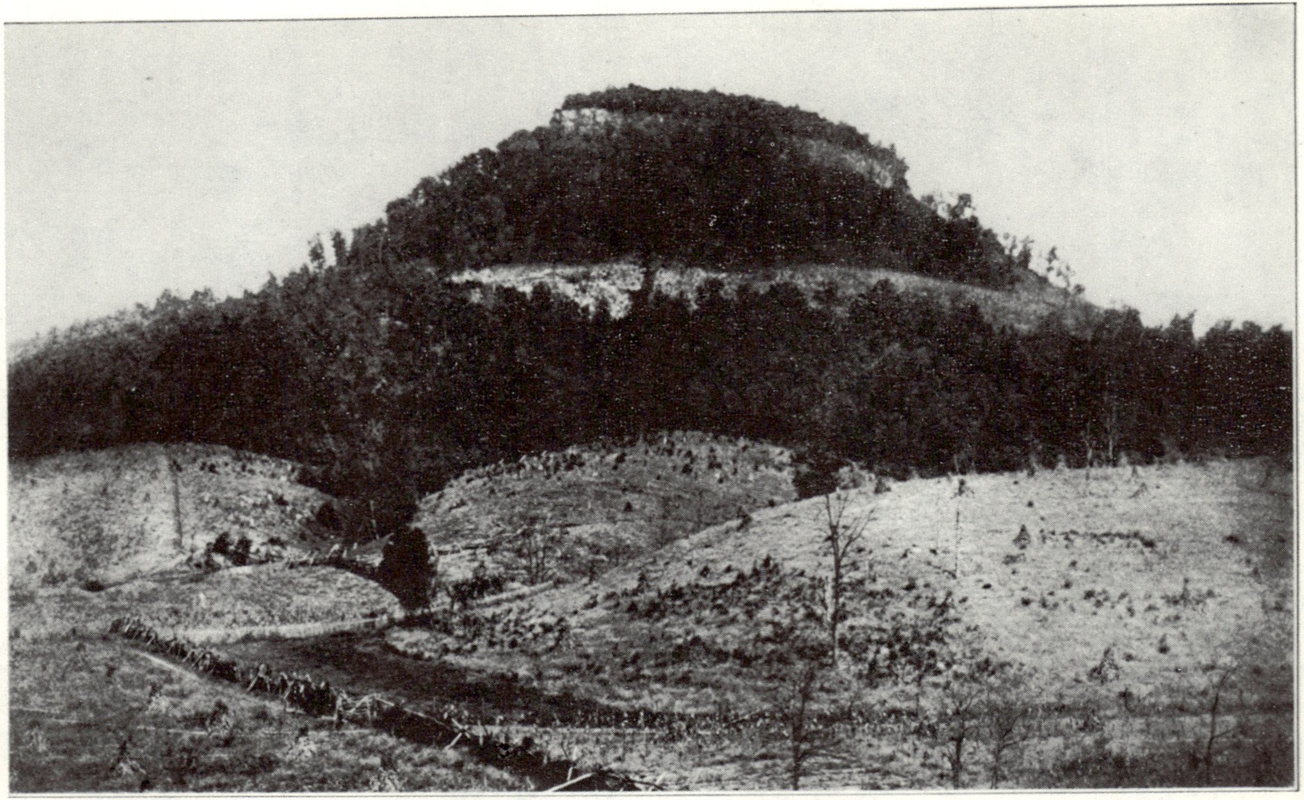

TYPICAL "KNOB.'

Note layer of limestone near the top.

# THE NUTRITION AND CARE OF CHILDREN IN A MOUNTAIN COUNTY OF KENTUCKY.

## INTRODUCTION.

### PURPOSE OF STUDY.

This report covers the findings of the first nutrition survey undertaken by the Children's Bureau in a rural district. Other rural studies have dealt with maternity and infant care, and the general conditions surrounding young children,[1] and some of them have revealed data of interest in connection with the nutrition of children, but in none was nutrition the chief object of the investigation. The study was made in a community in Kentucky in response to an appeal from the Kentucky State Board of Health to help find "why a State famous the world over for its prosperity should turn out so large a percentage of physically defective men as the draft records showed." Its purpose was to ascertain the physical condition of children of selected ages and to discover, if possible, the chief factors responsible for the conditions found. The field work was done in the winter of 1919–20.

### THE COMMUNITY STUDIED.

Kentucky is distinctly a rural State, its urban population, according to the 1920 census, being 633,543, while its rural population was almost three times that number. The State board of health suggested a study of five typical counties in different parts of the State in order to secure a representative picture. Unfortunately, such an extended survey could not be undertaken. Instead a county was chosen which had two distinct types of country, a blue-grass section and a mountain section, and later it became necessary to limit the survey to the latter only, a section embracing an area of about 30 square miles. Every home within this area having a child between 2 and 11 years of age was visited. These years were chosen because it was desired to exclude the periods of infancy and puberty, which

[1] Maternity and Infant Care in a Rural County in Kansas, U. S. Children's Bureau Publication No. 26, Washington, 1917; Rural Children in Selected Counties of North Carolina, U. S. Children's Bureau Publication No. 33, Washington, 1918; Maternity Care and the Welfare of Young Children in a Homesteading County in Montana, U. S. Children's Bureau Publication No. 34, Washington, 1919; Maternity and Infant Care in Two Rural Counties in Wisconsin, U. S. Children's Bureau Publication No. 46, Washington, 1919; Maternity and Child Care in Selected Rural Areas of Mississippi, U. S. Children's Bureau Publication No. 88, Washington, 1921.

involve special problems it was not deemed expedient to consider. In all, 123 families, with 256 children of the selected age, were interviewed.[a]

In a nutrition study in a rural community, the physiography and soil assume great importance not only because the food supply is directly dependent on them but also because they almost entirely determine economic status. Rich farming land presupposes an abundant food supply and financial prosperity, while hilly, stony soil usually means uncertain, meager crops and a struggle to obtain the necessities of life.

The county in which the area studied is located contains within its borders extremes of richness and of poverty of soil. The greater part of the county is in the blue-grass section where the soil is of great fertility, but a small portion of it extends into "the knobs," or "the mountains," as the rocky cone-shaped hills are called, where the soil is for the most part exceedingly poor. It was this small, mountainous part which constituted the area studied.

The farms of the area are of three types, depending on their location. The lowland just at the foot of the mountains is the poorest soil in the district. It rests upon a bed of shale only a few feet from the surface. This land is wet and sour and needs drainage, ground limestone, and phosphorus. Plenty of limestone lies near at hand, for "the knobs" are composed largely of limestone and near their tops are found massive outcroppings of the rock; if this rock could be pulverized and put on the land below it would be the greatest possible boon to the soil. Up to the time of this study, however, rock crushers were not available. On the sides of the mountains between the limestone and the lower shale land are farms far better than those of the lower land. The soil is better drained, and is enriched by washings from the limestone areas above. The third type of farm is found on the tops of some of the knobs. Here the soil is more nearly comparable than any other in the surveyed area to the soil of the blue-grass region, since it rests upon a limestone bed which by slow disintegration supplies the needed lime. As a rule, therefore, the better farms in this section are the upland farms, although similar to these in fertility are the patches of bottom lands with rich productive soil which has been formed by overflows of creeks and the consequent deposition of sediment. It is evident that the economic status of a family in the area studied can be predicted fairly accurately from the location of its farm.

Although the chief crop of the section is corn, only enough is produced for local needs. The average yield is about 15 bushels per

---

[a] In discussion of material based upon these interviews, cases not reported as to the particular item under consideration, usually not more than two or three in number, are omitted. The per cents are based upon the total number of cases.

acre, though some farms in the section yield considerably higher than this average, and some yield as little as 5 bushels. Other crops include tobacco,[2] oats, and rye in limited amounts, cowpeas, and sorghum. The upland soil is adapted to fruit culture, and a few of the progressive farmers of the section have planted orchards. In spite of the fact that frosts may kill the crop for a number of years in succession, a good yield once in five or six years, in the opinion of experts, makes fruit growing well worth while.

That poor roads and lack of development in a community go hand in hand is probably nowhere better illustrated than in the locality studied. The roads over which the majority of the people have to travel to get to market are almost universally poor. Although none of the families visited lived farther than about 7 miles from a fair-sized town, many were as isolated as if the distance were several times as great. For them to get to town was at certain seasons not only a long, laborious task, but often for prolonged periods an absolutely impossible one.

The 123 families visited in this survey were all native white and with very few exceptions were of mountain stock. Poor roads had tended to isolate them, although they lived within a few miles of a small town with railroad and educational advantages, which no doubt had influenced them to a certain extent. Their natural shyness and reserve, a heritage from many generations of mountain ancestors, has made them slow in responding to outside influences.

A visitor to the mountains never fails to be impressed by the premature ageing of the majority of the people, particularly the women. The early age at which the women marry and assume the cares of a home and family doubtless offers a partial explanation of this fact.

## METHOD OF STUDY.

A nutrition survey necessarily consists of two parts: First, a study of the physical condition of the children to determine their state of nutrition and to discover any clinical factors which may be either the result or the cause of poor nutrition; second, an examination into the factors of diet and care responsible for the condition of health in which the children are found. In the present study the children's physical condition was ascertained by means of a medical examination made by a doctor on the staff of the Children's Bureau, and information concerning their diet and care was gathered through interviews with the mothers in their homes by agents who were specialists in food and nutrition. A schedule covering the information to be

---

[2] Although the soil in general is not adapted to raising tobacco, the farmers had found in their barn lots and dooryards small plots of 1 to 1½ acres which could be used temporarily for this crop.

sought from a mother regarding the diet and care of her children was prepared, and general items of importance in a consideration of the nutrition and general health of the children were also included.[3] The visiting of the homes was done first, because this part of the study required more time, and because it also gave opportunity to explain to the mothers the purpose and value of the physical examination which formed the second part of the inquiry.

It was usually the mother but sometimes the father who was interviewed by the agent of the Children's Bureau. Often, indeed, the two answered the questions together, the mother supplying the information about the child's personal habits and the father contributing facts about the garden, the milk, and general farm matters. As a rule the agent's visit was expected, for contact had already been made with the children through the school, and word concerning the purpose of the inquiry and the intention of the agents to visit the parents had been carried home. The reception of the agents in the homes was invariably courteous, and answers to all the questions were freely given.

Whatever difficulties arose in securing accurate data came not from unwillingness on the part of the mothers to give the information but from the fact that they did not know their children's habits, particularly in regard to food. "I put the food on the table; I don't pay no 'tention to what nobody eats," was a not infrequent response. The mother, however, always knew what she had cooked, and she usually knew what the younger children ate, and the older children could supply the needed data regarding their own food. Since the agents were specialists in nutrition, they were able to supplement the schedule inquiries by further questions regarding essential points. It is believed, therefore, that the information secured is as accurate as can be obtained by the schedule method.

After the home visits were completed, the Children's Bureau "Child-Welfare Special" came to the locality in order that the children studied might be physically examined. The "special" is a large automobile truck fitted up as a health center and equipped with scales, measuring devices, and other facilities needed by a physician in giving a complete physical examination. A doctor, a nurse, and a clerk travel with the car.[4]

The "special" visited certain schoolhouses in the district, and the mothers were notified in advance, by letter usually, when and where to bring their children. Most of them when visited had seemed interested in having their children examined when the car should arrive, but persistent rain, muddy and impassable roads, lack of

---

[3] See schedule, following p. 41.

[4] The Child-Welfare Special. U. S. Children's Bureau Publication No. 69. Washington, 1920.

conveyance, illness, and, in some cases, inadequate clothing for the children kept many of them away. However, 149 children—a little more than half the number for whom schedules were obtained—reported for examination. Of those who arrived not a few struggled through great difficulties. One mother walked several miles in the rain carrying a baby, while the three older children trudged along in the mud beside her; another was obliged to walk to town for soap to wash the clothes her children were wearing, before she could bring them; and a third also found it necessary to make a trip to town on foot in order to purchase clothing for the occasion. Even then she had to borrow from a neighbor in order to have enough. Such are a few of the efforts which the mothers are known to have made in order that their children might have the benefit of the examination.

The examination was made in the presence of the mother or other person who accompanied the child to the car, and since each mother was told the special needs of her child as disclosed by the examination, it became of immediate personal value as well as serving the purpose of the study.

## THE PHYSICAL CONDITION OF THE CHILDREN.

One hundred and forty-nine children, 58 per cent of the total number between 2 and 11 years of age for whom information regarding home care was obtained, received physical examinations.[5] It is, therefore, only to these 149 children that the findings with reference to physical conditions relate.

### RESULTS OF WEIGHING AND MEASURING.

The children were weighed without clothes and the height was taken without shoes or stockings. In the absence of a standard of stripped weights with which to compare the weights of these children, a table derived from the Bowditch figures was used.[6] According to this scale, 20 per cent of the children were found to be 7 per cent or more underweight. A considerable number of this group were markedly below—from 15 to 23 per cent under the average

### CLINICAL FINDINGS.

#### Number of Defects.

The total number of physical defects found in the children, without regard to the relative seriousness of the kinds of defects, is shown

---

[5] See p. 39.

[6] A table of average stripped weights was derived by subtracting Bowditch's figures of estimated weights of clothing from his averages including weights of clothing. Bowditch, H. P.: Eighth Annual Report of the State Board of Health of Massachusetts, 1877.

in Table I. Thus, abnormal tonsil conditions count as one defect, decayed teeth as another, any heart defect as a third, and so on. Only five of the children examined were found to be free from physical defect of any kind; the greater number had from 3 to 5 defects, but a number had 6 or 7, and a few even had from 8 to 10. The total number of defects found in the 149 children studied was 621, an average of more than 4 to each child. The younger children—those under 6—averaged 3.2 defects each; the children between 6 and 11 years of age averaged 4.6 defects. This difference may be partly explained by the greater prevalence of decayed teeth among the older children.

TABLE I.—*Number of physical defects, by age; children 2 to 11 years of age given physical examinations.*

| Number of defects. | Children given physical examinations. | | | Number of defects. | Children given physical examinations. | | |
|---|---|---|---|---|---|---|---|
| | Total. | 2–5 years of age. | 6–11 years of age. | | Total. | 2–5 years of age. | 6–11 years of age. |
| Total | 149 | 45 | 104 | 5 | 29 | 8 | 21 |
| | | | | 6 | 10 | 1 | 9 |
| None reported | 5 | 4 | 1 | 7 | 13 | 2 | 11 |
| 1 | 13 | 9 | 4 | 8 | 6 | 1 | 5 |
| 2 | 12 | 3 | 9 | 9 | 4 | 1 | 3 |
| 3 | 20 | 7 | 13 | 10 | 2 | 1 | 1 |
| 4 | 31 | 5 | 26 | Number not reported | 4 | 3 | 1 |

Total number of defects reported for all children, 621.

It was evident that many of these defects were due to lack of proper care, and that nearly all needed early attention if permanent injury to the children was to be avoided. Comment will be made regarding only a few defects the relation of which to nutrition is of special importance.

## Tonsils and Adenoids.

Seventy-four children, 50 per cent of the total number examined, were found to have enlarged or diseased tonsils. Symptoms indicative of adenoids were found in 27 per cent of the children.

## Teeth.

More than three-fourths of the children examined (78 per cent) were found to have carious teeth. Even in the preschool group over half the children, 25 of 45, had decayed temporary teeth; 91 of 104 children 6 to 11 years of age, inclusive, had decayed teeth either permanent or temporary, and nearly one-third of the children in this age group had one or more permanent teeth decayed.

That lack of care may have been a factor in producing this condition is indicated by the fact that 122 of the children (82 per cent) were reported by the examining physician to have dirty teeth, and 26 children (17 per cent), inflammation of the gums.

**Nutrition.**

Weight in relation to height affords a rough indication of a child's general nutritive condition. It is customary, indeed, to class as undernourished all those who fall a certain per cent (usually 7 or 10 per cent) below the average weight for their height. In the present study it was desired in determining the nutrition to consider other criteria than weight alone, and also to show more gradations of nutrition than two—those corresponding to the undernourished and the well nourished. Five grades of nutrition were established—ex-

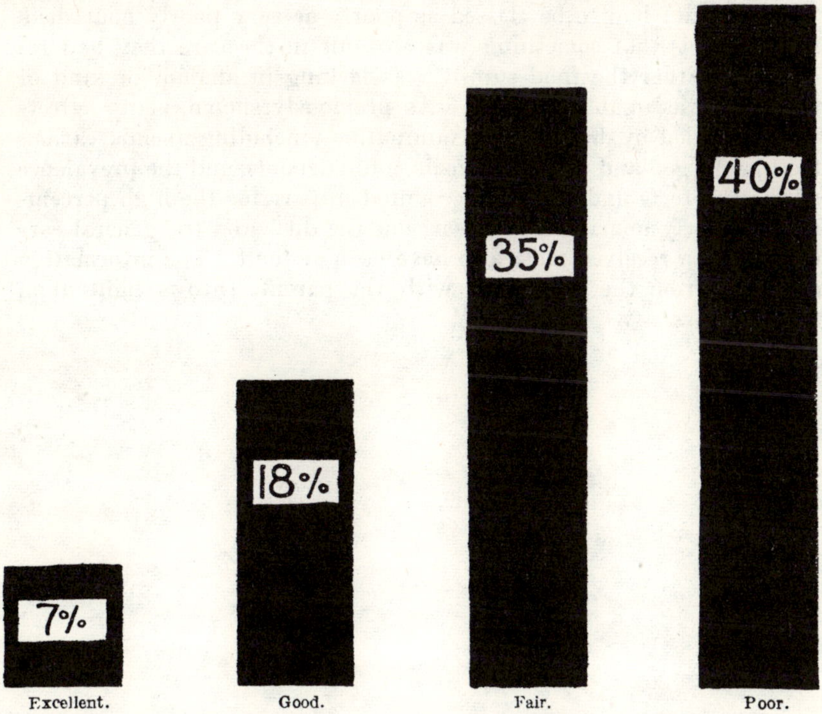


CHART I.—Per cent of children in each grade of nutrition.

cellent, good, fair, poor, and very poor—and the grade of each child was determined by the physician who made the physical examination. The weight was used as a guide, but it was not allowed absolutely to determine a child's grade of nutrition. As it happened, practically all the children 7 per cent underweight by the standard used were graded poor by the physician, but the converse was not always the case. A fat, flabby, anemic child was rated poor even though he measured well up to the average in weight, as was also a child who was unmistakably thin and undernourished. Every available factor, indeed, was taken into consideration in classifying the children.

It was found that only 10 children (7 per cent) could qualify as "excellent," and but 27 children (18 per cent) as "good." Two-thirds were classed either "fair" (35 per cent) or "poor" (34 per cent), and 9 children (6 per cent) were so much below par as to be rated "very poor." The significance of these figures becomes more apparent when it is borne in mind that with proper care and adequate and suitable diet maintained continuously from birth, every child should have been in the "excellent," or certainly in the "good," group. When only one-fourth of the children could be definitely graded as in excellent or good nutrition and when almost two-fifths (39 per cent) had to be classed as poorly or very poorly nourished, it is obvious that something was at fault in the care they had received. Either the food supply was lacking in amount or kind or the body was unable to use it. As previously shown, many defects were revealed by the physical examinations, including anemia, carious teeth, enlarged and diseased tonsils, and adenoids, and the prevalence of these defects undoubtedly accounted in part for the high percentage of poorly nourished children; but the diets and the general care the children received must also have been at fault. The information obtained from the interviews with the parents throws light upon these factors.

## HOME CONDITIONS DETERMINING THE CARE GIVEN THE CHILDREN.

### ECONOMIC STATUS OF THE FAMILY.

Most of the homes visited—103 of the 123—were the homes of small farmers; that is, the economic head of the household was working at least 3 acres of land, either owned or rented.[8] Where the land is extremely fertile and farming is intensive, 3 acres may furnish a good livelihood for a family; but, in sections like the one studied, where the soil is poor and the farms largely unimproved, a small farm can not possibly yield an adequate living. Forty-four of the 103 heads of families classed as farmers supplemented their income obtained from that source by earnings from some other occupation.

Information necessary to a fair judgment of the financial condition of each family was ascertained—regarding, for instance, in the case of those managing farms, the size of the farm, the acres cultivated, and the amount of stock; and in the case of those hired by the day or working at trades, their wages. On the basis of the information thus obtained the families were classed into three economic groups—A, B, and C—according to their ability to furnish the essentials of adequate living. In Group A are included the families whose ability to provide adequate food, shelter, and clothing could not be doubted; in Group B, those less certainly able so to provide for themselves; and in Group C, those who were unquestionably poor.

According to this classification 25 families containing 42 children between 2 and 11 years of age fell into Group A; 45 families with 95 children, into Group B; and 53 families with 119 children, into Group C. In other words nearly half the children (47 per cent) were living in homes in which the income was so small as to make even a minimum standard of care appear impossible, while but 16 per cent belonged to families clearly able to provide the modest requirements of adequate living.

Of the 25 families with the best economic status, 13 reported obtaining their living entirely from their farms, the average acreage of which was about 47; the others reported additional sources of income. Twenty-five of the 45 families in the B income group and 21 of the 53 in the C group reported that they were wholly dependent upon income from their farms.

---

[8] This classification is in accord with that used by the U. S. Bureau of the Census. See Thirteenth Census of the United States, Vol. V, Agriculture, 1909 and 1910, pp. 22-24.

## HOUSING.

Housing bears an important relation to nutrition, since it affects directly the family's health and general welfare. On the whole the homes of the families studied seemed pitifully poor. Some were no more than board sheds with open cracks in the walls and floors, and no boards or banking at the base to keep out the wind; some, equally poor, were timeworn, one- or two-room log cabins with ample space between the logs and flooring and around the doors and windows to allow the air to enter freely; some were new shanties with one small window or perhaps with none at all. The old log houses, though often picturesque, were commonly far from desirable habitations. In many the chinking had fallen from the cracks, the floor was sagging, and the doors and windows were loose, so that at a dozen or more places the cold air had free access.

Only 3 of the 123 houses visited had a foundation; 37 were built on high, uninclosed piles, and 81 were placed either directly on the ground or on low piles or blocks with the space between the floor and the ground boarded up. Wide spaces were usually left between the boards. Only 27 houses had moderately close-fitting doors and windows. Broken window panes, unreplaced or stuffed with rags or covered with pasteboard, were common. Only 45 houses had at least one room that was plastered or ceiled. The kitchen was usually the coldest room in the house, being frequently little better than a shed. The mild climate made these conditions less serious than they would otherwise have been, but even so the majority of the children studied were living in houses that did not adequately afford protection from the weather.

A few modest but comfortable homes were found in the community. Several new log houses and some older ones that had been kept in good repair, together with a very small number of clapboarded, ceiled, or plastered frame houses, were adequate and comfortable dwellings.

In view of the poor construction of many of the houses, their heating was a problem. A fireplace with its open fire of logs added much to comfort and cheerfulness, but even a rousing fire on the hearth failed utterly to warm a house so open as were many of those visited. A small stove was not much more effectual. Of the 123 houses 63 were heated by fireplaces, 51 by stoves, and 7 had both a stove and a fireplace. The cooking in the homes was usually done on a kitchen stove, though many families also utilized the fireplace to some extent for cooking.

## SANITATION.

The method of disposal of human waste in the district studied was most insanitary. Considerably over half the families, 56 per

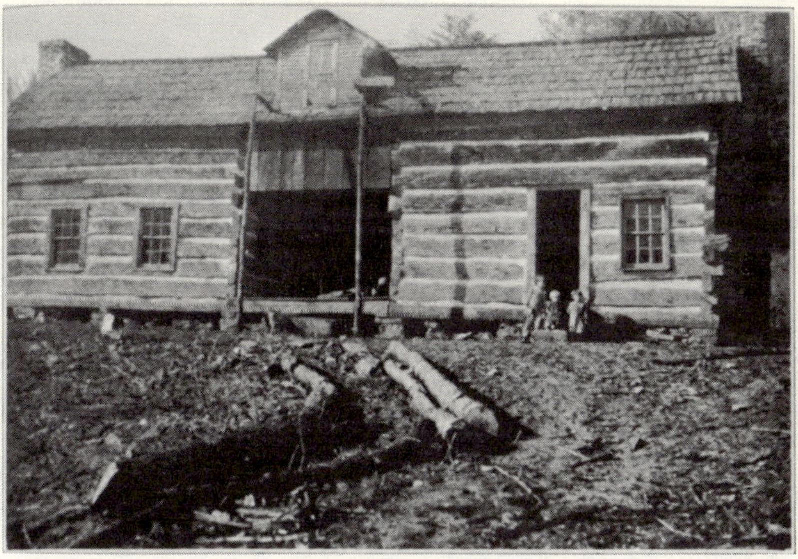

A NEW LOG HOUSE OF BETTER TYPE.

Note the base.

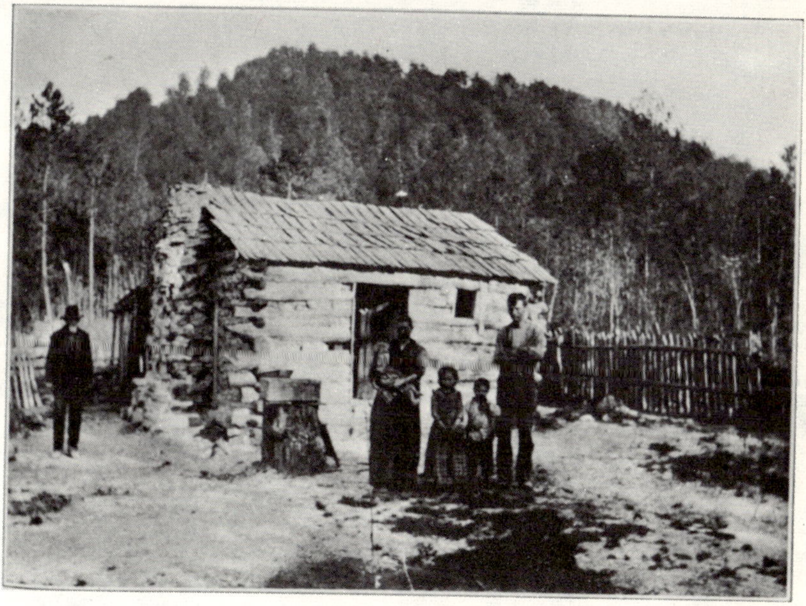

A TYPICAL CABIN.

cent, had no toilet of any kind, but used the barn, the chicken house, the yard, or the woods. Only one family had a water-flushed toilet; 51 had some kind of a yard privy. More than one of these privies, however, because of broken walls or missing doors failed to offer even privacy, and others were distinctly insanitary, because easily accessible to animals and flies. The general attitude seemed to be that a privy was nonessential.

## WATER SUPPLY.

More than half the families, 55 per cent, secured water from a spring, a stream—the "branch" it was usually termed—an open well, or some other unprotected source. The remainder obtained their supply from either a drilled well or a hydrant. Although undoubtedly the drilled well was a much safer source than the open well or the stream, the type used in this section appeared less safe than the term would imply. The well was not fitted with a tight cover nor the water drawn by a pump. Instead, the pipe, five or six inches in diameter, extended above the surface of the ground and was left open at the top. The water, which could be seen in the pipe a few feet below ground level, was drawn by means of a small bucket fitting into the pipe. The bucket hung by the well or sat on the ground when not in use. This, together with the fact that the pipe was uncovered, made contamination possible, though certainly less probable than in water secured from the other sources.

## AVAILABLE FOOD SUPPLY.

The chief concern of this survey was to secure all the information possible regarding the diet of the children. In order to do this in a rural area, it was necessary to investigate the source of supply, since the kind, amount, and variety of the children's food depend upon the food supply and food habits of the family. In addition, therefore, to learning the habits of the individual child with reference to diet, a detailed study was made of the foods which were grown or purchased for family use. Thus information was obtained concerning the production, preservation, and use of milk, butter, eggs, fruit, vegetables, cereals, breads, and meat—the chief foods in any dietary.

### Cereals and Bread.

Since corn was practically the only grain crop in the area, it was not surprising to find corn meal universally used for food. Most farmers took their corn to a local mill and had the whole grain ground into meal. This meal contained the bran layer and the germ, as well as the starchy endosperm—the part from which the usual market product is made. Eighty-six families, representing 72 per cent of the children, used whole corn meal exclusively; 34 families purchased their meal at the store and so obtained only the bolted meal, while 3 families used some of both kinds. There can be no doubt of the distinct superiority of the whole meal over the bolted kind, especially if it is used as the main constituent of a rather restricted diet; most of the mineral matter of the grain as well as the vitamines which protect the body against the so-called deficiency diseases are contained in the bran and germ.

Wheat flour to some extent in all the homes supplemented corn meal. This flour was almost always the patent, highly milled variety, 118 families using only that made from bolted wheat. The remaining 5 families used some whole wheat or graham flour in addition. Oatmeal was used to a greater or less extent by 85 families.

Corn bread was the most common type of bread. Biscuits, however, occupied a place in the dietary second only to that of corn bread. Many families had biscuits for breakfast and corn bread for the other two meals, and frequently both were served at the same meal. A company meal, it seemed, demanded both, for apologies were offered when corn bread without biscuits was set before a guest. Yeast bread—or "light bread," as it is usually called—occupied a very minor place in the dietaries of the families. In 85 homes, 69 per cent, corn bread and biscuits were used exclusively; only 37 families reported using any light bread. Some families who lived nearer town than the others bought light bread frequently, but in most homes it was purchased only on rare occasions. A single exception to the general practice was found in a home where the mother made light bread regularly and used corn bread and biscuits for occasional variation. The general relative use of these breads was strikingly shown by the local application of the term "bread," which, it was soon discovered, always referred to corn bread.

This bread was usually made of corn meal, buttermilk, soda, and salt. Water was substituted for part of the milk if the milk supply was short. The bread was either baked in a sheet or fried in a skillet.

The biscuits observed in the school lunches and in the homes were usually large, underdone, and frequently yellow from excess of soda, and they were as a rule less palatable than the corn bread. They were most often made with soda and buttermilk, with water added if the amount of milk was insufficient.

**Meat.**

Meat was commonly regarded as a necessity and eaten at every meal. It was the custom for a farmer to keep at least one hog to fatten during the summer and kill in the fall. In general, it might be said that the more prosperous the farmer the more hogs he killed. For example, 6 of the 9 families who killed five or more hogs belonged to the A income group, 2 to the B group, and 1 to the C group; while of the 27 families who killed but one hog, 12 were of the C group, 8 of the B group, and but 1 of the A group.

A little more than 80 per cent of the families killed at least a part of their own meat. Of these 101 families, 28 killed all they used, while 73 bought some meat to supplement their own. Twenty-one families purchased all their meat.

In the majority of families only salt meat was eaten, except during a short period immediately following butchering. The weather was not uniformly cold enough to make preservation by freezing practicable, and so the meat had to be preserved by means of salt. In addition to this, the meat which was purchased when the home supply gave out was usually salt.

In the section studied, hog killing was done in the late fall. The meat was usually salted on the day of the killing or very shortly afterwards. It was spoken of as fresh,[9] however, for some time after it had been laid down in salt. This study was made during "hog-killin'" time, and so the majority of the families were having "fresh hog meat" three times a day.

It may readily be seen that a family which depended entirely upon its own butchering had to eat salt meat most of the time. This meat was bound to be fat salt "middlings" (the side meat) for a considerable part of the year; the fresh meat—ribs, backbones, and sausage—was eaten first, then the hams and shoulders, and lastly the middlings. When the middlings gave out more was purchased.

Some families bought fresh meat in small amounts the year round, and most of them occasionally killed chickens, though these were much less commonly used than might be expected in a farming community.

In order, in the discussion of the diet, to distinguish between families living almost entirely on salt meat and those having appreciable amounts of fresh meat with some regularity, the families have been separated into two groups—those having a salt meat diet for as much as eight months of the year and those having fresh meat as often as weekly for more than four months, no matter whether the meat was beef, pork, chicken, or rabbit. It will be seen, therefore, that even the families classed as "fresh meat users" were not necessarily having any large amount of such meat. Yet only 24 per cent of the families could qualify for this group, while 60 per cent be-

---

[9] The use of this term varied among the families. Some called meat fresh until it was hung up to dry, after it had been in salt two, three, or even six weeks; others, only while it had not yet absorbed enough salt to give it a salty taste, at the most two or three weeks after salting.

longed definitely in the "salt meat group." Sufficient data to classify the remainder were not obtained.

These facts are significant from the dietary standpoint. Although meat was served the year round three times a day, it consisted to such an extent of fat salt middlings that it made on the whole a questionable addition to the protein of the diet, the chief requisite that meat is supposed to supply. It is probable, moreover, that the vitamines which are present in fresh lean meat to a certain extent, and which are capable of protecting the body against certain nutritional disorders, were almost if not completely destroyed by the salting process. On the whole, therefore, the only food requirement which the meat supply in this section could be expected to contribute was that of energy.

**Vegetables.**

Every family visited except two had a garden. The yield of vegetables, however, was very limited in variety and amount. The vegetables most commonly raised were beans, white potatoes, tomatoes, and onions; next to these came corn, cabbage, lettuce, peas, beets, sweet potatoes, and squash, or pumpkin; much less common were cucumbers, radishes, turnips, parsnips, and rhubarb. Carrots, cauliflower, asparagus, and celery were almost unknown; while greens, such as chard, collards, and spinach—with the exception of mustard, which six families reported raising for greens—were not grown at all.

The list of vegetables raised, while it shows restricted variety, makes the situation as regards vegetables appear much better than it really was; the amounts of all but a few of those raised were commonly found to be so small as to be almost negligible. In many cases the garden might have been disregarded because of the small contribution it made to the family's food. Sometimes it "burned out" so early in the summer that it furnished nothing at all. "Our ground's plumb wore out," commented one woman in explanation of their garden's failure. Even in homes where gardens did better, not more than a few vegetables were raised in any amount.

Of the 123 families, only 13 reported having any vegetables to sell. This does not necessarily signify that even these families had an abundant crop; more probably it indicates a need for ready money in the fall. To secure money at that season a few beans or potatoes were sold, though to do so might mean the buying of these same foods in late winter or spring at a higher price.

Comparatively few vegetables were stored for the winter. Eight families stored no vegetables at all; 28 families stored one or two; and 87 families a little more than two, but not many. More than four-fifths of the families canned some tomatoes; one-half of them stored white potatoes; somewhat more than three-fifths stored dry beans; only one-third stored cabbages and onions, and fewer than this, beets or turnips.

Again it must be stated that this list, meager as it is for a farming community, makes the situation appear much better than the reality. One or two dozen cans of tomatoes might be all that a family had, or a bushel or two of potatoes and a few beans might be the winter supply. It was common to find that the few vegetables which had been stored were already used by the end of January. During the remainder of the winter the family must either buy more or go without. Except for beans, which the family usually purchased, if possible, when its own supply was exhausted, to go without was the general custom.

It is thus seen that beans were the principal winter vegetable. In some families they were practically the only vegetable for the greater part of the year. Some had beans every day—much as people in other sections have potatoes—and it was an exceptional family that did not cook them at least as often as twice a week. To use local terminology, only two kinds appeared to be used, "soup beans" and "shuck beans." The former term is used to designate any kind of dry shelled beans—the navy bean, the red kidney, or any other variety. The navy bean is the one most raised, though specialists say that the red kidney bean would probably do much better. The "shuck" beans are the same beans dried with the shells on—string beans they are in reality—though the seeds are much larger than it is usual to let them become. The beans may be broken into pieces and dried, but more often they are strung on a thread and hung to dry in the kitchen. They are cooked with pork for a long time until both pod and seeds are tender.

**Fruit.**

In spite of the claim of agricultural specialists that this section is well adapted to fruit culture, very little fruit is grown. Fully 80 per cent of the families visited were found to raise no fruit at all, while the remaining 25 families raised a small number of apples or peaches, or, in a few cases, both.

This scarcity of orchard fruit was somewhat alleviated by the fact that large quantities of blackberries grow wild in the mountains and may be had for the picking. As proof of their abundance may be cited the record of three women who were out but "four hours and picked 14 gallons." Every family in the section was found to depend on wild blackberries to add fresh fruit to the diet. The blackberry season, however, lasts not more than a few weeks at the best, and so this fruit, which was the only one available in a large percentage of the homes, could influence the diet for but a short period unless it was canned. Practically every family (95 per cent), however, canned or preserved some blackberries for the winter, though in many cases the amount put up was known to be very small.

The extent to which these families depended on blackberries for fruit is further shown by the fact that no other fruit was canned by nearly two-thirds of them (63 per cent). Somewhat less than a third (32 per cent) put up a few apples or peaches in addition, while six families canned or preserved no fruit at all, not even blackberries.

It may readily be seen that fruit, either fresh or preserved, was far from being a daily article of diet. Indeed it appears certain that a considerable number of families must have been without fruit of any kind for more than half the year—from the time the few canned blackberries gave out (in October, November, or December) until the next blackberry season the following summer.

**Eggs.**

In spite of the fact that 85 per cent of the families kept chickens, eggs were comparatively little used throughout the section. This was accounted for, in part, by the small production. The number of hens kept by a family was ordinarily not large, and the yield of eggs was unusually small. At the time this study was made, in late fall and early winter, 105 families were keeping a total of 3,004 hens, and the total daily yield of eggs was 215. The yield was not high, moreover, even in the most productive season of the year.

The explanation of the poor yield lay in the lack of care which was given the hens. Very poor shelter or none at all, even during the winter, was the usual lot of a flock, and their food was quite on a par with their housing. They ran wild the year round, and received practically no food but corn.

The few eggs produced were usually sold. "We can't eat eggs when every egg is worth 5 cents!" exclaimed one woman, voicing thereby the common sentiment. The daily consumption of eggs at the time of this study averaged less than one per family.

**Sorghum.**

In the community studied farmers customarily either raised enough sorghum for their own use or purchased it from their neighbors. Butter and "lasses," as the sorghum was locally called, was a favorite combination. The butter was stirred into the sorghum and the mixture eaten with biscuit. Children sometimes carried glasses of it in their school lunches. Sorghum appeared to be used somewhat less widely than usual during the year this study was made, due probably, at least in part, to its higher price. Many families were using a commercial corn sirup instead.

**Milk and Butter.**

Milk, throughout the area studied, was regarded as a necessity, and keeping a cow, if it could be afforded, was taken as a matter of course. Eighty per cent of the families had one or more cows at the time of the study. Of the 24 families without them, 9 were purchasing a regular and apparently adequate amount of milk, 4 were buying an irregular or an inadequate supply, while 11 families had very little or none.

Fifty-seven of the 99 families keeping one or more cows had no period when they were without milk of their own. Of these families those with more than one cow planned to have them go dry at different times, while the others traded the cow about to go dry for a fresh one.[10] Thirty-four families, when the cow was dry, either bought milk or received it as a gift from neighbors. The milk secured was usually buttermilk and varied in amount and regularity. Eight families went without milk when their own cows furnished none.

Only one family in the whole district used condensed milk, and milk powder was unknown. To summarize, 100 families, or 81 per cent, were having a fairly steady milk supply, while 19 per cent either had no milk at all or were without it for considerable periods.

In many places milk figures little in the diet of children and perhaps not at all in the diet of adults. In this community, on the contrary, it was regarded as a staple article of diet and whenever obtainable, was drunk regularly by children and adults alike. When it was plentiful great pitchers of it were put on the table at every meal. "Milk," said one mother, "is what I've raised my family on. My family here uses buttermilk like it was water." A number of families testified to using milk "for water;" and many a strong man was pointed out proudly as having been reared on milk and corn bread.

Milk was alike the best feature of the better diets and the salvation of many of the poorer ones. Indeed, as later will be more fully apparent, it was the one redeeming feature of the whole food situation.

Seventy-one per cent of the families visited were accustomed to making all their own butter. Of the remainder, 13 families bought all they used, 4 supplemented their home supply by purchase, and 18 (15 per cent) used no butter. The amount that was made was frequently inadequate and the making of butter was necessarily discontinued in many homes during the period of decreasing milk supply as well as during the time when the cow was dry. At such times the families who depended entirely on their home supply of butter

[10] There were traders in this section who made a regular business of buying up dry cows and selling them at a higher price when they became fresh.

substituted drippings. Some families, to be sure, that had more than one cow could manage so that their own supply never failed. It is certain that a far larger number than the 15 per cent who did not use butter at all must have had a very limited supply or lacked this food entirely during an appreciable part of the year.

Absence of butter from the diet is of small consequence, providing plenty of whole milk is used, as it customarily was in the homes of this section whenever available. But, unfortunately, when the milk supply diminished or failed entirely and the family could no longer make butter, it was skim milk or buttermilk rather than whole milk which was usually secured. Thus the families who were most in need of butter, those using skim milk, were the ones without it, while the families having plenty of whole milk were also those who had butter.

**Adequacy of food supply.**

It has been seen that the diet of families in this section was much restricted. Vegetables and fruits, which are usually relied upon to lend variety and flavor to the diet, were little used, while even potatoes, a staple food, did not figure very largely in the dietary. Fresh meat, eggs, and butter, all of which add much in the way of flavor and general palatability as well as food value, had but limited use. The diet may indeed be described as one of corn bread, milk, and fat salt meat, while in some diets milk was lacking or limited in amount during at least a part of the year. Adding to this list beans, sorghum, and biscuits, with butter when the cow was fresh, and blackberries and a few vegetables for a short season, there results the usual diet at its best. Only a limited number of families fared better than this, their supply of milk and butter being more plentiful, fresh meat bought fairly frequently, and vegetables and fruit used more extensively.

So restricted a diet is unquestionably monotonous. A hopelessly monotonous diet, however, may be a perfectly adequate one if it is capable of supplying all the body's needs. The diet of corn bread and milk on which a considerable number of mothers stated they had reared their families is probably capable of barely meeting all the needs of the body, provided that the milk is whole and is taken in liberal amounts, and provided that the corn meal is made from the whole grain. Both of these conditions were often met in the diets studied in this district.

To suggest the advisability of living on a diet of these two foods is not for a moment, of course, intended. It can not be doubted that the addition of fruits and vegetables would render such a diet more surely safe as well as distinctly more palatable. Nevertheless the fact remains that it would be difficult to find two other foods which together would be better able to provide an adequate diet. Any other whole cereal, or potatoes, might take the place of the corn meal, but if the milk is dropped out, decreased in amount, or changed to skim milk or buttermilk, as was all too frequently done in this section, the effect is disastrous.

The corn-bread and fat-meat diet which was the common one when milk was omitted is deficient in calcium, adequate protein, and vitamine content. Add any one or more of the foods used in the community—beans, biscuits, sorghum, potatoes, sweet potatoes, or fresh meat—and though the diet is bettered it still remains inadequate in some respect, notably in calcium and in the fat-soluble vitamine. Restore milk and all the deficiencies are covered. Small wonder, then, that milk is called a "protective" food. It is veritably the salvation of the diets of this community.

## THE DIET OF THE CHILDREN.

In the discussion of the family food supply, the possibilities for the children's diet in the families studied have to no small extent been indicated. Diet is of such importance in relation to nutrition, however, that an effort was made to secure more detailed information concerning the feeding of the children between 2 and 11 years of age. The actual diet of a child on the day preceding the interview was learned,[11] and to supplement this information his food habits were ascertained—the amount of milk he drank; the frequency with which he ate fruits, vegetables, meat, and eggs; his likes and dislikes for important foods; his custom with reference to eating between meals; his indulgence in candy and other sweets: and his use of coffee and tea. As a result a fairly clear picture of the child's dietary was obtained. and what is believed to be a tolerably safe judgment regarding its adequacy was in most cases possible.

The feeding of the children during the period of infancy will first be discussed, after which consideration will be given to the use of the different classes of food and the adequacy of the diets as a whole.

### INFANT FEEDING.

No study of the factors responsible for a child's nutritive condition would be complete without some inquiry as to his care and feeding during infancy. In this survey a detailed study was impossible, but a few important questions were included in the schedule. Information was secured as to whether or not a child was breast fed, the age at which he was weaned, and the time at which he was given solid food.

**Breast feeding.**

Practically all the children in the survey had the very distinct advantage of having been breast fed; 221, or 86 per cent, were reported to have been nursed for 6 months or longer, 4 less than this time, and only 9 had never been breast fed. For 22 children, no reply as to infant feeding was obtained. It was indeed fortunate that so many had had the benefit of breast feeding, for a breast-fed child has not only a better chance of living beyond infancy but can withstand much more in the way of unwise care and feeding than can an artificially fed child.

---

[11] If the diet on the day preceding varied from the ordinary one, a more typical day's diet was ascertained instead.

**Age of weaning and age at which solid food was given.**

Not only was breast feeding common but prolonged nursing was not at all unusual. Of the 221 children who were nursed for six months or longer only 22—10 per cent—were weaned before they were a year old. About half were weaned when they were between 1 year and 18 months of age and 44 per cent were nursed for 18 months or longer. Indeed, more than a fourth were not weaned until the age of 24 months or even later.

The prevalence of this custom of late weaning would be of greater significance had the children received no other food than breast milk before weaning. It was a common practice, however, to give tastes of food to very young babies. Thirty-four children (13 per cent) were given solid food before they were 1 month old, and fully two-thirds of the children were receiving it when they reached the age of 6 months. By solid food is meant food from the family table. The common belief and practice in respect to early feeding was probably summed up by the mother who stated that at about one month she began giving her babies " mighty nigh anything " that was soft, and at 5 months the whole family diet, because " a great big baby 5 months old can eat anything."

The feeding of babies, as the foregoing discussion indicates, was rarely according to plan, but followed rather the line of least resistance. A baby was nursed because it was the custom; he was taken to the table in his mother's arms and given tastes of whatever the mother ate; he was nursed whenever he cried; and he weaned himself when he grew big enough to prefer other food to breast milk or when another baby had usurped his place.

## MILK.

Where the family food supply is as limited as in the locality studied the rôle which is played by milk becomes a doubly important one. Especial effort was therefore made to gather information regarding its use by the children. The amount of the family supply, taken in connection with the number in the family, afforded some indication of the amount available for each child, but further effort was made to learn how much each child consumed. The daily amount was usually reported by the mother as so many " cups." Since a " cup " might hold from a fourth to a half of a pint, the agent asked to see the cup which the child used and then approximated the amount. Inquiry was also made regarding frequently used foods containing milk, such as corn bread and milk gravy. From the amount consumed by the entire family, the number in the family, the amount which was taken as a beverage by the child, and the amount consumed in other food, a conservative estimate of the total amount of milk consumed by the child was made.

On the basis described above, it was judged that nearly three-fourths of the children, 72 per cent, consumed at least a pint of milk daily, the amount commonly regarded as the minimum for children of the ages covered by the study. The majority in this group, 57 per cent, had daily as much as one and one-half pints, a quart, or even more. Eighteen children were receiving well over a quart of milk a day, some of them nearly 2 quarts.

Not all were so fortunate, however; 63, or 25 per cent, of the children fell below the standard of a pint a day, and 24 of these, or 9 per cent of the total, had no milk at all—a serious situation for any children but doubly so for those in this section where the diet was so restricted in other respects.

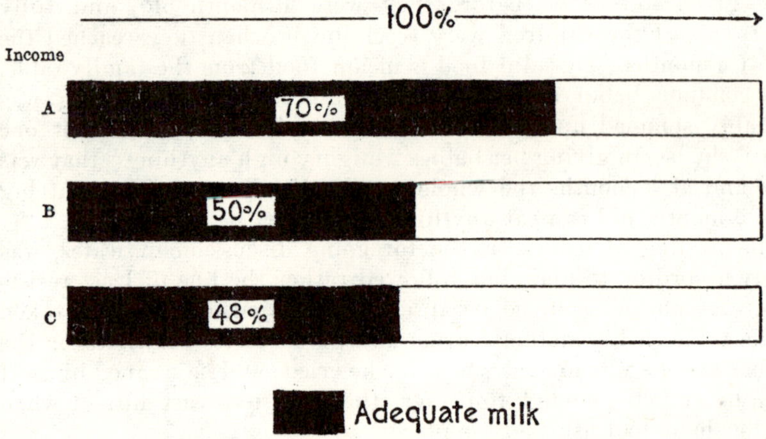


CHART II.—Adequate use of milk in relation to income.

The failure of these children to have sufficient milk was evidently not to any large extent the result of dislike for it, since only 16 children, or 6 per cent, were said not to care for milk, while a fourth of the children were getting less than the minimum amount. That milk was so generally liked by the children was probably due, in part, to the monotonous diet common in the community, and to the absence of highly flavored foods which tempt the appetite and make a bland, mild-flavored food like milk unpalatable. The fact that milk drinking by old and young was a community custom undoubtedly helped also.

Chart II shows how the proportion of children whose milk supply was adequate varied in the different income groups. Seventy per cent of the children in families with A incomes—the highest income group—had an adequate supply, and only about 50 per cent in the B or C groups.

A child's physicial condition, however, depends not only on his present use of milk but on what he has had throughout his life. An effort was made, therefore, to secure for each child as complete a milk history as possible. In the belief that sufficient data were thus obtained to warrant forming a judgment as to whether or not a child had an adequate milk supply for practically all his life, the children have been classified as follows:

Class A: Those who undoubtedly had always had an adequate supply of milk.

Class B: Those who had experienced periods of ample and of scant supply, or children the adequacy of whose milk supply was doubtful.

Class C: Those who undoubtedly had not had an adequate supply.

More than half the children, 52 per cent, were considered as belonging in class A; nearly a third, or 31 per cent, were placed in class B; and about one-eighth, or 17 per cent, in class C.

### EGGS.

Since eggs were not plentiful in this community they could not figure very largely in the diet of the children. Even during the period of maximum yield only 159 children, 62 per cent, had eggs twice a week or oftener—with sufficient frequency, that is, to influence their diet to any extent. Of the remainder, 24 were given an egg about once a week, 7 about once in two weeks—or even less frequently—and 64, or 25 per cent, had no eggs at all.

In the winter eggs were practically never eaten; 208 children, or 81 per cent, did not have any during that period; 7 had them as rarely as once in two weeks; only 17, about weekly; and only 23, or 9 per cent, twice a week or oftener.

Occasionally a mother said her child did not eat eggs because he disliked them, or because they disagreed with him. But usually the reason for the infrequency of eggs in the diet seemed to be that they were regarded as money.

### VEGETABLES.

Vegetables other than beans did not figure largely in the family food supply and hence played but small part in the diet of the children. During the very short time the gardens produced, nearly all the children had access to fresh vegetables and ate them almost daily, but throughout the remainder of the year there was little opportunity for any variety. True, during the winter two-fifths of the children, 41 per cent, were reported to have some kind of vegetable as often as five or six times a week; a somewhat larger number, 47 per cent, as often as two, three or four times a week; and only 27 children, or 10 per cent, ate no vegetables at all. But if it is recalled how few vegetables were raised, how short the garden period was, what limited amounts were canned or stored, and how restricted the purchase of them was, practically the only vegetable purchased being beans, it is clear that beans were often of necessity the only vegetable the children had during the winter and until the next garden season.

Children apparently failed to eat vegetables not because of distaste for them but rather because of the meagerness of the supply; 214 children, 84 per cent, were reported as eating and liking all the kinds they had had opportunity to try, and more than half the remainder, 22, were said to like all but one. It would appear that, on the whole, they ate willingly whatever was offered them.

## FRUIT.

Plenty of fruit is commonly regarded as essential in the diet of children and fruit of some kind at least once a day is practically always considered a minimum requirement. Only 35 children included in this study, 14 per cent, customarily had fruit every day; 80 children, 31 per cent, had it several times a week; and more than half, 55 per cent, had little or none.

Fifty-four per cent of the children almost never had any other fruit than wild blackberries. The remainder occasionally had in addition an orange or a few canned or dried apples. A very limited number of those having fruit every day were known to be receiving a moderate variety.

## MEAT.

Although meat was usually served three times a day in the community studied, the children did not necessarily eat it at every meal. The figures show that 94 children, or 37 per cent, were eating meat two or three times a day; 102, or 40 per cent, were eating it once a day; while 58 children, 23 per cent, ate it less frequently than daily and six of these ate no meat.

Although these figures seem to show that the children's meat consumption was rather high and that, therefore, they were securing a liberal supply of protein, this was not the case. During "hog-killin' time," to be sure—the period during which the study was made—many children were having fresh meat with a fair proportion of lean in it three times a day. One could tell which families had butchered by observing which children had fresh hog meat in their dinner pails at school. This period lasted but a short time. Considerably more than half the children were known to belong to families in which the meat supply was practically all salt middlings and in the families of most of the remainder fresh lean meat was by no means common. If, as was true in many cases, the children had no other lean than the "little lean streak" in the middlings they could not be regarded as securing much protein even though they ate a "streak" or two of lean at each meal. Meat therefore made on the whole but a negligible contribution to the protein of the children's diets. With eggs little used, it may be seen that milk was the only food which could be relied upon to supply the needed animal protein.

### BREAD AND CEREALS.

Biscuits made of bolted white flour and corn bread made in the majority of cases out of whole corn meal were the only bread eaten by 70 per cent of the children (179). The remainder had some yeast bread in addition, though usually as a rare treat rather than as a customary part of the diet. Only one child included in the study had light bread most of the time.

### CANDY.

The candy habit, though not so extreme as among city children, was still a problem with which to reckon. Only 47, or 18 per cent, of the children had no candy at all or had it very infrequently; 17 had it almost daily; 80 (31 per cent) several times a week; and 111 (43 per cent), about once a week. More important than the frequency of eating, however, is the time at which candy is eaten. At the close of a meal a piece or two is probably harmless for children past early childhood, but eaten between meals it certainly can not be so regarded. The candy eaten by the children studied was almost invariably eaten between meals, for only five were said to have it at the end of meals.

The younger the child, the greater the harm which may be done by injudicious eating of unsuitable foods. The candy habit, like the coffee habit, is often started very early in life. Nearly half the children here considered (42 per cent) began eating it before they were six months' old, and all but 32 of the remainder who had candy at all were given it by the time they were 1 year of age. One mother said that long before they could sit alone her children had candy, while another knew that one of her children was given his first candy when only a few days old, for, as she explained, "it was while I was still a layin' in the bed, for I remember callin', 'Maw, do come and see Andrew Jackson eat this stick of candy!'"

The amount of candy consumed and the frequency of eating it probably depended more upon accessibility to a source of supply and financial ability to purchase it than upon any convictions the parents had as to its harmful effects. Thirty-four of the forty-seven children who had little or no candy belonged to families in the C income group. Six children, however, were refused it because their parents felt it was not good for them. The fathers of these children brought from town fruit instead of candy for their treat. Of the 17 children who had candy almost daily 7 passed a store on their way to school; the parents of 2 others were in town every day; and 5 were "only children" and were humored by their parents.

Over two-fifths of the children, as has been noted, had candy about once a week. The father usually went to town on Saturday, and, apparently, did not feel that he had done his duty unless he brought home candy for the children. When the family was large and the income small, the amount each child received was not sufficient to do much harm, though eaten, as it was, between meals; but sometimes the amount was greater and a child was allowed to eat all he wanted, to the extent of interfering with his appetite for wholesome food. "He refuses his grub," observed the mother of a 2-year-old boy, whose father, to use the mother's words, "is a sight to buy candy."

Although undoubtedly some of the children were eating too much candy for their good, the majority probably did not receive enough to do them much harm. It is probable, however, that candy would have been as great a menace to the children's health in the locality studied as it is in any other if stores had been nearer at hand, and the money more easily spared.

## COFFEE AND TEA.

No attempt has been made in this study to distinguish between coffee and tea, as their effect on children is about the same. In the following discussion, therefore, the use of the term "coffee" should be interpreted to mean either coffee or tea. As a matter of fact, it was coffee rather than tea which was generally used.

Coffee drinking was common among the children, though not to the extent that it frequently is among children in other localities. Of the children studied 45 per cent drank neither coffee nor tea. Four of these had previously done so, but had discontinued the habit, one because his mother thought it "made him nervous" and two of the others—in one family—because their mother, who had first given them tastes at about 6 months of age, decided that coffee was affecting one child's kidneys, and so stopped giving it to both. A few mothers were found who had never allowed their children coffee, because they believed it was not good for them, but usually when children did not drink coffee it was because they did not want it.

There were 142 children (55 per cent) who drank coffee, 64 irregularly, but 78, or 30 per cent, at least once a day. This is more significant in view of the fact that the coffee which the children drank was not as a rule diluted with water or a large amount of milk. Of the children who used coffee at all 85 per cent drank it as strong as the adults in their families, and only 13 per cent had it diluted to any extent.

A second consideration which increased the probability of harm was the early age at which coffee drinking started. Of the 124 children whose age at beginning to drink coffee was ascertained all but 9 had started before they were 6 years of age. Sixteen had been given coffee before they were 6 months old and 50 more by the end of their first year. An early start seems to establish the habit; of the children who began at 1 year of age or younger 46, or 70 per cent, were having it daily or oftener. One small boy revealed that coffee had already become a necessity to him by his statement that it "hurt him in the head" if he did not have it.

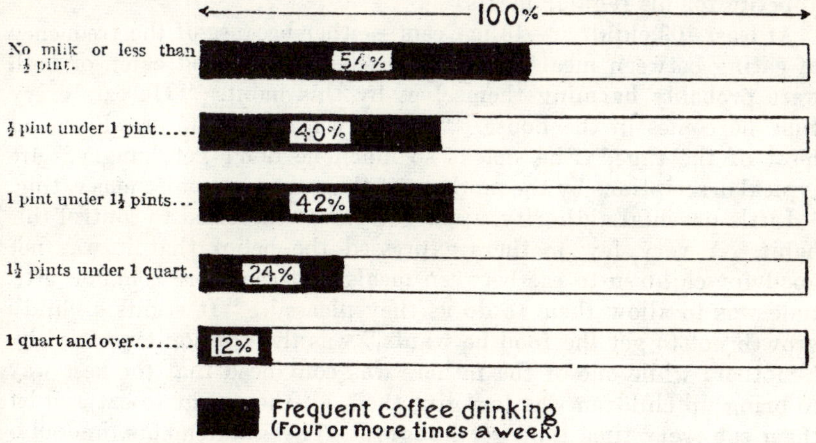


CHART III.—Coffee drinking in relation to the use of milk.

The custom is often begun when the mother takes the baby to the table in her arms and gives him tastes from her cup, just as she gives him tastes of potatoes and other foods. The custom of allowing small children to drink coffee is also in accord with the belief that they are competent to choose their own foods and to eat anything which the rest of the family have.

The consumption of coffee was apparently greater when the use of milk was small. Half the children who drank no milk drank coffee four times a week or oftener, while only 29 per cent of those who drank a pint or more of milk a day drank coffee to this extent. "If he has milk, he doesn't care for coffee," was a comment not infrequently made by mothers. One mother explained that her child drank coffee only when the family were using buttermilk, which the child disliked. Increasing the milk supply in this locality would probably decrease the use of coffee by the children.

## EATING BETWEEN MEALS.

Among the children in the district eating between meals was not so serious a problem as it usually is among city children. Nevertheless, the habit of "piecing" was indulged in to a greater extent than can be considered wise. Only 10 of the children were said not to eat between meals, while 142 habitually did so at least once a day. The seriousness of the habit, however, depends not only upon its frequency but also upon the kind of things which are eaten. Simple foods, like bread and butter, milk, and fruit, eaten as an extra meal after school or as a midmorning lunch, are commonly regarded as harmless and sometimes even as advisable; but promiscuous indulgence in candy or other sweets or haphazard eating of any food, however harmless in itself, is fairly sure to interfere with a child's appetite for his regular meals.

At least 109 children—43 per cent—either because of the frequency of eating between meals or the character of the food eaten or both were probably harming themselves by this habit. "He eats every time he comes in the house." "he carries a piece of bread around most of the time," "he snacks so much he don't get hungry," are typical descriptions by the mothers of this sort of promiscuous eating.

Little parental authority, apparently, was exercised to control this habit. A very few mothers expressed the belief that it was not good for children to eat between meals, but the more common attitude was to allow them to do as they pleased. "It stunts a child's growth not to get the food he wants," was the opinion expressed by a mother; while one of the fathers was convinced that the best way to bring up children was to "give them all they want to eat and let them eat every time they get hungry." These statements, undoubtedly, sum up the current belief and practice in the locality.

## ADEQUACY OF THE DIETS.

Owing to the method employed in this study only a very rough estimate of the quantity of food eaten was obtainable, and it was not possible to secure much definite information concerning the factors which determine the digestibility and assimilation of this food. Hence, in formulating judgments concerning the adequacy of the diets these two factors have been disregarded and the judgment in each case has been based upon whether or not the diet, assuming that enough was eaten and the body was able to utilize it, probably contained the constitutents necessary to nourish the child. It is evident that a judgment thus arrived at does more than justice to the diets, for it is known that an insufficient amount of food and inability to utilize food eaten are two important causes of malnutrition in children; and even with these factors eliminated the evidence still remains that the majority of the children studied were living on diets which were very far from meeting their requirements for growth.

In order to facilitate discussion and make possible the relation of diet to other conditions, the children have been placed in three groups according to the adequacy of their diets. Class A comprises all children whose diets it seemed fairly certain included the constitutents required to nourish the growing body: class C includes

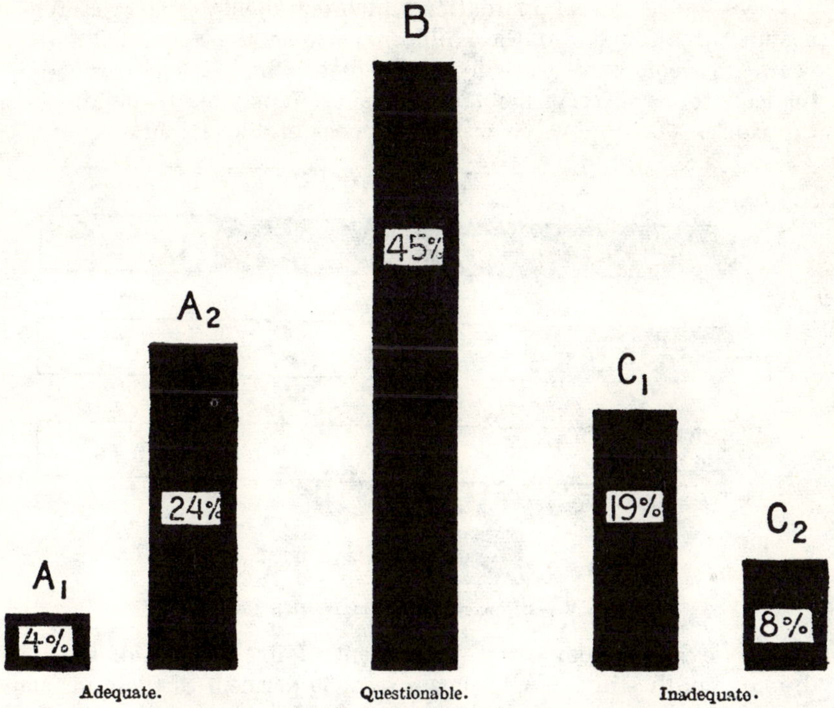


CHART IV.—Per cent of children in each grade of diet.

children whose diets just as certainly failed to meet these needs; and class B includes the children whose diets could not clearly be assigned to class A or class C. Classes A and C have been further subdivided into $A_1$ and $A_2$, $C_1$ and $C_2$, to show gradations of adequacy and inadequacy. The distinction between $A_1$ and $A_2$ diets is merely that the latter consist very largely, if not exclusively, of milk and corn bread made of whole meal, and so are very monotonous; while the former contain in addition fruit, vegetables, and in general a better variety. In the same way $C_1$ diets, though plainly inadequate, may have some redeeming feature, while those designated as $C_2$ are practically "deficiency diets."

According to this classification, 28 per cent, or more than a fourth of the children, had class A diets; 10 of these could be ranked as $A_1$, while 62 were on diets of $A_2$ grade. Nearly the same proportion of the children—27 per cent—were found to be receiving class C diets, 48 of them being considered $C_1$, while the diets of 20 were so exceedingly poor that they were classified as $C_2$. The remainder of the children—45 per cent—were in the group having class B diets.

These figures reveal a situation which is undeniably grave. When nearly three-fourths of the children between the ages of 2 and 11 years in a community are living on diets which are either plainly inadequate or of very doubtful adequacy, it is time to inquire into the cause. That poverty was to a considerable extent responsible

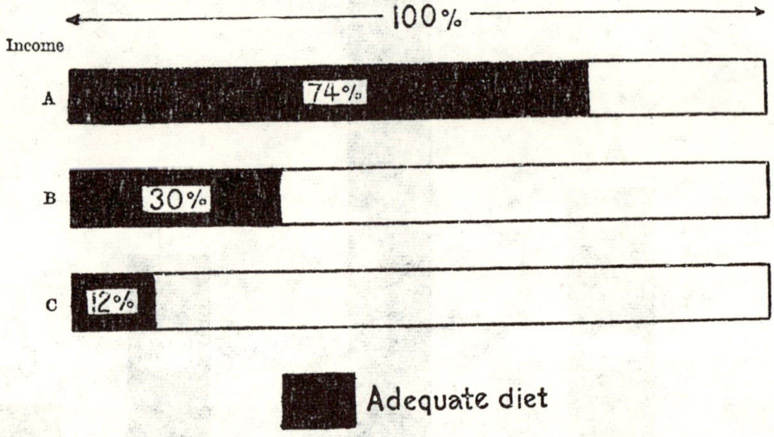


CHART V.—Adequacy of diet in relation to income.

appears evident from Chart V. Seventy-four per cent of the children of families in the A income group, 30 per cent of those in families with B incomes, and but 12 per cent of those in families with C incomes were receiving diets judged as adequate (class A). That ignorance and lack of control were also responsible can not be doubted. Little knowledge existed of children's food needs and little or no control was exercised over their diets. Even though poverty might be relieved, and improvement in the dietary follow, there would still remain the need of education in the food requirements of children.

Milk, as has already been stated, was the salvation of the diets in this section. Of the children having less than a pint of milk a day practically all had an unquestionably inadequate diet. No child having less than a pint of milk daily had a class A diet, and even of those securing this amount only half could be so classified. This indicates what was actually the fact, that the diets on the whole were so lacking in all other important foods that their only chance of attaining adequacy was the inclusion of a liberal amount of milk. With no dependable supply of vegetables, fruit, eggs, butter, or lean

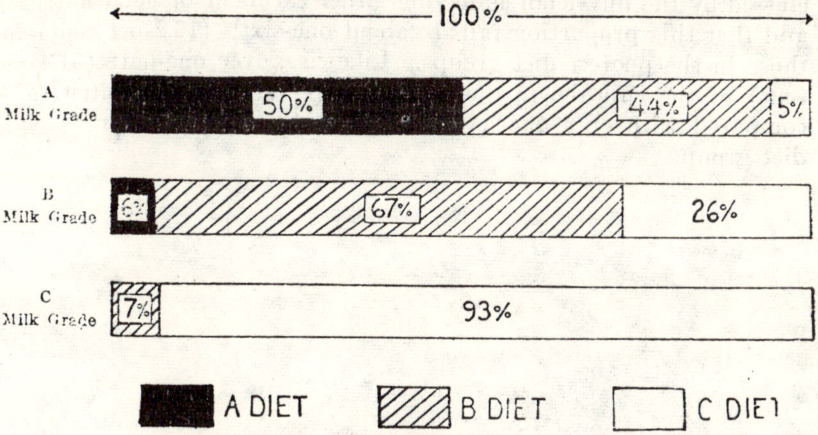


CHART VI.—Grade of diet in relation to use of milk.

meat, the sole food which could be counted on to any extent to furnish vitamines, minerals—particularly calcium—and adequate protein, was milk.

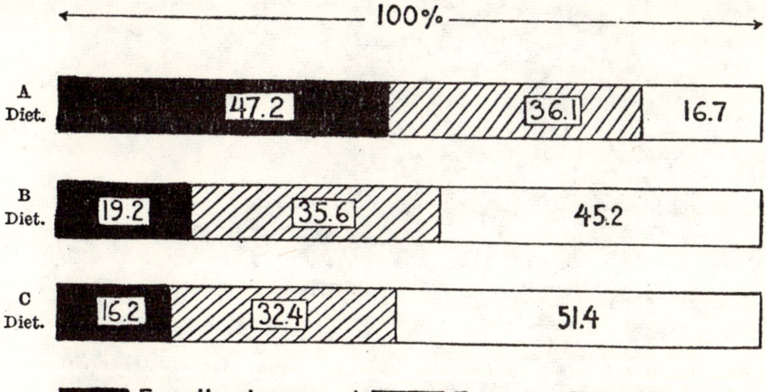


CHART VII.—Grade of nutrition in relation to grade of diet.

## RELATION OF DIET TO NUTRITION.

The nutrition of the children, as determined by the medical examination, has already been discussed,[12] and the children have been classified into five groups—those with excellent, good, fair, poor, and very poor nutrition. It is of interest to compare the distribution

---

[12] See p. 7.

of the children according to the adequacy of their diets with their classification by grades of nutrition. Chart 7 shows that nearly one-half (47.2 per cent) of the children with the best type of diet were classed by the physician as having either excellent or good nutrition and that this proportion falls to about one-sixth (16.2 per cent) for those in the poorest diet groups. Likewise, over one-half (51.4 per cent) of the children in the latter group were in poor nutrition as compared with only one-sixth of those (16.7 per cent) in the best diet group.

## OTHER ITEMS OF CARE AFFECTING THE CHILD'S NUTRITION AND GENERAL WELFARE.

Although the chief emphasis in the survey was placed on the food problem. other factors of hygiene known to affect the nutrition and general well-being of children were likewise studied. These included sleep, fresh air. habits of cleanliness, adequacy of clothing. and conditions of schooling.

### SLEEP.

Aside from diet there is probably no factor which has a greater influence than sleep on the physical well-being of a child. The bedtime and rising time, the number of hours of sleep. and the conditions under which the children slept were therefore ascertained.

Bedtime was found to be, on the whole. commendably early. but because of the early hour of rising the total sleep in the majority of cases was less than the needed amount. Almost two-thirds of the 100 children under 6 years of age were in bed by 7 o'clock—the latest hour usually advised for children of this age—while all but 7 of the remaining third were in bed by 8 o'clock. Unfortunately, however, the time of rising was correspondingly early, since nearly two-thirds of this group were up by 5 o'clock, and 23 of them by 4 o'clock. Only 4 of the children under 6 got up later than 6 o'clock.

It is impossible to state the exact number of hours of sleep which are needed by children of these ages; no doubt the amount varies with different children and with the quality of the sleep. Various authorities advocate different amounts—some, 12 or 13 hours; others, a minimum of 11. The majority of the children under 6 years of age included in the study were found to fall below any of these standards; 65 of the 100 were having less than 11 hours sleep, and 38 were having even less than 10 hours.

The condition was much the same among the children 6 to 11 years of age. The bedtime, as with the younger children, was early, for nearly 90 per cent of them were in bed by 8 o'clock and half by 7 o'clock; but again the early rising hour cut short the amount of sleep. Only 7 of the 156 children in this group got up later than 6 o'clock in the morning, while almost seven-tenths were up by 5 and 29 arose as early as 4. The number of sleeping hours, therefore. in spite of the early bedtime, was less than it should have been. Almost half the children in this group fell below a 10-hour minimum, the least amount estimated as sufficient for children 6 to 11 years of age.

A popular impression exists that sufficient sleep is not a problem for children in rural communities because of the habit of early retiring. This study shows that the "early-to-bed" habit was by no means a sure indication that a child was getting sufficient sleep. In spite of the fact that the large majority of the children in the district studied were going to bed early, more than half—55 per cent—were securing less sleep than the amount required, according to the lowest standards for their respective ages.

It is difficult to understand why little children should be required to get up so early. The explanation seems to be that all the members of the family—adults, children, and babies—follow the same hours, both for retiring and rising. A 7-o'clock bedtime for an adult means that by 3 or 4 o'clock in the morning he is ready to get up. The children may be required to conform to the hours of their elders, or if the whole family sleeps in the same room the children are disturbed when their parents rise, so get up with them.

It is probable that one mother gave the explanation for others as well as herself when she said of her 4-year-old child: "Sometimes he gets up at 3 o'clock when I do; but if he isn't up by 4 o'clock, I wake him, because I want to learn him to be smart." There seemed to be a general belief that a child who was not up to eat breakfast with the family, no matter how young the child nor how early the breakfast hour, would never amount to anything.

A separate bed in a separate room is usually considered the ideal sleeping arrangement for a child. Few of the children in this study were thus provided for. Only 18 of the 256 included slept alone; 106 slept two in a bed; while more than half (132) slept three or four in one bed. Rooms were crowded as well as beds. Only 4 children slept in rooms by themselves, while half (128) shared rooms with four or more other persons. Thirty-six children were sharing rooms with 5 others, 15 with 6, 26 with 7, and 4 with 8.

This does not necessarily indicate crowding as determined by the number of cubic feet of air per person. The room was often large enough to accommodate two or three beds and yet give ample space to be used as a sitting room; not infrequently, however, it was small and distinctly crowded. But disregarding the size of the room altogether, it can not be doubted that the sleeping conditions of many children were not conducive to either their physical or their moral well-being. A child sleeping one of four in a bed, in a room with as many as eight occupants, can scarcely have peaceful, undisturbed rest. Moreover, six, seven, eight, or nine persons—adults, small children, grown boys and girls—can not be thus herded in one sleeping room without endangering moral standards.

In the winter season, when this study was made, 205, or 80 per cent, of the children either removed only a few outer garments at night or slept in all their clothes except their shoes. Only 51 children, or 20 per cent, had some sort of night garment, and but 17 of these customarily removed all their day clothing. Not more than about 7 per cent of all the children, therefore, were sleeping in a suitable night garment with all day clothing removed.

The cold houses, the lack of privacy, and bedding frequently inadequate accounted for this at least in part. "Yes," answered one mother when this question was put to her, "the children sleep in all their clothes. If they didn't they would freeze to death." Not all the failures to attain the standard in this particular can be accounted for on these grounds, however. It was evident that provision of suitable sleeping garments did not enter into the ordinary standard of living of the locality.

## FRESH AIR.

Fresh air in abundance day and night is requisite to the proper care of children. In the district studied it was the requirement most commonly fulfilled, but from compulsion and not from choice. It is probable that most of the children would not have had any fresh air at night if it had not been for poor housing, for 93 per cent of them were sleeping in winter in rooms the windows of which were not opened. On account of the poor construction of houses, however, resulting in cracks in floors and walls and loose-fitting doors and windows, most of the children were receiving abundant fresh air. Only about 6 per cent, in fact, were to be regarded as having insufficient fresh air at night; these children belonged to the families who lived in the better houses and were able to exclude fresh air by keeping windows closed. Improvement in the housing conditions of the community, therefore, sorely needed as it is, must be accompanied by education concerning the value of fresh air.

The greater number of children spent considerable time out of doors, even in the winter. More than three-fourths—79 per cent—averaged at least 2 hours a day in winter and 6 hours daily in summer. Some of the younger children, and older ones who had inadequate clothing, were out of doors less in the wintertime.

## HABITS OF CLEANLINESS.

Somewhat more than half the children, 52 per cent, customarily washed their hands before meals; 47 per cent had neck and ears, face and hands washed daily. In the summer, when many of the children went swimming, bathing was more frequent; in winter, slightly more than three-fifths, 62 per cent, had a weekly bath. Of the remainder, 35 bathed once in two weeks in winter, 28 about once a month, and 33 even less than monthly. Twenty-six did not bathe at all in the wintertime. "No, I don't wash them plumb off nary time, all cold weather," answered one mother. "I wash their feet, neck, and ears once a week." Another mother's answer to the question regarding winter bathing was, "I don't never do that in cold weather! I wash their feet when they are going somewhere." Still another explained that when she had had a fireplace she had made it a rule to bathe the children twice a week, but now that they were living in a "little old open house" it was not easy and they were bathed less frequently.

It is easy to censure a community for upholding no higher standard of personal cleanliness, but in view of the cold houses, the lack of privacy, and all the difficulties involved in carrying and heating water for bathing, that so much was accomplished under such conditions seems surprising.

## CARE OF TEETH.

The children's teeth were very generally neglected. Eighty-two per cent of the children, 211, did not own a toothbrush, and only 15 of the 45 who did, brushed their teeth as frequently as once a day; 29 brushed them irregularly, and one confessed that although he had a brush he never thought to use it. A very few who owned no brushes made some attempt to clean their teeth occasionally in other ways. Three children of one family about weekly used dogwood brushes of their own making; two other children cleaned their teeth with cloths. Such irregular and ineffectual attempts are far from adequate, however, and may for the most part be disregarded. Less than 6 per cent of the children, the 15 who brushed their teeth as often as daily, may be considered as giving their teeth even a minimum of care.

The teeth were found to be in the condition which might be expected from this lack of care. Of the 149 children who were given physical examinations, 82 per cent had conspicuously dirty teeth. The 27 children not so described were chiefly the younger ones whose teeth had not had time to become much coated, and the few who regularly brushed their teeth.

Not only was lack of care shown by dirty teeth, but by decayed teeth as well. Of the children examined, 77.8 per cent were found to have one or more teeth decayed; 31 per cent of those 6 to 11 years of age had one or more permanent teeth in this condition.

## CONDITION OF THE CHILDREN'S BOWELS.

In a consideration of nutrition the condition of the bowels is important. Constipation not only may be the result of an unsuitable diet, but also may operate as a direct cause of undernutrition by decreasing the appetite and the total amount of food eaten.

It is interesting to note that not one mother reported that her child was constipated. Ten children were reported to be somewhat irregular, but 245, or 96 per cent of all the children studied, were, according to their mothers' statements, absolutely regular. The extremely plain diet, which often consisted largely of whole corn meal containing the bran, and was therefore laxative, together with abundant exercise in the open air and the simple, regular habits of living probably helped in no small measure to make constipation uncommon. It is also probable, however, that many mothers in reality knew little about their children's habits in this respect and that children became constipated without the mothers' knowledge and eventually began to feel sick from the effects. Then mothers, for the "sickness," not for constipation, gave some medicine—"black draught," perhaps to correct the evil. While fully 70 per cent of all the children were never given any medicine to assist bowel movement, 69 children—27 per cent—whenever they were sick were given a cathartic.

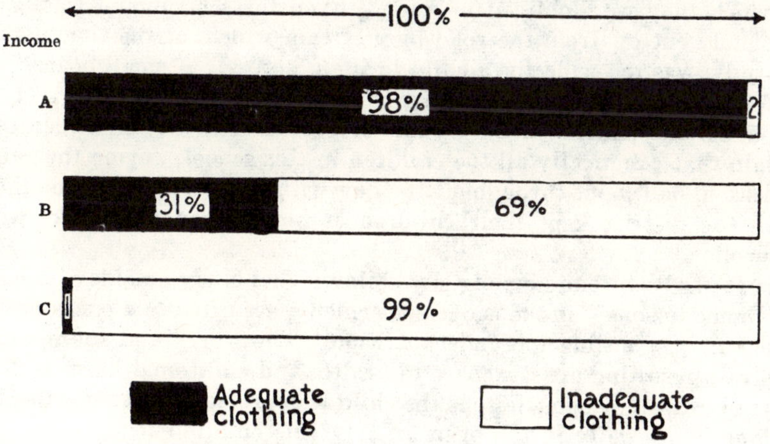


CHART VIII.—Clothing in relation to income.

## CLOTHING.

Inquiries regarding clothing were made to discover whether the children had garments which gave them adequate protection from the weather. Only three-fifths of the children were found to have at least the following: Shoes, an overcoat or other extra wrap, and some kind of winter underwear. Sometimes, however, the garments were so poor and thin that they could not possibly afford much warmth. Only about one-fourth of all the children, 27 per cent, were found to have clothing which could furnish adequate protection from the elements.

That poverty was largely responsible for this situation seems evident from Chart VIII, for it will be noted that almost all the children (98 per cent) in the highest income group had adequate clothing, while practically the whole (99 per cent) of the lowest income group had clothing which was totally inadequate for winter wear.

## SCHOOLING.

The area studied comprised five school districts. Terms were short and attendance poor. Cold weather, inadequate clothing, distance from school, and the bad condition of the roads contributed to this poor attendance.[13] Many children lived a mile or more back in the mountains and the lanes which led to their homes were bad beyond description. It was often literally impossible for a child to trudge a mile or more in the thick, wet clay of the roads. Moreover, the numerous streams were commonly without bridges, and when swollen were too deep for a child to cross on foot.

In one school district the only way for about half the children to get to school was by a road down which for some distance ran a creek, which they were obliged to wade. Even the schoolhouse was completely cut off from the road by a stream which, at the time of the study, was too wide for a child to jump across. A small board or a few stepping stones would have made it possible to cross dry shod, but no one had taken the trouble to provide either. It seemed certain that practically all the children in this school, during the rainy season, had to sit throughout the day with wet feet. Many mothers in the district kept their children at home when the creeks were swollen.

It has been found among city children that study outside of school, "home lessons" and music lessons chiefly, are often to a considerable extent responsible for undernutrition. The worry and the nervous strain resulting are a menace to health, and additional harm is done if by reason of home lessons the child is deprived of his right to play long hours daily in the open air. Of the children included in this investigation, only 45 were doing any studying at home, and these studied voluntarily and for short periods only.

---

[13] The compulsory school attendance law of Kentucky in effect in rural school districts at the time of the study required all children between the ages of 7 and 12 years, inclusive, to be enrolled in and to attend some public or private day or parochial school each school year for the full term of said school, exempting only children taught at home and given equivalent instruction, and those not in proper physical or mental condition to attend school. The penalty for a parent's failure to cause his child to attend school as required by this law was a fine of not less than $5 nor more than $20 for each offense. The law also required that the school term should be not less than six months (120 days).

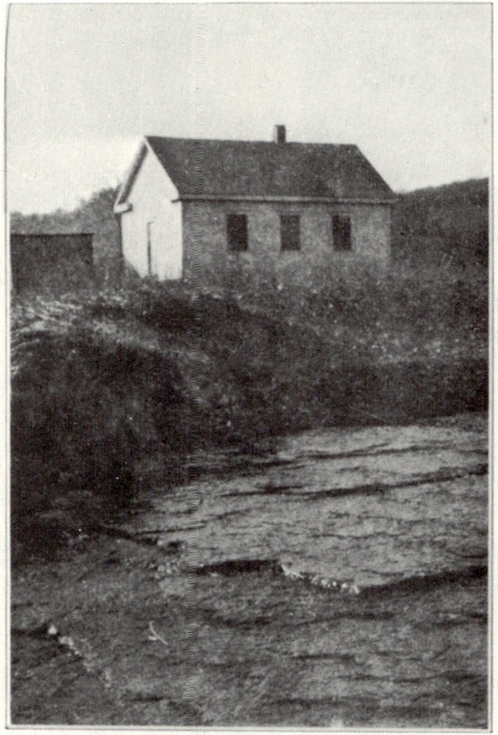

SCHOOL CUT OFF FROM ROAD BY CREEK.

Children must wade this "moat" to get to the school-house.

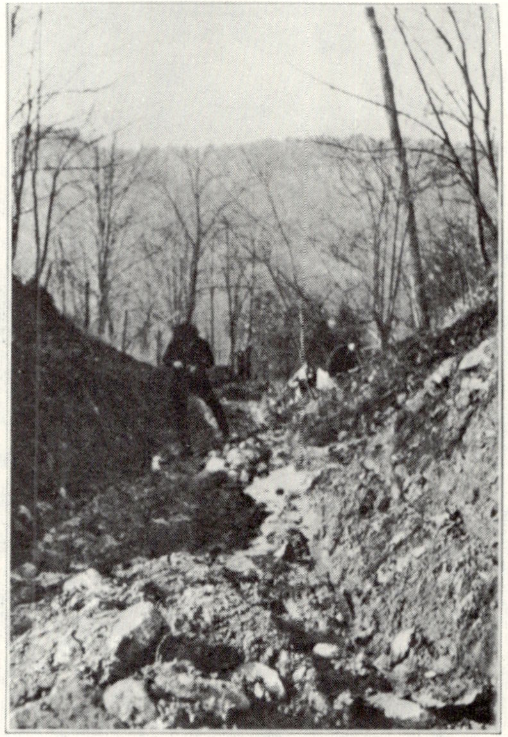

VIEW OF A ROCKY MOUNTAIN ROAD.

The road referred to over which the produce from an adjoining county must be hauled to market.

## SUMMARY AND CONCLUSIONS.

This study of a small mountain section of Kentucky included 123 families in which lived 256 children from 2 to 11 years of age. The heads of households in 103 families were farmers, but only 59 were occupied in farming alone, while 44 supplemented work on their farms by some other occupation.

### PHYSICAL CONDITION OF THE CHILDREN.

A total of 149 children were given physical examinations. Half this number had enlarged or diseased tonsils; more than a fourth showed symptoms of adenoids; over three-fourths had carious teeth. Only 7 per cent of the children were ranked excellent in nutrition; 18 per cent, good; 35 per cent, fair; 34 per cent, poor; and 6 per cent, very poor.

### HOME CONDITIONS.

The income in the homes of 42 children was considered adequate; in the homes of 95, its adequacy was doubtful; 119 children, or 47 per cent, were living in homes clearly incapable of providing the essentials of a simple standard of living. Sanitary facilities were poor; 56 per cent of the families had no toilet. More than half the families (55 per cent) depended for their water supply upon a spring, stream, open well, or other source which might suffer pollution.

The family food supply was restricted both in kind and amount and the family diet was in consequence monotonous and sometimes so limited as not to furnish all the elements necessary. Milk and whole corn meal were the redeeming features of the diet, but in many homes even the supply of milk was too limited, especially at certain periods, to insure an adequate diet, though 80 per cent of all the families kept one or more cows.

### THE DIET AND CARE OF THE CHILDREN.

Only 28 per cent of the children were having a diet which probably included all the constituents necessary to nourish their bodies, provided enough was eaten and the body was able to utilize it. The diets of 27 per cent were clearly inadequate for the needs of growing children. In other words, nearly three-fourths of the children were living on diets of either doubtful adequacy or certain inadequacy.

Fruit and vegetables occupied a minor place in the children's dietary; beans were the predominating vegetable; wild blackberries were practically the only fruit, either fresh or canned, 54 per cent of the children had. Eggs were almost entirely absent from the winter diet and even at the time of greatest yield were eaten by only 62 per cent of the children as often as twice a week. Seventy-seven per cent of the children had meat daily or oftener, but since meat in this community was usually fat salt meat it made a very questionable contribution to the protein in the dietary. It was estimated that 72 per cent of the children had at least a pint of milk daily; 70 per cent had corn bread made of whole corn meal or biscuits made of bolted white flour. Coffee was used by 55 per cent of the children, though only 34 per cent drank it four or more times a week. Eating between meals was indulged in by 43 per cent to such an extent as probably to be harmful.

Of the children in the highest income group, 74 per cent, as compared with only 12 per cent in the lowest, were receiving diets which could be considered adequate. The diet grades corresponded closely to the nutrition grades as revealed by the physical examinations.

Chiefly because of the early rising hour, but 45 per cent of the children were having sufficient hours of sleep. Only a little more than a fourth of the children had clothing which could be considered sufficient to furnish adequate protection from the elements. Care of the teeth was very generally neglected

## POSSIBILITIES OF IMPROVEMENT.

There is urgent need in the community studied for improvement in the conditions affecting the health and welfare of children. In order to better the physical condition of the children, adequate diets, improved housing, more adequate clothing, and higher standards of general hygiene are essential.

If the diet of the children is to be improved, the family food supply must be enlarged. This will involve increase in the amount and quality of milk; improvement of gardens; raising and canning or drying more vegetables; greater utilization of the wild blackberries, until fruit culture can be developed; and increase in the yield of eggs until enough are available both for family consumption and for selling. The use of meat could in many cases be restricted without harming the diet. The use of sorghum and the use of beans, particularly those dried without removing the pods, could well be extended.

Soil improvement and education in better farming methods would improve economic conditions and dietaries. Better housing, more adequate clothing, and generally higher standards of living would follow. Instruction of the mothers and fathers in the health needs and care of children is also essential.

In such a program a county agricultural agent, a county home demonstration agent or nutrition specialist, and a county public health nurse could render valuable service. Education in diet and hygiene through the public school would also be of assistance. At the time of the study the county had an agricultural agent on part time, and much had been accomplished through his efforts. The territory covered was too large, however, and a full-time agent could be employed with advantage.

UNITED STATES DEPARTMENT OF LABOR
FRANCES PERKINS, Secretary

CHILDREN'S BUREAU
GRACE ABBOTT, Chief

# MATERNAL DEATHS

## A BRIEF REPORT OF A STUDY MADE IN 15 STATES

Bureau Publication No. 221

UNITED STATES
GOVERNMENT PRINTING OFFICE
WASHINGTON : 1933

## CONTENTS

CHART 1.—STATES INCLUDED IN MATERNAL-MORTALITY STUDY.

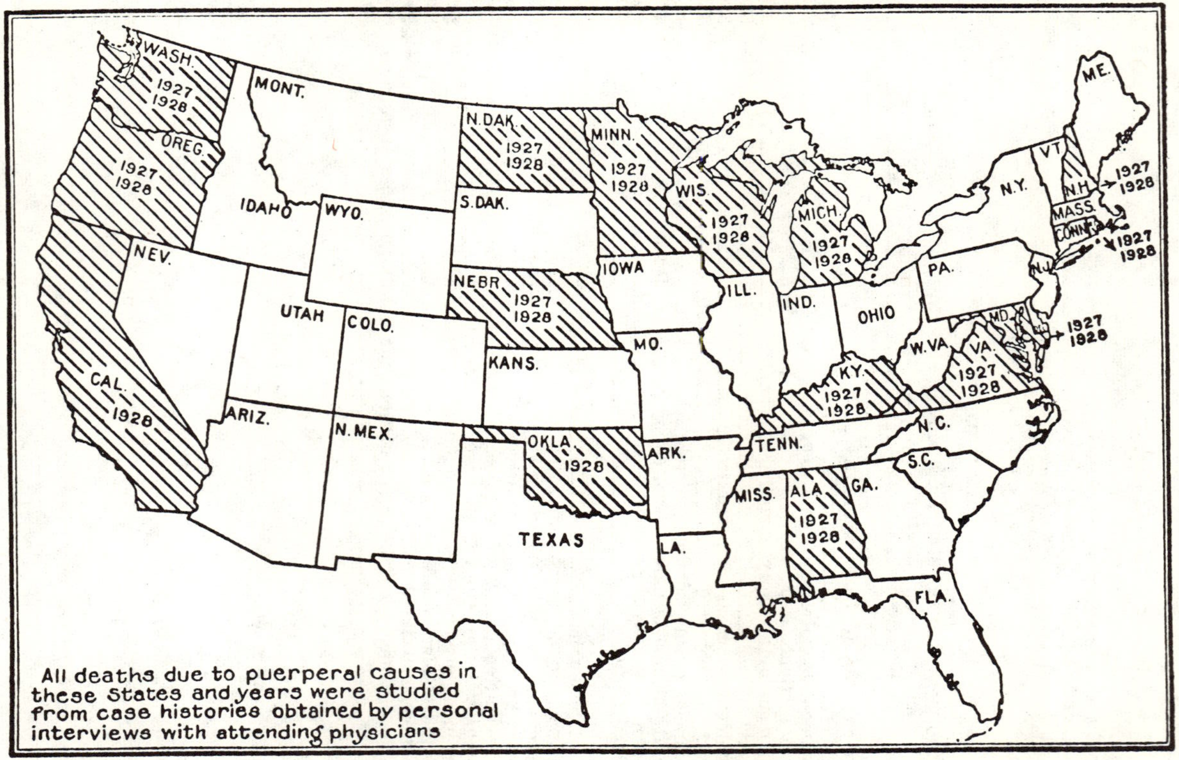

# MATERNAL DEATHS

## SCOPE AND METHOD OF THE STUDY

The maternal mortality rate in this country is generally recognized as high, and it has shown comparatively slight changes over a period of years. Moreover, information hitherto available concerning maternal deaths consisted only of such limited data with regard to all deaths in a given area as are contained in death and birth certificates and more detailed studies of selected groups. The former were not sufficiently detailed nor the latter sufficiently general to give a picture of the conditions contributing to the 16.000 deaths assigned annually in the United States to causes that are associated with pregnancy and childbirth. At the 1926 conference of State directors in charge of the Maternity and Infancy Act, the chairman of the Children's Bureau obstetric advisory committee [1] presented a plan for a comprehensive study of maternal mortality. It was decided to undertake such a study only in States which were included in the birth-registration area and in which both the State board of health and the State medical society made formal request for it. The United States Children's Bureau undertook to prepare, with the assistance of its obstetric advisory committee, a schedule for use in all the States studied, and to report the findings.[2] In the preparation of the schedule standards of prenatal care previously set up by the obstetric advisory committee were considered,[3] as were hospital standards and standards of obstetric care in hospitals approved by the American College of Surgeons.[4]

The material here presented is an abstract of the full report,[5] with tables and careful analyses, of the resulting study made by the United States Children's Bureau of all the maternal deaths which occurred in 13 States in 1927 and in these same States and 2 others in 1928. The States in which the study was conducted for both years were Alabama, Kentucky, Maryland, Michigan, Minnesota, Nebraska, New Hampshire, North Dakota, Oregon, Rhode Island,

[1] The members of the obstetric advisory committee are: Dr. Robert L. DeNormandie, instructor in obstetrics, Harvard Medical School, chairman; Dr. Fred L. Adair, professor of obstetrics and gynecology, University of Chicago; Dr. Rudolph W. Holmes, professor of obstetrics, Northwestern University Medical School, Chicago; Dr. Frank W. Lynch, professor of obstetrics and gynecology, University of California Medical School; Dr. James R. McCord, professor of obstetrics and gynecology, Emory University School of Medicine, Atlanta; Dr. C. Jeff Miller, professor of gynecology, Tulane University of Louisiana School of Medicine, New Orleans; Dr. Otto H. Schwarz, professor of obstetrics and gynecology, Washington University School of Medicine, St. Louis; Dr. Alice N. Pickett, assistant professor of obstetrics, University of Louisville School of Medicine, Louisville.

[2] The study was made under the supervision of Dr. Blanche M. Haines, formerly director of the maternity and infant hygiene division of the Children's Bureau. The taking of the schedules in the different States was coordinated by Dr. Frances C. Rothert, of the Children's Bureau, who also analyzed the material and wrote the complete report, with the cooperation of members of the obstetric advisory committee.

[3] Standards of Prenatal Care; an outline for the use of physicians. U.S. Children's Bureau Publication No. 153. Washington, 1925.

[4] American College of Surgeons. Fourteenth Year Book. 1927, p. 71.

[5] Maternal Mortality in Fifteen States. U.S. Children's Bureau Publication No. 223. Washington, 1933.

Virginia, Washington, and Wisconsin. California and Oklahoma were included in the 1928 study only. In Michigan, Wisconsin, Minnesota, North Dakota, California, and Oklahoma all or most of the schedules and in Alabama some of them were taken by physicians on the staffs of the State departments of health. In the remaining States the schedules were taken by physicians on the staff of the Children's Bureau.[6]

The States of the study are fairly well distributed geographically and fairly typical of the sections in which they are located. The composition of the population for the group of States conforms very closely to that of the entire United States according to the census of 1920.

In these 15 States, during the years of the study, the deaths of 7,537 women were assigned to puerperal causes by the United States Bureau of the Census in accordance with the International List of Causes of Death. This number of deaths was 26 percent of the 29,298 deaths from puerperal causes in the entire United States birth-registration area for these 2 years. In the States of the study 3,546 (47 percent) of the maternal deaths were urban and 3,991 (53 percent) rural; in the birth-registration area for these 2 years 54 percent were urban and 46 percent rural (rural including towns of less than 10,000). Eighteen percent of the deaths in this study and 19 percent of the maternal deaths in the birth-registration area were of colored women. Colored women, according to the definition used by the Census Bureau, include Negroes, Japanese, Indians, and Chinese.

As there were 1,176,603 live births in the States during the years of the study, these 7,537 deaths gave a maternal mortality rate of 64 per 10,000 live births; in the birth-registration area for 1927 and 1928 together the maternal mortality rate was 67. Conditions as regards maternal mortality were evidently better in the States studied. The four States admitted to the birth-registration area in 1928 all had higher rates than the area as a whole for that year; if they had been in the area in both years of the maternal-mortality study the rate for the area for the 2 years would probably have been higher.

The regions studied, then, are probably fairly representative of the United States as a whole, with some overemphasis on the Pacific Coast and North Central States, and some underemphasis on the Rocky Mountain regions, the far South, and the eastern industrial centers. Conditions as regards maternal mortality were apparently better in the regions studied—they were certainly not worse—than those obtaining in the United States as a whole.

The collection of data was begun in February 1927, and most of the schedules were completed before July 1, 1929. All the finished

[6] The following persons made the interviews in the different States: Alabama—Dr. Wade H. Garner, Dr. Charles M. Lacy, Dr. Robert A. Berry, Dr. William H. Abernathy, and Margaret Murphy, R. N.; Kentucky—Dr. Frances C. Rothert, Dr. Frances M. Hennessy, and Dr. Janice Rafuse; Maryland—Dr. Margaret Swigart; Michigan—Dr. Joseph H. Curhan, Dr. Dorothy L. Green, and Dr. Florence Knowlton; Minnesota—Dr. William H. Rumpf and Dr. Ruth G. Nystrom; Nebraska—Dr. Herman M. Jahr and Dr. MaBelle True; New Hampshire and Rhode Island—Dr. Hennessy; North Dakota—Dr. Maysil M. Williams, Dr. M. May Allen, and Dr. Iva Stevens Merritt; Oregon—Dr. Mildred McBride; Virginia—Dr. Swigart, Dr. Rothert, Dr. Hennessy, and Dr. Rafuse; Washington—Dr. Harold L. Kennedy, Dr. Harvey J. Felch, and Dr. Paul W. Spickard; Wisconsin—Dr. Charlotte J. Calvert; California—staff physicians of the State department of health under the supervision of Dr. Ellen S. Stadtmuller and Dr. Swigart; Oklahoma—Dr. True, Dr. David M. Cowgill, Dr. Margaret Dubois, and Dr. Louise Smith King.

schedules were sent to the Children's Bureau for statistical examination, and tabulations were made there. A very close contact between the interviewers and the Bureau was maintained in order to keep the interpretation of the schedules uniform.

The routine used was as follows: All certificates of deaths assigned to puerperal causes as reported to the State departments of health were copied. Birth certificates were matched when possible. The physicians or other persons signing the death certificates were then interviewed. The families were not visited, except where there were no physicians. The hospitals and clinics in which the patients had received care were visited, and the case records were studied with the consent of the attending physician. In some cases in which the interview was delayed the physician had forgotten many of the details of the case. Very few of the physicians kept case histories, and usually no laboratory work other than a urinalysis and a blood-pressure examination had been done. However, most of them remembered the cases vividly. The physicians interviewed cooperated most heartily, giving freely of their time and helping in every possible way.

# GENERAL CONSIDERATIONS

## CAUSE OF DEATH

### Classification of deaths according to international list

The International List of Causes of Death (edition of 1920)[7] was used as the general basis for the analysis of these deaths. The titles included in the group "the Puerperal State" are as follows:

143. Accidents of pregnancy. This includes (*a*) abortion, (*b*) ectopic gestation, and (*c*) others under this title. ("Abortion" will be referred to throughout this report as "abortion or premature labor." The word "abortion" as generally used in this report does not have the same meaning as it does in the international classification, but is defined as the termination of a uterine pregnancy before the period of viability, i.e., in the first two trimesters.)
144. Puerperal hemorrhage, which includes (*a*) placenta previa, (*b*) others under this title—postpartum hemorrhage, accidental hemorrhage, etc.
145. Other accidents of labor.
    (*a*) Cesarean section.
    (*b*) Other surgical operations and instrumental delivery.
    (*c*) Others under this title.
146. Puerperal septicemia.
147. Puerperal phlegmasia alba dolens, embolus, sudden death.
148. Puerperal albuminuria and convulsions. This title also includes pyelitis, nephritis, tetanus, and uremia.
149. Following childbirth (not otherwise defined).
150. Puerperal diseases of the breast.

When more than one puerperal cause appears on a death certificate, the death is assigned to one of them in accordance with definite rules published in the Manual of Joint Causes of Death,[8] which the Children's Bureau has followed literally in all cases. It is well to realize what the general rules of the classification are. If one of the more serious acute infectious diseases, such as typhoid fever, smallpox, diphtheria, or if cancer or syphilis, or if an external cause such as an accident or homicide, appears on a woman's death certificate with a puerperal cause, her death is assigned to that cause and not to the puerperal cause. (Influenza, however, takes precedence over no puerperal cause except "other accidents of pregnancy", "following childbirth (not otherwise defined)", and "puerperal diseases of the breast.") Puerperal septicemia takes precedence over all puerperal and nonpuerperal causes except the ones mentioned. Tuberculosis in most forms takes precedence over all puerperal causes except puerperal septicemia. Other serious chronic diseases, such as cardiac valvular disease and chronic nephritis, take precedence over all puerperal causes except the most severe complications of childbirth. The term "pregnancy" on a death certificate causes a death

---

[7] Manual of the International List of Causes of Death, 1920. U.S. Bureau of the Census. Washington, 1924.

[8] Manual of Joint Causes of Death Showing Assignment to the Preferred Title of the International List of Causes of Death When Two Causes Are Simultaneously Reported. U.S. Bureau of the Census. Washington, 1925.

to be classified as puerperal only when it appears alone or with a term denoting a mild disorder or with a cause implying a complication of pregnancy.

**Comparison of causes originally assigned and those found through interviews**

The 7,537 deaths classified by the United States Bureau of the Census as due to puerperal causes include not only those originally so certified by the physician but those added as a result of the answers to queries by the Bureau of the Census and by State bureaus of vital statistics. Of this total 7,380 were found, by means of the interviews in connection with the study, to have been actually puerperal in the meaning of the international classification, and 157 were found to have been nonpuerperal. The detailed tabulations and the analyses that are in the complete report are based on these 7,380 puerperal deaths.

TABLE 1.—*Cause of death*[1] *as given on the death certificate and as shown by interview, and mortality rate among women whose deaths were assigned to puerperal causes*

| Cause of death[1] | Deaths from causes as given on death certificate | | | Deaths from causes as shown by interview | | |
|---|---|---|---|---|---|---|
| | Number | Percent distribution | Rate per 10,000 live births | Number | Percent distribution | Rate per 10,000 live births |
| All causes | 7, 537 | | | 7, 537 | | |
| Puerperal | **7, 537** | **100** | **64. 1** | **7, 380** | **100** | **62. 7** |
| Accidents of pregnancy | 770 | 10 | 6. 5 | 719 | 10 | 6. 1 |
| Abortion, premature labor | *368* | *5* | *3. 1* | *353* | *5* | *3. 0* |
| Ectopic gestation | *264* | *4* | *2. 2* | *248* | *3* | *2. 1* |
| Others | *138* | *2* | *1. 2* | *118* | *2* | *1. 0* |
| Puerperal hemorrhage | 758 | 10 | 6. 4 | 791 | 11 | 6. 7 |
| Other accidents of labor | 812 | 11 | 6. 9 | 652 | 9 | 5. 5 |
| Cesarean section | *155* | *2* | *1. 3* | *136* | *2* | *1. 2* |
| Other surgical operations and instrumental delivery | *76* | *1* | *. 6* | *109* | *1* | *. 9* |
| Others | *581* | *8* | *4. 9* | *407* | *6* | *3. 5* |
| Puerperal septicemia | 2, 827 | 38 | 24. 0 | 2, 948 | 40 | 25. 1 |
| Puerperal phlegmasia alba dolens, embolus, sudden death | 337 | 4 | 2. 9 | 344 | 5 | 2. 9 |
| Puerperal albuminuria and convulsions | 2, 006 | 27 | 17. 0 | 1, 900 | 26 | 16. 1 |
| Following childbirth (not otherwise defined) | 24 | [2] | . 2 | 23 | [2] | . 2 |
| Puerperal diseases of the breast | 3 | [2] | [3] | 3 | [2] | [3] |
| Nonpuerperal | | | | 157 | | |

[1] According to the Manual of the International List of Causes of Death, 1920.
[2] Less than 1 percent.
[3] Less than one tenth per 10,000.

The causes of death of the cases excluded from this study because they were found to be nonpuerperal were: Chronic nephritis, 32; lobar pneumonia, 18; tuberculosis, 17; other infectious disease, 8; appendicitis, hernia, intestinal obstruction, 12; chronic cardiac valvular disease, 13; salpingitis and pelvic abscess, 21; other diseases of the female genital organs, 17; and all other diseases, 19. Sixty-eight of these 157 women had not been recently pregnant.

179179°—33——2

**Changes in classification within the puerperal group**

As a result of the interviews changes in classification were made in many of the 7,380 cases (table 1). Clerical errors had led to erroneous classification. Lack of knowledge of the International List of Causes of Death had led to the omission of statements which, if present, would have caused a different classification. Moreover, some of the 558 autopsies in the group of 7,380 deaths were performed after the death certificates had been signed.

Deaths will be spoken of throughout the report as having been "assigned" or "attributed" to the individual causes of death. The term "assigned" is used of the official classification by the Bureau of the Census, as in the first three columns of table 1; the term "attributed" is used as referring to the classification after interview, for purposes of this study, as in the last three columns of table 1.

The International List of Causes of Death was revised by the international commission late in 1929. The chief changes are: (1) Puerperal septicemia (no. 146) is divided into Abortions with septic conditions (no. 140), Ectopic gestation with septic conditions specified (no. 142a), and Puerperal septicemia not specified as due to abortion (no. 145); (2) Puerperal albuminuria and convulsions (no. 148) is divided into Puerperal albuminuria and eclampsia (no. 146) and Other toxemias of pregnancy (no. 147), which also includes chorea and pernicious vomiting of pregnancy from the old subtitle 143c; (3) the title numbers of 143a, b, and c are changed to 141, 142b, and 143, respectively; title 147 becomes 148, and 145 becomes 149, without change of name or content; (4) Following childbirth not otherwise defined (no. 149) and Puerperal diseases of the breast (no. 150) are combined into Other and unspecified conditions of the puerperal state (no. 150).

Although analysis in this report was based largely on the 1920 list, which was in use at the time these deaths were classified, the subdivisions of the topics follow very closely the subdivisions in the 1929 list.

## AUTOPSIES

Autopsies were known to have been performed in 571 of the 7,537 deaths certified as puerperal. They were performed in 130 (36 percent) of the 362 cases in which the coroner signed the death certificate and in 441 (6 percent) of the 7,046 cases in which a physician other than the coroner signed the death certificate. Thirteen of the autopsies were included in the 157 cases in which the death was certified as puerperal but was found at the interview with the attending physician to have been nonpuerperal. The remaining 558 constituted only 8 percent of the 7,380 cases found on interview to have been puerperal.

## SIGNATURE ON DEATH CERTIFICATE

Death certificates were signed in 7,046 cases by physicians, in 362 cases by coroners, in 62 cases by others (a few by irregular practitioners not listed in the medical directory and some by husbands or parents), and 67 certificates were not signed. Of the 188 cases of women who had no medical attention, the death certificate was signed in 65 cases by physicians, in 47 cases by coroners, and in 76 cases it was signed by some other person or was unsigned.

## RACE AND NATIVITY

Deaths of colored women made up 18 percent of those included in the study. *The maternal mortality rate of colored women in the years of the study was nearly twice that of the white women* (table 2). The maternal mortality rates were significantly higher among colored women for every main cause of death except puerperal phlegmasia alba dolens, embolus, sudden death. For Cesarean section, other surgical operations and instrumental delivery, and "others" under the title "accidents of pregnancy" the differences were insignificant. The greatest difference was in the deaths from puerperal albuminuria and convulsions, which caused more than twice as many deaths per 10,000 live births among the colored women as among the white women.

TABLE 2.—*Cause of death[1] as shown by interview, and mortality rate among white and colored women dying from puerperal causes*

| Cause of death [1] as shown by interview | Women dying from puerperal causes | | | | | | |
|---|---|---|---|---|---|---|---|
| | | White | | | Colored | | |
| | Total | Number | Percent distribution | Rate per 10,000 live births | Number | Percent distribution | Rate per 10,000 live births |
| **All causes** | **7,380** | **6,072** | **100** | **57.5** | **1,308** | **100** | **108.5** |
| Accidents of pregnancy | 719 | 613 | 10 | 5.8 | 106 | 8 | 8.8 |
| *Abortion, premature labor* | *353* | *301* | *5* | *2.9* | *52* | *4* | *4.3* |
| *Ectopic gestation* | *248* | *210* | *3* | *2.0* | *38* | *3* | *3.2* |
| *Others* | *118* | *102* | *2* | *1.0* | *16* | *1* | *1.3* |
| Puerperal hemorrhage | 791 | 670 | 11 | 6.3 | 121 | 9 | 10.0 |
| Other accidents of labor | 652 | 525 | 9 | 5.0 | 127 | 10 | 10.5 |
| *Cesarean section* | *136* | *123* | *2* | *1.2* | *13* | *1* | *1.1* |
| *Other surgical operations and instrumental delivery* | *109* | *97* | *2* | *.9* | *12* | *1* | *1.0* |
| *Others* | *407* | *305* | *5* | *2.9* | *102* | *8* | *8.5* |
| Puerperal septicemia | 2,948 | 2,437 | 40 | 23.1 | 511 | 39 | 42.4 |
| Puerperal phlegmasia alba dolens, embolus, sudden death | 344 | 314 | 5 | 3.0 | 30 | 2 | 2.5 |
| Puerperal albuminuria and convulsions | 1,900 | 1,493 | 25 | 14.1 | 407 | 31 | 33.8 |
| Following childbirth (not otherwise defined) | 23 | 17 | (2) | .2 | 6 | (2) | .5 |
| Puerperal diseases of the breast | 3 | 3 | (2) | (3) | ------ | ------ | ------ |

[1] According to the Manual of the International List of Causes of Death, 1920.
[2] Less than 1 percent.
[3] Less than one tenth per 10,000.

Of the 6,072 white women whose deaths were included in the study, 5,109 were native born and 805 were foreign born; the nativity of 158 was not reported.

## DEATHS IN URBAN AND RURAL AREAS

The Vital Statistics Division of the United States Bureau of the Census includes in urban areas all cities of 10,000 or more population as shown in the 1920 census. The maternal mortality rate was higher in urban areas (75 per 10,000 live births) than in rural areas (55 per 10,000 live births). The rates for the groups "accidents of pregnancy", "other accidents of labor", "puerperal septicemia", "puerperal phlegmasia alba dolens" were significantly higher in urban than in rural areas. There was no significant difference in the other main groups. The greatest difference was in the mortality

CHART 11.—MATERNAL MORTALITY RATES, BY CAUSE

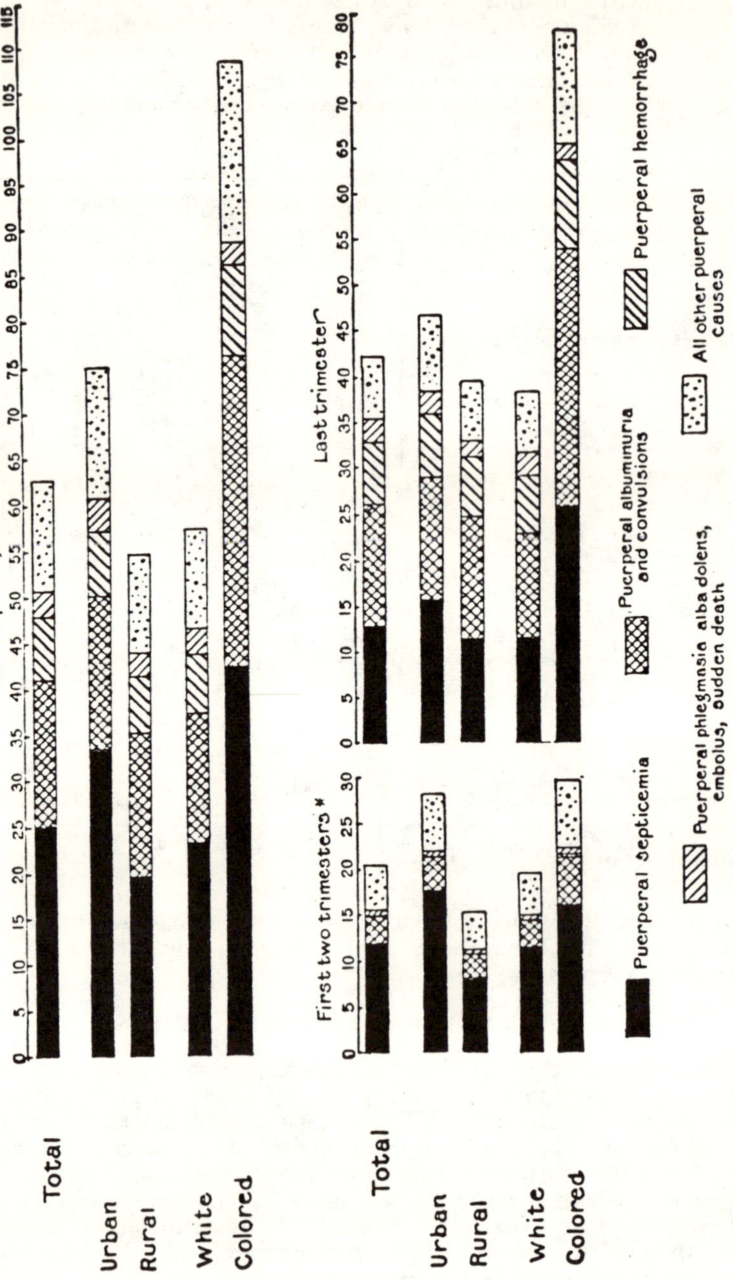


* In the bars showing rates for total, urban, rural, and white, the rate for puerperal hemorrhage (1 tenth per 10,000 live births) is too small to appear.

rates from puerperal septicemia. and the difference in this rate was largely due to the higher rates from septic abortion in the cities than in the rural areas. The urban rates are undoubtedly raised by the deaths of nonresidents who are brought to hospitals after delivery and who die there.

## LACK OF MEDICAL ATTENTION AND INACCESSIBILITY

Nine percent of all the deaths were of women who had had no medical care or care only when dying. In strictly rural areas the distance from a physician may become an important cause for lack of early and sufficient medical attention. partly because of the actual distance and partly because of the charge for country travel on a mileage basis in addition to the usual medical fees. Lack of medical attention was not always associated with inaccessibility of the

CHART III.—MATERNAL MORTALITY RATES BY CAUSE AND BY TRIMESTER OF PREGNANCY

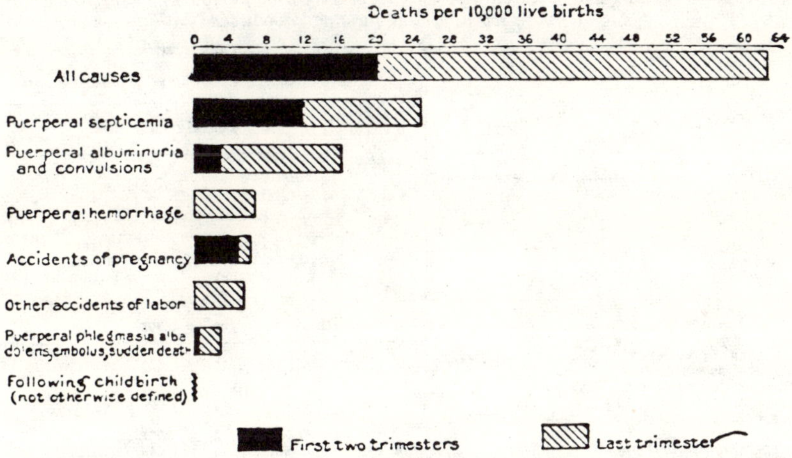


physician, but it was more frequent when there was no physician living in the vicinity. Yet even in cases of women having a physician nearby, 7 percent of the number for whom medical attention was reported had no care or care only when dying. Poor roads and slow transportation are greater factors in inaccessibility than mere distance, for apparently more patients are really inaccessible in the Kentucky and Virginia mountains than in the western States where the distances are very much greater.

## HOSPITALIZATION

Of the 7,380 women included in the study there was a report on hospitalization for all but 14. More than half were hospitalized at some time during their final illness. The deaths of 4,066 occurred in hospitals, but the deliveries or abortions of only 2,629 occurred in hospitals. *Relatively few of these patients who died in hospitals had planned hospitalization.* Of the 4,066 women whose deaths occurred in hospitals, 2,501 had reached the last trimester; 1,558 had not reached the last trimester; and for 7 the period of gestation was not reported. Of the 2,501 who were known to have reached the last trimester of pregnancy, only 1,893 were in the hospital for delivery, and less than half of these (845) were known to have had planned hospitalization. Hospitalization was less frequent and more of it was of an emergency nature among the colored women than among the white women.

## PERIOD OF GESTATION

*About one third of the women included in the study died before they reached the last trimester of pregnancy.* Puerperal septicemia was the most important cause of death prior to the seventh month and accounted for 59 percent of the deaths in this period. But puerperal albuminuria and convulsions equaled puerperal septicemia in importance in the last trimester, to each being attributed 31 percent of the deaths (table 3). (See charts II and III.)

TABLE 3.—*Cause of death as shown by interview, and period of gestation among women dying from puerperal causes*

| Cause of death as shown by interview | Women dying from puerperal causes | | | | | |
|---|---|---|---|---|---|---|
| | | Period of gestation | | | | |
| | Total | First two trimesters | | Last trimester | | Not reported |
| | | Number | Percent distribution | Number | Percent distribution | |
| All causes | 7,380 | 2,381 | 100 | 4,965 | 100 | 34 |
| Accidents of pregnancy | 719 | 575 | 24 | 142 | 3 | 2 |
| Puerperal hemorrhage | 791 | 11 | (1) | 779 | 16 | 1 |
| Other accidents of labor | 652 | 1 | (1) | 651 | 13 | |
| Puerperal septicemia | 2,948 | 1,403 | 59 | 1,529 | 31 | 16 |
| Puerperal phlegmasia alba dolens, embolus, sudden death | 344 | 53 | 2 | 291 | 6 | |
| Puerperal albuminuria and convulsions | 1,900 | 338 | 14 | 1,549 | 31 | 13 |
| Following childbirth (not otherwise defined) | 23 | | | 22 | (1) | 1 |
| Puerperal diseases of the breast | 3 | | | 2 | (1) | 1 |

1 Less than 1 percent.

## LIVE BIRTHS AND STILL BIRTHS

Only 3,091 (43 percent) of the 7,226 women for whom the type of issue was reported gave birth to living children. Twenty percent were delivered of still-born children (that is, children born dead at 7 or more months' gestation). Twenty-nine percent had nonviable issue (born dead at less than 7 months' gestation), and 8 percent died undelivered. (See chart IV.)

## PARITY AND AGE

Primiparæ made up one third and multiparæ two thirds of the 6,854 women in the study for whom the number of pregnancies was reported.

This study shows, as do other published figures, that the risk of childbearing is comparatively great for mothers under 15 years of age, that the most favorable age is from 20 to 25 years, and that from that age onward the maternal mortality rate increases, reaching a maximum in the age period 45 years and over. This is true both for white and for colored women.

## ILLEGITIMACY

The deaths of 509 unmarried women are included in the study. Approximately one half (51 percent) of the deaths, as compared with 39 percent of the deaths of married women, were from puerperal septicemia. Of the deaths from septicemia, almost two thirds occurred before the women reached the third trimester. Puerperal albuminuria and convulsions also caused a larger proportion of deaths of unmarried (32 percent) than of married women (25 percent). The other deaths of unmarried women were due to accidents of pregnancy (7 percent), other accidents of labor (5 percent), puerperal hemorrhage (3 percent), and puerperal phlegmasia alba dolens, embolus, sudden death (2 percent). More than one half of

CHART IV.—TYPE OF ISSUE AMONG WOMEN DYING FROM PUERPERAL CAUSES

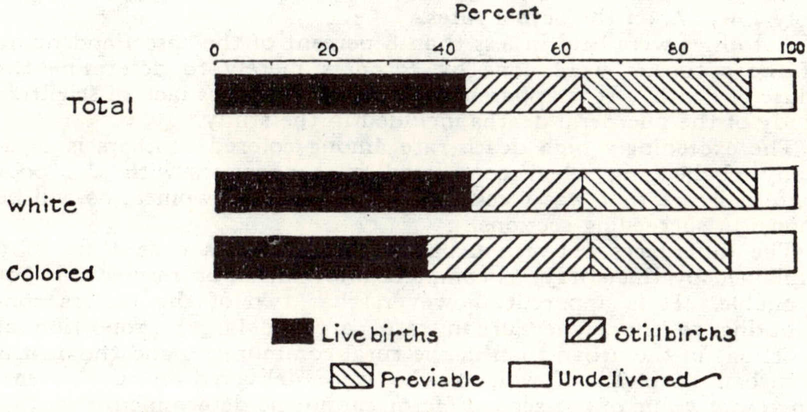


the unmarried women were colored, as compared with 18 percent colored in the total group. Of the 506 unmarried women for whom the period of gestation was reported 219 (43 percent) died at less than 7 months' gestation, as compared with 2,152 (32 percent) of the 6,819 married women for whom this was reported. This larger proportion of early terminations of pregnancy among the unmarried women who died was confined, however, to the white women. Among the white women for whom the period of gestation was reported, 60 percent of the unmarried and 32 percent of the married women died before reaching the last trimester of pregnancy.

The maternal mortality rate for unmarried mothers in the States included in the study (except California, where data on legitimacy do not appear on the birth certificate) was 143 per 10,000 illegitimate live births; for married mothers it was 60 per 10,000 legitimate live births.

## COMMENT BY ADVISORY COMMITTEE

This study apparently represents a fair sampling of maternal deaths throughout the registration area.

In this study the International List of Causes of Death together with the Manual of Joint Causes in use by the United States Bureau of the Census has been used as the chief basis of classification. While this procedure was not entirely satisfactory from a medical point of view, the inherent disadvantages seemed counterbalanced by the fact that it provides a definite and understandable classification and that its use would assist the comparison of the findings with those of other investigators.

Certain changes in classification resulted after the interviews. These alterations, which were made necessary by various causes, emphasize the dependence of the official statistics on the original death certificate and the apparent unavoidability of a small percentage of error. A relatively small number of cases were excluded as nonpuerperal. These cases are easily equaled or exceeded by those that were actually puerperal but that were classed in the vital statistics as nonpuerperal and so were not included in the study. Therefore, maternal mortality rates as given in this study are probably *lower* than the actual rates.

Autopsies were held in less than 8 percent of the cases, and many of the autopsies were done by coroners merely to determine the cause of death. It is apparent that there was gross lack of scientific study of the puerperal deaths included in the study.

The exceedingly high death rate among colored mothers is especially challenging when considered in connection with the poor maternal care that was received by these colored women, as will be shown in succeeding sections.

The differences between urban and rural rates cannot be fully explained by this study, as complete information on residence is not available. It is apparent, however, that two of the factors contributing to the higher urban rates are the larger proportion of abortions in the urban than in the rural communities and the deaths in urban hospitals of women who were delivered in rural areas. The exact value of the second factor cannot be determined from this study for reasons given in the report.

Nine percent of the women had no medical attention whatsoever, or else had attention only when they were actually dying. Only part of this was due to physical inaccessibility. Inaccessibility due to distance and bad roads, however, was a serious problem in certain localities of the States studied. The part played by inaccessibility in the lack of *early*, as distinguished from *any*, medical attention was not measured; but the larger proportion of deaths from hemorrhage and the toxemias in the less accessible groups is suggestive, especially when considered in conjunction with the lack of prenatal care among women who died in the rural areas.

It is impossible to draw conclusions as to the relative safety of deliveries in hospitals and homes from a study of deaths alone. Data regarding the total number of deliveries in hospitals and homes were lacking. Many hospital deaths followed home deliveries, and many of the hospital deliveries were emergency cases. However, there were too many deaths (899) of women who had planned hospital deliveries in the last trimester.

The figures relative to still births and live births indicate strikingly the appalling loss of fetal life associated with maternal deaths; 37 percent were either undelivered or previable infants, 20 percent were of viable age but stillborn, and only 43 percent are credited as being live births. The number of these infants who died or were damaged survivors was not possible to determine from this investigation.

One third of all the deaths were of women who had not reached ihe last trimester of pregnancy. Duration of pregnancy is a most tmportant consideration in the evaluation of any statistics on maternal mortality.

Illegitimacy contributes to maternal mortality, as 7 percent of the deaths in this study were of unmarried women, and the mortality rate is much higher for unmarried than for married mothers. There was a larger proportion of abortions among the unmarried, and the deaths from such preventable causes as sepsis and toxemia were relatively more numerous among the unmarried mothers. Social and economic factors doubtless play an important role in creating this mortality and they should be adjusted to prevent this loss of life.

179179°—33——3

## MATERNAL CARE

Maternal care in the fullest sense includes very many factors—the woman's food, her living conditions, her mental condition, the conditions under which her confinement takes place, how she spends the lying-in period. Of particular importance is the type of medical and nursing care that she obtains. In this study attention was confined largely to the medical aspects of maternal care.

Of the 7,380 women whose deaths are included in this study only 933 were known to have had no complication of pregnancy. Six hundred and sixteen of these women were reported to have had no intercurrent disease. Only 263 of the 616 were known to have had normal spontaneous deliveries in the last trimester, and only 199 of

CHART V.—PRENATAL CARE AMONG WOMEN DYING FROM PUERPERAL CAUSES[1]

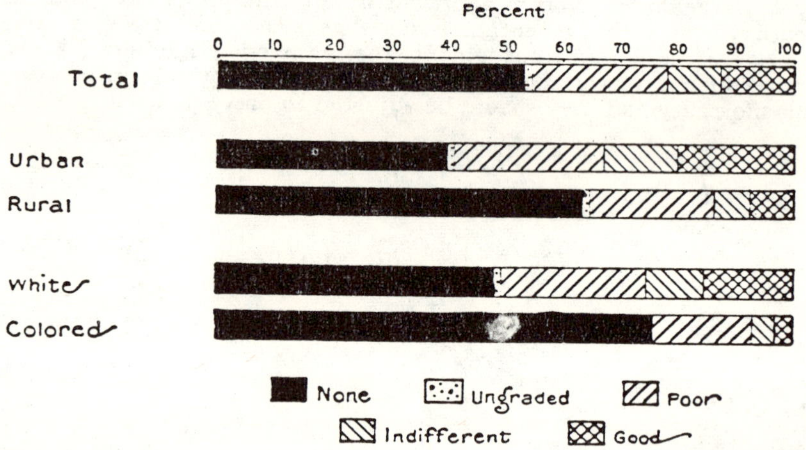


the 263 were reported to have had a normal third stage of labor and no postpartum hemorrhage. And yet 100 of these 199 women with apparently normal pregnancy and labor died of puerperal sepsis, 55 of puerperal phlegmasia alba dolens, embolus, sudden death, 23 of other accidents of labor, 15 of puerperal albuminuria and convulsions, and the other 6 of other puerperal conditions. It should be borne in mind in connection with these figures that a large number of women who had no prenatal care or about whose care during pregnancy nothing was known were not included in the discussion.

### PRENATAL CARE

All pregnant women should receive prenatal care. In practice prenatal care is seldom sought before the third month of pregnancy. Also, it is not sought by women who are sufficiently hostile to their pregnancy to resort to self-induced or criminal abortions. As 1,154

[1] Excludes women for whom pregnancy terminated before the third month and women who had induced abortions.

of the 7,380 women in this mortality group had pregnancies which terminated before the third month, either spontaneously or intentionally, or had later induced abortions other than therapeutic, there were 6,226 to whom it might reasonably be expected that prenatal care would have been given.

A report on prenatal care was obtainable concerning only 5,636 of the 6,226 who might be expected to have had such care. Of these 5,636, 3,025 (54 percent) had had no prenatal examination by a physician. For the most part, physicians had no opportunity to give prenatal care to these women, for they were not consulted.

Prenatal care was much more frequent among the white than among the colored women, and in both groups prenatal care was more frequent in the urban areas than in the rural areas (table 4).

TABLE 4.—*Prenatal care received by white and colored women dying in urban and rural areas from puerperal causes*

| Grade of prenatal care | Women dying from puerperal causes | | | | | |
|---|---|---|---|---|---|---|
| | Total | | In urban areas | | In rural areas | |
| | Number | Percent distribution | Number | Percent distribution | Number | Percent distribution |
| Total | 7,380 | | 3,462 | | 3,918 | |
| Report on prenatal care | **5,636** | **100** | **2,452** | **100** | **3,184** | **100** |
| Grade I | 725 | 13 | 484 | 20 | 241 | 8 |
| Grade II | 449 | 9 | 320 | 13 | 179 | 6 |
| Grade III | 1,337 | 24 | 630 | 26 | 707 | 22 |
| Ungraded | 50 | 1 | 32 | 1 | 18 | 1 |
| None | 3,025 | 54 | 986 | 40 | 2,039 | 64 |
| No report on prenatal care | **590** | | **313** | | **277** | |
| Inapplicable [1] | **1,154** | | **697** | | **457** | |
| **WHITE** | | | | | | |
| Total | 6,072 | | 2,951 | | 3,121 | |
| Report on prenatal care | **4,568** | **100** | **2,061** | **100** | **2,507** | **100** |
| Grade I | 694 | 15 | 463 | 22 | 231 | 9 |
| Grade II | 458 | 10 | 291 | 14 | 167 | 7 |
| Grade III | 1,157 | 25 | 540 | 26 | 617 | 25 |
| Ungraded | 45 | 1 | 28 | 1 | 17 | 1 |
| None | 2,214 | 48 | 739 | 36 | 1,475 | 59 |
| No report on prenatal care | **458** | | **248** | | **212** | |
| Inapplicable [1] | **1,046** | | **644** | | **402** | |
| **COLORED** | | | | | | |
| Total | 1,308 | | 511 | | 797 | |
| Report on prenatal care | **1,068** | **100** | **391** | **100** | **677** | **100** |
| Grade I | 31 | 3 | 21 | 5 | 10 | 1 |
| Grade II | 41 | 4 | 29 | 7 | 12 | 2 |
| Grade III | 180 | 17 | 90 | 23 | 90 | 13 |
| Ungraded | 5 | (2) | 4 | 1 | 1 | (2) |
| None | 811 | 76 | 247 | 63 | 564 | 83 |
| No report on prenatal care | **132** | | **67** | | **65** | |
| Inapplicable [1] | **108** | | **53** | | **55** | |

[1] Induced abortions and cases in which pregnancy terminated before the third month.
[2] Less than 1 percent.

**Prenatal care in the different States**

The quality and amount of prenatal care given varied greatly in the different States included in the study. Of the women who might be expected to have had prenatal care, 71 percent in Oregon and 70 percent in Rhode Island had had some care, but only 22 percent in Alabama and 30 percent in Oklahoma. In every State except one, more of the women who died in cities than of those who died in the rural areas had had prenatal care. In general, the States in which more of the women who died had had grade I care had lower mortality rates from puerperal albuminuria and convulsions.

**Grading of the prenatal care received**

The prenatal care given was divided into three grades:

*Grade I* includes (1) a complete physical examination, (2) pelvic measurements, internal and external, except in pregnancies terminating before the eighth month and for multiparæ who had had a previous normal delivery, and (3) regular monthly visits to a physician, beginning with or before the fifth month, with examination of urine and blood pressure at each visit. This care, which is on the whole good, although not up to highest standards, was received by 725 women (13 percent). *Only 42 women (less than 1 percent) had adequate care* as described in Standards of Prenatal Care (Children's Bureau Publication No. 153). This includes chiefly, in addition to the above, a Wassermann test and visits beginning with the second month.

*Grade II* includes a general physical examination, regular monthly visits to the physician, beginning not later than the seventh month, with examination of the urine and blood pressure; this can be classified only as indifferent care. Four hundred and ninety-nine women (9 percent) had had this care.

*Grade III* included in some cases only a single visit to the physician; in some cases there were repeated visits, but blood pressure was not taken or other essentials of the better grade of care were omitted. Care of this kind must be classified as poor. There were 1,337 women (24 percent) included in this group. (See chart V.)

*More than three fourths had had poor or indifferent care, or none at all. Only 16 percent had had a Wassermann test.*

Of the 1,478 women who first consulted the physician before or during the fifth month of pregnancy, 725 (49 percent) received grade I care, 243 (16 percent) received grade II care, and 501 (34 percent) received grade III care; for 9 the grade was not reported.

In the grading of prenatal care no account was taken of the treatment given, for the methods of treatment are not so standardized as are the methods of examination.

**Prenatal care and trimester of pregnancy**

Fifty-five percent of the women who died before they reached the last trimester died too early in pregnancy to have been expected to have prenatal care, or they had induced abortions, or else information concerning their care was not obtained. But of the remaining 1,064 women 17 percent had had grade I care, 3 percent had had grade II care, 14 percent had had grade III care, 1 percent had had care that was ungraded, and 66 percent had had no care.

Of the 4,570 women who died after reaching the last trimester and for whom a report was obtained concerning prenatal care, 12 percent had had grade I care, 10 percent grade II care, and 26 percent grade III care; 1 percent had had care that was ungraded, and 51 percent had had no care. Twenty-four percent of those who died following grade I care and 34 percent of those who had had no care died of puerperal albuminuria and convulsions.

**Prenatal care and number of pregnancies**

Of the 2,334 known primiparæ whose deaths were included in this study, a report as to prenatal care is available and applicable for 1,924. Of these 14 percent had had grade I care, 14 percent grade II care, 24 percent had had poor care (grade III), and 46 percent had had no prenatal care whatsoever. Of those in their second pregnancy 22 percent had grade I care, 11 percent grade II care, 27 percent grade III care, and 39 percent no care. After the second pregnancy the percentage of those who had good prenatal care decreased, and the percentage of those who had no prenatal care rose with the number of pregnancies.

**Prenatal care in relation to live births and still births**

Among the 4,843 cases of women who had reached the last trimester in which there was a report on the character of issue, 70 percent were live births for the mothers who had had grade I and grade II prenatal care, 63 percent for those who had had grade III care, and 58 percent for those who had had no prenatal care.

## DELIVERY CARE

The paramount importance of adequate care at the time of delivery is conceded by all. Adequate delivery care requires the careful management of normal labor, the maintenance of aseptic technique, and the proper handling of any abnormalities. These in turn imply an attendant who has not only skill but patience and good judgment, sufficient trained assistants, and clean surroundings with facilities for dealing with emergencies. The actual evaluation of all these factors is obviously difficult. In this study no attempt was made to grade the types of delivery care given. The simplest and most objective of the factors involved were merely studied separately.

**Hospitalization at delivery**

Of the 4,965 women who reached the last trimester of pregnancy, 1,971 were in hospitals for delivery or at the time of death if they died undelivered. The hospitalization of 899 of these 1,971 women was planned, but for 1,018 it was an emergency measure, and for 54 there was no report as to whether it was planned or not. Two thousand nine hundred and ninety women were delivered or died undelivered outside of hospitals, and for four women the place of delivery was not reported. The hospitalization of white women was much more frequent than of colored women. Maternal mortality rates for hospitals and for homes cannot be given, because data regarding the total number of deliveries in hospitals and in homes are not available; but even if there were such data, the large and varying proportions of complicated cases among those delivered in hospitals invalidate comparisons.

### Attendant at confinement

Information on the attendant at delivery or at death if the patient died undelivered was obtained for 4.903 of the 4.965 women who died after reaching the last trimester. Of these 4.903, 4.065 (83 percent) were attended exclusively by physicians, internes, or medical students (3.915 by physicians only, 87 by physicians preceded by internes or medical students, 63 by internes or medical students only). Midwives attended 550 (11 percent) of the 4.903 women, including 193 for whom physicians (in 2 cases internes) were called in before the delivery was completed. Nonmedical attendants such as relatives attended 172 women (4 percent), including 47 for whom a physician was called in before the delivery was completed, and 116 women (2 percent) were said to have been unattended.

Practically all the midwives who cared for these women were untrained, although there were a few foreign-trained midwives. All cases in which the patient was delivered by a midwife and all cases in which a midwife was known to have been in attendance for the purpose of delivering the patient, even if the physician made the actual delivery, were classified as having been attended by midwives. Four hundred and sixty-two of the five hundred and fifty women attended at confinement by midwives died in Alabama, Kentucky, Maryland, and Virginia, and these 4 were the only States of the 15 in the study in which the number of deaths of women attended by midwives constituted 10 percent or more of the total number of deaths of mothers who had reached the last trimester. In 3 of these 4 States (Alabama, Maryland, Virginia) the proportion of midwife-attended confinements among the women who died was very slightly smaller than the proportion of midwife-reported births among the total live births of the State. In these 4 States the midwives were employed rather than physicians because the patients were not accustomed to the services of a physician at childbirth or could not afford a physician's care. The inaccessibility of a physician was also an important factor.

### Technique of the principal physician

The technique of the principal physician at confinement was reported in 3.619 of the 4.305 cases in which a physician attended women in the last trimester. In 1.740 cases (48 percent) an aseptic technique was said to have been used. This included shaving, scrubbing, sterile drapes, instruments, and rubber gloves, and adequate assistance at delivery. In 510 cases (14 percent) the technique was not so good and was classed as attempted aseptic. In 1.099 cases (30 percent) the technique was classified as clean but not sterile. This meant only ordinary cleanliness and usually sterilization of any instruments used. In many cases the principal physician whose technique was assigned to 1 of these 3 classes was preceded by someone whose technique was less careful. In 270 cases (7 percent) not even ordinary cleanliness was used. The technique as described may not coincide in some cases with that which was actually used, for the grading was based on the physician's subsequent description of his technique as he remembered it.

The principal physician made vaginal examinations in 2.765 cases and made no vaginal examination in 1.089 cases: in 451 cases there was no report on this matter: and in 660 cases no physician was in attendance. The principal physician had made 1 vaginal examination in 871 cases, 2 in 565 cases, and 3 or more in 771 cases; in 558 cases the number was not given. Of the 2,765 cases in which the principal physician made vaginal examinations, rubber gloves were reported used in 2,188 cases, not used in 484 cases, and there was no report on their use in 93 cases. Rectal examinations were reported as having been made by the principal physician in 778 cases; in 326 of these he made 1 or more vaginal examinations also.

There was a report on the use of pituitrin in 3,718 of the 4,305 last-trimester cases with a physician in attendance. Pituitrin was said to have been used before the delivery of the child in 711 cases, after the delivery of the child only in 1,004 cases, and at an unreported stage of labor in 24 cases. In 1,979 cases pituitrin was said not to have been used. In the group of cases in which pituitrin had been used before the delivery of the child larger proportions of the deaths were from puerperal septicemia and puerperal hemorrhage and a smaller proportion was from puerperal albuminuria and convulsions than in the group in which no pituitrin had been used.

## COMMENT BY ADVISORY COMMITTEE

This section shows clearly what a serious situation exists in regard to the quality of the maternal care that many women receive in this country during their pregnancy. Although this study covered but 15 States, they represent a fair cross section of the country, and therefore it is probably fair to assume that the findings in this section are applicable to the country as a whole.

It is discouraging to find that of the women on whom a report as to prenatal care could be obtained and who could reasonably have been expected to have such care, 54 percent had had no prenatal examination by a physician. In only 1 percent was the care given up to the standard that it is the right of every pregnant patient to have and to demand.

For the deaths of the women who had had no prenatal examination the attending physician could hardly be held responsible, for he was not consulted until an emergency had arisen. Gross ignorance, carelessness, and sociological and economic problems all had a share in this responsibility. However, in those cases in which the physician was consulted he was responsible for providing adequate maternal care; and in many of these cases physicians failed in their responsibility, for half the women who did consult a physician had poor prenatal care.

Although the question of prenatal care was considered for only 45 percent of the women who died before they reached the last trimester of pregnancy, 80 percent of these 1,064 women had no care or poor care. Furthermore, many of the 20 percent who had good or indifferent care already had troublesome symptoms before they consulted a physician. Of those women who died after reaching the last trimester and for whom a report was obtained, 78 percent had poor prenatal care or none.

Evidence of the value of prenatal care may be found in the fact that smaller proportions of the women who died after good prenatal care than of those who died after poor prenatal care died of puerperal albuminuria and convulsions. Further evidence may be found in the larger proportion of live births in those cases in which there had been good prenatal care, and in the fact that those States with more good prenatal care, even among the women who died, had lower death rates from albuminuria and convulsions.

Primiparæ and the mothers of many children particularly need prenatal care, but many of these women failed to receive it.

Prenatal care, such as it was, was much more frequent among the white than among the colored women, and in both groups it was more frequent in the urban than in the rural areas. In the rural areas among the colored women there was practically no prenatal care, for 83 percent had none and 13 percent had grade III, which is poor care.

Delivery care, though as important as prenatal care, was more difficult to evaluate, but certain facts were noted. For more than half the women who died in hospitals after reaching the last trimester, hospitalization was an emergency measure. Among the colored women emergency hospitalization was much more frequent than among the white women. Eighty-three percent of the women were attended by physicians, internes, or medical students, 11 percent by midwives, 4 percent by nonmedical attendants; 2 percent of the women had no attendant at the delivery or at the death if the patient died undelivered.

Figures given in the report would indicate that, though the midwives played a part in the mortality, they could not have been responsible for any large proportion of the deaths because they attended a relatively small percentage of the cases.

No study of the qualifications of the individual physicians or midwives was attempted. As it was known, however, that the majority of the midwives were ignorant "grannies", it may safely be assumed that these midwives did not use a satisfactory aseptic technique at delivery. In 48 percent of the cases the physicians described their technique, as they remembered it, in such a way that it was classified as aseptic; but obviously this is not a sure way of determining how good this technique was. The point to be noted is that the physicians themselves admitted it was unsatisfactory in more than 50 percent of the cases. The frequency of vaginal examinations, often times without gloves, is clear, and the relatively small number of rectal examinations must be noted.

Although the data on the use of pituitrin are incomplete, its use is shown to be common and to be associated with serious accidents. Higher percentages of maternal deaths from sepsis and from hemorrhage occurred among those who had it than among those who did not have it. The percentages of ruptured uterus and of stillbirths also were higher.

The almost total lack of adequate prenatal care and the relative infrequency of any prenatal care were outstanding. Besides permitting the unchecked development of unfavorable factors during pregnancy, this situation led to delivery care that was unsatisfactory because given without previous knowledge of the case and frequently in circumstances that necessitated emergency hospitalization.

## OPERATIONS

*In this study more than half of the women had had some operative procedure before death.* Of the 7,234 women concerning whom there was a report on this point, 3,370 (47 percent) had had no operations, while 2,649 (37 percent) had had an operation directed toward delivery and 1,131 (16 percent) had had some operation other than for delivery. By an operative delivery is meant an operation for the purpose of delivering the fetus or for the immediate removal of the placenta. Attempts at these operations, as well as completed operations, are included. Other operations were secondary, usually on account of sequelæ of the delivery.

### OPERATIONS IN THE LAST TRIMESTER

#### OPERATIONS FOR DELIVERY

Of the 4,965 women who reached the last trimester of pregnancy, 2,225 (45 percent) were known to have had an operative delivery or

CHART VI.—OPERATIONS FOR DELIVERY IN THE LAST TRIMESTER OF PREGNANCY AMONG WOMEN DYING FROM PUERPERAL CAUSES

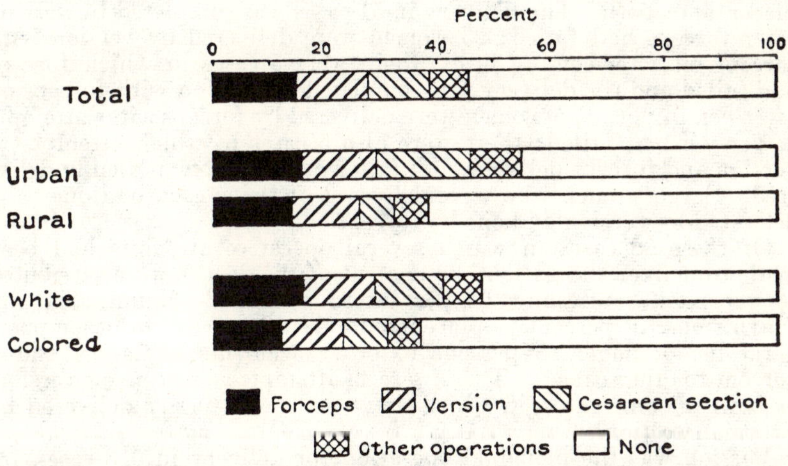


an attempt at operative delivery. Forceps operations were performed 718 times. In addition, there were 98 cases of forceps and version combined. Usually when forceps failed the delivery was completed by version. In 150 of the 718 cases the application of forceps followed induction of labor or artificial dilatation of the cervix.[1] In 24 cases the use of forceps was followed by manual removal of the placenta. In 12 cases all 3 procedures were used. In 14 cases forceps were used in combination with some other opera-

[1] Throughout this report "artificial dilatation of the cervix" includes mechanical induction of labor.

tion. In 162 cases, including 12 with manual removal of the placenta, the use of forceps followed induction of labor or artificial dilatation of the cervix. Of these women 106 were not in labor when the artificial dilatation of the cervix was begun; in 56 cases of women in labor the dilatation of the cervix was done to facilitate delivery. The 718 cases include 2 in which the forceps operation failed and the women delivered themselves spontaneously later, and 13 in which they died undelivered after unsuccessful attempts at delivery by forceps.

The deaths of 35 percent of these 718 women who had forceps operations were attributed, according to the international classification, to puerperal albuminuria and convulsions, 26 percent to puerperal septicemia, 7 percent to embolus and sudden death, 5 percent to placenta previa, 11 percent to other puerperal hemorrhage, 15 percent to other accidents of labor, and 1 percent to other puerperal causes.

Of the 162 cases in which artificial dilatation of the cervix preceded the use of forceps, the deaths were attributed to puerperal albuminuria and convulsions in 62 percent, placenta previa in 10 percent, other puerperal hemorrhage in 9 percent, septicemia in 9 percent, sudden death in 2 percent, and other causes in 8 percent.

In 98 cases attempts at both forceps and version were made, in some cases with dilatation of the cervix or manual removal of the placenta, or both. The delivery in 51 cases was completed by version after forceps had failed; 25 women were delivered by version with forceps on after-coming head; there were 5 cases in which forceps had failed and the delivery was completed by version with forceps on after-coming head; 5 women were delivered by forceps after attempts at version had failed; there were also 5 cases in which attempts at version and forceps delivery both failed and the woman died undelivered. Seven women who were delivered of twins each had one baby delivered by version and one by forceps.

Of these 98 cases in which several operative attempts had been made to deliver the patient, 32 percent of the deaths were attributed to puerperal septicemia, 20 percent to puerperal albuminuria and convulsions, 12 percent to placenta previa, 12 percent to other puerperal hemorrhage, 18 percent to other accidents of labor, and 5 percent to other causes. There were 44 attempts at forceps or version, or both in some cases, in which the woman was finally delivered by Cesarean section.

Version was the principal operation for delivery in 618 cases, including the cases in which a forceps operation was used in conjunction with version—or 520 cases in addition to the 98 already discussed. *In 272 of these 520 cases version followed artificial dilatation of the cervix;* in 48 of these 272 cases it was also followed by manual removal of the placenta. In 26 cases version was followed by manual removal of the placenta, and in 4 cases it was accompanied by some other operation or a combination of operations. In 172 of the 272 cases in which version was preceded by dilatation of the cervix the dilatation was done to induce labor as well as to facilitate delivery. Six of the 520 women died undelivered after attempts at version had failed.

Of these 520 deaths following version, 32 percent were attributed, according to the international classification, to placenta previa, 10 percent to other puerperal hemorrhage, 28 percent to puerperal albuminuria and convulsions, 19 percent to puerperal septicemia, 2 percent to embolus and sudden death, and 9 percent to other causes.

In addition to the cases of dilatation of the cervix performed with some other operation for delivery, the cervix was dilated manually, by bag, or by other artificial means in 112 cases. Eighty-nine women later delivered spontaneously, but 23 women died undelivered without further attempts at delivery. Four of the 89 women who delivered spontaneously after dilatation of the cervix also had manual removal of the placenta. There were also 87 women who had manual removal of the placenta following an absolutely spontaneous labor and delivery.

Sixty-five women were delivered by breech extraction. Eight of these had labor induced, 55 went into labor spontaneously, and for 2 the type of onset was not reported.

Fifty-seven women were delivered by craniotomy or embryotomy. Two of these had labor induced. Eight women with abdominal pregnancy were delivered by laparotomy in the last trimester. Twenty women had had some operation or combination of operations for delivery other than those already mentioned. Nine women had some operation for delivery, but its type was not reported. For 133 women no report could be obtained as to whether or not there had been an operative delivery.

Cesarean section preceded the deaths of 531 women who had reached the last trimester. For 62 of them attempts had been made at some other method of delivery. The Cesarean-section cases are discussed later (p. 29).

The technique of the operating physician as regards asepsis was analyzed. The term "aseptic" is used to indicate the usual good hospital delivery or operating-room technique without reported breaks. This was applicable in 1,328 cases. The term "attempted aseptic" is applicable to 275 cases, indicating that conditions as regards asepsis were not so good. Four hundred and fifty cases were assigned to the classification "clean, not sterile." "Dirty" indicated usually no preparation of the patient and sometimes no preparation even of the physician's hands; 89 cases were so assigned.

Table 5 shows the duration of labor of primiparæ and multiparæ who had reached the last trimester of pregnancy and whose deaths were preceded by various operations for delivery. *Two hundred and eighty-six primiparæ and 1,170 multiparæ were in labor less than 6 hours.* Three hundred and seventy-three primiparæ and 538 multiparæ were in labor 6 but less than 12 hours. Cesarean sections were performed 56 times on primiparæ and 31 times on multiparæ after 36 hours or more of labor. Almost all these operations were of the classical type.

### Onset and termination of labor

Artificial onset and artificial termination of labor were more frequent among the white than among the colored women who died. Not only did a larger proportion of colored women die undelivered, but a larger proportion died before the onset of labor.

Of the 1,990 women who died following operative termination of labor in the last trimester of pregnancy, there was a report as to

**Table 5.**—*Hours in labor and type of principal operation for delivery performed on primiparæ and multiparæ dying from puerperal causes who had reached the last trimester of pregnancy*

| Type of principal operation for delivery | Total | Primiparæ: Total | Primiparæ: None | Primiparæ: Less than 6 | Primiparæ: 6, less than 12 | Primiparæ: 12, less than 24 | Primiparæ: 24, less than 36 | Primiparæ: 36 and more | Primiparæ: Not reported | Multiparæ: Total | Multiparæ: None | Multiparæ: Less than 6 | Multiparæ: 6, less than 12 | Multiparæ: 12, less than 24 | Multiparæ: 24, less than 36 | Multiparæ: 36 and more | Multiparæ: Not reported | Parity not reported |
|---|---|---|---|---|---|---|---|---|---|---|---|---|---|---|---|---|---|---|
| | Women dying from puerperal causes who had reached last trimester — Hours in labor | | | | | | | | | | | | | | | | | |
| **Total** | **4,965** | **1,746** | **204** | **286** | **373** | **306** | **130** | **184** | **263** | **3,041** | **229** | **1,170** | **538** | **282** | **90** | **151** | **581** | **178** |
| Forceps (without version) | 718 | 408 | ...... | 59 | 93 | 111 | 58 | 53 | 34 | 301 | ...... | 93 | 66 | 59 | 23 | 32 | 28 | 9 |
| With dilatation of cervix | *162* | *86* | ...... | *35* | *19* | *12* | *6* | *9* | *5* | *76* | ...... | *43* | *8* | *10* | *4* | *5* | *6* | ...... |
| Cesarean section | 531 | 292 | 133 | 15 | 20 | 27 | 19 | 56 | 22 | 231 | 116 | 23 | 14 | 21 | 13 | 31 | 13 | 5 |
| Version | 618 | 164 | ...... | 49 | 31 | 23 | 19 | 33 | 9 | 415 | ...... | 196 | 68 | 56 | 27 | 39 | 50 | 9 |
| With dilatation of cervix | *296* | *74* | ...... | *39* | *16* | *6* | *4* | *7* | *8* | *218* | ...... | *137* | *24* | *15* | *11* | *9* | *22* | *4* |
| Dilatation of cervix only | 108 | 37 | 2 | 11 | 14 | 3 | 2 | 3 | 2 | 70 | 5 | 34 | 13 | 6 | 3 | 3 | 6 | 1 |
| Manual removal of placenta only | 87 | 26 | ...... | 3 | 4 | 9 | 4 | 3 | 3 | 60 | ...... | 35 | 8 | 2 | ...... | 1 | 14 | 1 |
| Craniotomy or embryotomy | 57 | 22 | ...... | 1 | ...... | 7 | 4 | 8 | 2 | 35 | ...... | ...... | 7 | 9 | 5 | 11 | 3 | ...... |
| Breech extraction [1] | 65 | 15 | ...... | 3 | 4 | 2 | 4 | 2 | .. | 48 | ...... | 15 | 12 | 10 | 1 | 4 | 6 | 2 |
| Other operation [2] | 32 | 7 | 2 | ...... | ...... | ...... | 1 | 3 | 1 | 25 | 5 | 9 | 4 | 1 | 1 | 2 | 3 | ...... |
| Type not reported | 9 | 1 | ...... | ...... | ...... | ...... | ...... | ...... | 1 | 4 | ...... | ...... | ...... | ...... | ...... | 1 | 3 | 4 |
| No operation for delivery | 2,607 | 747 | 67 | 145 | 207 | 123 | 19 | 23 | 163 | 1,757 | 103 | 764 | 345 | 114 | 17 | 25 | 389 | 103 |
| No report on operation for delivery | 133 | 27 | ...... | ...... | ...... | 1 | ...... | ...... | 26 | 62 | ...... | 1 | 1 | 1 | ...... | 2 | 57 | 44 |

[1] Includes 17 with dilatation of cervix.
[2] Includes 9 with dilatation of cervix.

prenatal care for 1,879. Of these, 807 are known to have had no prenatal care; that is, 43 percent of the operative deliveries were on women whom the physician had not seen before labor or before the acute emergency.

**Operative deliveries and parity**

The percentage of deaths preceded by version and version combinations increased with the number of pregnancies, from 10 percent in the first pregnancy to 16 percent for those with five pregnancies. It decreased slightly for the sixth and seventh pregnancies and rose again to 21 percent of those dying after eight or more pregnancies. Dilatation of the cervix preceding version was also more common in the later than in the earlier pregnancies. The frequency of forceps operations dropped rapidly from 24 percent in the first pregnancies to 11 percent in the second pregnancies, 9 percent in the third, and 8 percent in the fourth pregnancies, after which it rose slightly.

The incidence of operations for delivery increased with age both for primiparæ and for multiparæ. Among primiparæ there was a definite increase with age for Cesarean section. Among multiparæ there was a definite increase with age for forceps, version, and Cesarean section.

**Incidence of operative delivery**

The deaths of white women were more often preceded by operative deliveries than those of colored women, and the deaths were more often preceded by operative deliveries in the urban than in the rural areas. The proportion of maternal deaths that were preceded by operations for delivery varied in the different States. Some operation for delivery in the last trimester preceded 57 percent of the maternal deaths in California and Wisconsin but only 34 percent in Alabama.

## OPERATIONS OTHER THAN FOR DELIVERY

Some operation other than the actual delivery of the child or of the placenta was performed on 636 women who died after reaching the last trimester. Three hundred and one of these women also had an operative delivery. Most of these other operations were done for conditions resulting from the delivery. In 62 cases transfusion was the only operation. In other cases there was a curettage or incision and drainage for infection, packing of the uterus, or enterostomy. Packing of the uterus was recorded in 138 cases. In 73 cases packing followed an operative delivery, and in 65 cases it followed after a normal delivery. A curettage was done in 109 cases, usually on women who died from sepsis. It followed an operative delivery in 22 cases and a normal delivery in 82 cases. In 5 cases the type of delivery was not reported. Some of these women also had a blood transfusion. Incision and drainage of an abscess was reported for 45 cases. In 32 cases a laparotomy for drainage of peritonitis was done. Practically all these secondary operations were performed as a result of sepsis.

Fourteen women had appendectomies, 7 antepartum and 4 postpartum, 2 at Cesarean section, and 1 at laparotomy for abdominal pregnancy. In some cases the appendectomy had apparently little to do with the death; in other cases it was a factor of greater importance.

Another group of women had enterostomy operations done subsequent to the delivery. Still another group had hysterectomies for one cause or another. A few of these secondary operations were for accidental complications, but most of them were intended to relieve conditions arising from the delivery, and most of the deaths that were preceded by these operations were from sepsis.

## OPERATIONS IN THE FIRST TWO TRIMESTERS

Nearly all the operations for delivery performed on women who died before reaching the third trimester were classified either as therapeutic abortions or as laparotomies for ectopic gestation.

Laparotomies for ectopic gestation were performed on 195 women. In 3 cases abdominal pregnancies of 5 or 6 months were found. Various other operations were performed in conjunction with the operation for ectopic gestation or on account of sequelæ of the first operation. In 13 cases the appendix was removed at the time of the operation. Fifteen of the women were curetted before the laparotomy was performed, in some cases for diagnosis and in other cases because of mistaken diagnosis.

The deaths of 52 of these 195 women were attributed to puerperal septicemia. The other deaths in this group were attributed to ectopic gestation; in other words, the women died of hemorrhage and shock.

Only 26 of the 195 women who had had laparotomies for ectopic gestation had blood transfusions.

Of the 205 therapeutic abortions 84 were performed in the first trimester and 117 in the second trimester; the time at which the remaining 4 were performed was not reported. Pernicious vomiting was given as the principal indication for 112 of the 205 therapeutic abortions; other toxemias for 52; hemorrhage, placenta previa, or premature separation for 14; dead fetus for 12; and other causes for 15. Most of the therapeutic abortions were done from below, but in four cases a hysterectomy and in at least seven cases an abdominal hysterotomy was the method used.

Of these 205 women who had had therapeutic abortions, 38 had some other operation besides—a second curettage, a blood transfusion, or packing of the uterus because of hemorrhage. Fourteen of the 38 women had laparotomies subsequent to the therapeutic abortion. Most of the additional operations were for complications, and sepsis caused the death of most of these 38 women.

At least one curettage had been done on 585 women who had had a spontaneous or induced abortion other than a therapeutic abortion, and most of the deaths of these women were attributed to puerperal septicemia. Fifty-three of the women who died in the first two trimesters had had blood transfusions as their only operation. Most of these deaths also were due to sepsis. Another group (82) who had had no operation for delivery, had laparotomies performed for various complications, such as peritonitis or salpingitis, and the majority of these deaths were due to sepsis.

## COMMENT BY ADVISORY COMMITTEE

In this series of cases all the women died (and many of the babies), and, therefore, it is a record of failure. One cannot say that the operative procedures followed in many cases caused the deaths, but analysis of these procedures leads to many criticisms of the management of these cases.

The physicians who delivered these cases cannot be blamed in all cases for the results obtained, for in 43 percent of the operative deliveries they had not seen the women before labor or before the acute emergency had occurred. Under these circumstances it is a well-recognized fact that the operation of election is not always possible; the physician many times is forced to do something which he appreciates may not be the best but which, at the time, seems justifiable. This shows, from another point of view, the absolute necessity, if maternal mortality is to be lowered, of insisting upon continuous prenatal and adequate delivery care.

In a study of this type the physician's ability to do well the operation he has chosen can be evaluated only by the results, which show that many of the operations either were badly chosen or were poorly done. In nearly 40 percent of these operative deliveries it was admitted by the physicians that their technique was at least unsatisfactory with regard to asepsis. It is therefore not to be wondered at that 26 percent of the deaths following forceps deliveries and 19 percent of the deaths following versions were due to sepsis. Had those women whose deaths were assigned to eclampsia and placenta previa lived longer, many of them also would probably have died of sepsis. An operative delivery is a surgical procedure and should not be undertaken by physicians untrained in surgical technique. It is evident that many of these physicians did not have such training.

Many of these patients were operated upon after very little or no labor, and this explains the frequency of artificial dilatation of the cervix in both forceps and version deliveries. The number of cases in which manual dilatation of the cervix, forceps or version, and manual removal of the placenta occurred, or forceps failed and version was done, was deplorably large. From this it is evident that accouchement forcé was resorted to many times, and accouchement forcé is not regarded as good obstetrics today; it gives bad results and should not be performed.

That attempts at delivery by vagina were followed by Cesarean section in 62 cases is to be noted and condemned. (For further comment on the Cesarean sections done in this series see p. 31.)

That 57 women died following delivery by craniotomy or embryotomy shows clearly the lack of care these women had.

The frequency with which a curettage was done on women who had developed sepsis is surprising, for such treatment has long been condemned. Secondary operations for various conditions, usually of a septic nature, were much too common.

Most of the operative deliveries in the first two trimesters were classified either as therapeutic abortions or as laparotomies for ectopic pregnancy. The main comment on the deaths occurring from these two conditions is made in their respective sections, but a few comments may be made here. The removal of the appendix at the time of operation for an ectopic gestation is not good surgery. The fact that of the 195 women who had had a laparotomy for ectopic gestation only 26 had transfusion is to be noted. It must be recognized that preparation to transfuse is almost as essential as operation in ectopic pregnancy. That 52 women died of sepsis shows clearly how perfect one's technique should be if sepsis is to be avoided.

It is to be expected that the operative incidence would be higher in a group of fatal cases such as those included in the present study than among women who survived. Without having all the data for all areas studied it would be difficult to draw too many absolute conclusions. Necessarily the more serious operation would make up a higher percentage in a mortality study than the less dangerous operations.

## CESAREAN SECTION

Five hundred and thirty-seven of the maternal deaths included in the study followed Cesarean section. This is 7 percent of the 7,211 deaths for which information concerning operations was secured. Five hundred and thirty-one women whose deaths followed Cesarean section had reached the last trimester of pregnancy. A Cesarean section was done on 11 percent of the 4,832 women who died after reaching the last trimester and for whom there was a report on operation for delivery. Twenty-four percent of all operations for delivery on women who died after reaching the last trimester were Cesarean sections.

The percentages of maternal deaths that were preceded by Cesarean section in the last trimester ranged in the various States from 2 in North Dakota to 24 in California. Deaths following Cesarean section were twice as frequent in the urban as in the rural areas. For 8 percent of the white and 6 percent of the colored women death was preceded by Cesarean section. For those women who died following Cesarean section in the last trimester, the incidence was 17 percent among the urban white, 16 percent among the urban colored, 7 percent among the rural white, and 4 percent among the rural colored.

### CAUSE OF DEATH

For these women who died following Cesarean section the number of deaths from each cause, as given on interview by the attendant physicians and classified according to the international list was: Accidents of pregnancy, 3; puerperal hemorrhage, 42; other accidents of labor, 146 (including Cesarean section, 136); puerperal septicemia, 143; puerperal albuminuria and convulsions, 202; and embolus and sudden death, 1.

### INDICATIONS

The indications for Cesarean section were very numerous. Combinations of indications were very frequent; in one fourth of the cases more than one indication was given. Eclampsia was given alone or in combination in 165 cases. Contracted pelvis was given in 107 cases, but this probably does not represent the actual number of women with contracted pelves in the group, as in many cases the principal indication given was a long and difficult labor with no word about contracted pelvis. Preeclamptic toxemia was the indication in 47, uremia in 27, placenta previa in 38 cases. Twenty-five of the 537 women who had a Cesarean section are known to have had a previous Cesarean; but this fact was used as the sole indication for operation in only 6 cases, and as the principal indication in 17.

The following list shows the principal indications for Cesarean section:

| Indication for operation as given by attending physician | Women who died following Cesarean section |
|---|---|
| Total | 537 |
| Principal indication reported | 534 |
| Eclampsia | 165 |
| Preeclampsia | 47 |
| Uremia | 27 |
| Placenta previa | 38 |
| Premature separation of placenta | 15 |
| Ruptured uterus | 9 |
| Previous Cesarean section | 17 |
| Contracted pelvis | 28 |
| Contracted pelvis and other indication | 55 |
| Abnormal presentation | 33 |
| Disproportion and long or difficult labor | 61 |
| Other indication | 39 |
| Principal indication not reported | 3 |

### PARITY AND AGE

The deaths of 13 percent of primiparæ, 8 percent of secundiparæ, 5 percent of the women who had had three to five pregnancies, and 4 percent of those who had had six or more pregnancies, followed Cesarean section. When the percentages are based only on those women who died after reaching the last trimester, it appears that the deaths of 17 percent of all primiparæ and 33 percent of primiparæ of 30 years or older were preceded by Cesarean section.

### DURATION OF LABOR

The duration of labor was reported for 495 of the 531 women dying from Cesarean section in the last trimester of pregnancy. Two hundred and fifty of these were not in labor, and the cause of death in 59 percent of these cases was puerperal albuminuria, in 12 percent puerperal hemorrhage, and in 11 percent puerperal septicemia. Of the 245 women in labor for whom the number of hours was reported, 38 were in labor less than 6 hours; 35 from 6 to 12 hours; 51 from 12 to 24 hours; 32 from 24 to 36 hours; and 89 more than 36 hours. With increase in the duration of labor, the percentage of deaths that were attributed to puerperal septicemia rose rapidly from 29 percent for those in labor less than 12 hours to 51 percent for those in labor 36 hours or more.

### RUPTURE OF THE MEMBRANES

There was a report on rupture of the membranes for 491 of the 531 Cesarean-section cases occurring in the last trimester. In 324 cases the membranes had not ruptured. They were ruptured artificially in 34 cases and had ruptured spontaneously in 109 cases; there was no report on this point in 24 cases. Of the 324 women with unruptured membranes, 15 percent died of perperal septicemia, 51 percent of albuminuria and convulsions, 10 percent of hemorrhage, and the rest of other causes. Of the 167 women with ruptured membranes, 49 percent died of puerperal septicemia, 14 percent of albuminuria and convulsions, 4 percent of puerperal hemorrhage, and the rest of other causes.

### PLANNED AND EMERGENCY OPERATIONS

Eighty-two of the five hundred and thirty-seven Cesarean sections were planned, 452 were emergency, and in 3 cases there was no report.

### ATTEMPTS AT OTHER OPERATIONS

Cesarean section followed attempts at other forms of operative delivery in the cases of 62 women, 42 of whom were primiparæ.

### VAGINAL EXAMINATIONS

Vaginal examinations by the operating physician preceded the Cesarean section in 254 cases, or 52 percent of the 485 women dying in the last trimester for whom this information was secured. Of the 231 women who had had no vaginal examination by the operating physician, 20 percent died of sepsis, 43 percent of albuminuria and convulsions, and the rest from other causes; but of the 254 women who had vaginal examinations 34 percent died of sepsis, 30 percent of albuminuria and convulsions, and the rest of other causes.

### LIVE BIRTHS AND STILL BIRTHS

Live-born infants resulted from 393 (74 percent) of the 534 Cesareans for which the type of issue was reported. The largest proportion of stillbirths was obtained in those Cesareans for which the indication was premature separation of the placenta or ruptured uterus.

### ANESTHESIA

Ether was the most common anesthetic used. It was used alone in 275 of the 480 cases for which this information was obtained. In other cases nitrous oxide, ethylene, chloroform, or local anesthesia was used. Ether was used alone in 90 of the 150 cases in which Cesarean section was done on account of eclampsia and in which a report on the anesthetic used was obtained. Nitrous-oxide oxygen anesthesia was used alone in 56 cases, with ether in 62 cases, and in a few cases with local anesthesia. Ethylene was used in 41 cases, 1 of which was with spinal anesthesia. Chloroform was used in 14 cases, 7 of which were eclamptic. Local anesthesia was used in only 19 cases, in 5 of which it was supplemented by nitrous oxide or ether and in 1 of which it was used with sacral anesthesia. Spinal anesthesia was used in 8 cases.

## COMMENT BY ADVISORY COMMITTEE

The very fact that Cesarean section was done on one fourth of all the women who died following operation for delivery suggests that there had been unwise selection of cases for the operation, or of the types of operation, or both, as Cesarean sections constitute only a small percentage of all operative deliveries in general. Additional evidence to this effect is found in the causes of the deaths following Cesarean section.

According to statements of the physicians upon interview, 27 percent of the women died of sepsis, but careful study of each record indicates that 47 percent were probably septic. The conditions under which the operations were done may account for this high percentage of sepsis. Eighty-five percent of the operations had not been planned. In 34 percent the membranes were ruptured before the operation was done. Fifty-two percent of the women had had one or more vaginal examinations. Twelve percent had had attempted delivery from below. The number of sections done for various types of dystocia after long and exhausting labors is appalling. There was evident lack of recognition of the fact that the mortality from classical Cesarean section increases with the length of time the woman has been in labor and with attempts at delivery from below.

In any discussion of sepsis following Cesarean section it is to be remembered that the operating surgeon often does not have "first chance" with his patients. Yet this should be no reason for unwise selection of the operation to be performed. In many of these cases a Porro or low cervical operation should have been done instead of the classical Cesarean; in others no type of Cesarean operation should have been done.

Probably many of the surgeons could appropriately analyze the selection of their cases and study their operative technique and the surgical technique of their institutions, for death resulted from sepsis in many cases in which it apparently should not have occurred.

The most frequent indication for the Cesarean section was some toxemia—in many cases eclampsia. Although the mortality from eclampsia in Cesarean-section cases is known to be higher than in those treated conservatively, this fact was apparently not appreciated. Women with recognized toxemia were kept under observation for long periods of time and finally developed convulsions and were delivered by emergency Cesarean; women having convulsions were carried long distances to hospitals and operated on immediately upon arrival—both inexcusable procedures.

Many of the cases resulting in death from hemorrhage were equally mismanaged. In many cases the operation was done after great loss of blood when the patient was in shock, and without transfusion or other treatment for shock.

Unwise selection of anesthetic was frequent. In the cases of Cesarean section for eclampsia ether was the most common anesthetic, and even chloroform was occasionally used (7 cases). Ether was also used in the presence of acute respiratory infection. Local anesthesia was used in surprisingly few cases (19).

The tremendous mortality attending Cesarean sections throughout the United States warrants a careful review of the indications in the choice of operation.

## ABORTIONS

*Abortion as used in this study may be defined as the termination of a previable uterine pregnancy.* Attempted abortions and inevitable abortions are also included, even if the woman died without actual expulsion of the fetus. The term therefore includes all terminations of uterine pregnancy in the first two trimesters except the very few cases already spoken of that resulted in live births. Abortion thus defined is not the same as the title "Abortion" (no. 143*a*) in the International List of Causes of Death, which includes premature labor and does not necessarily denote previability.

Deaths certified as due to criminal abortion are assigned to homicide in the International List of Causes of Death, and therefore are not included in "maternal mortality." However, abortions not certified as criminal were not excluded from this study, even if the attending physician knew or was convinced that they were criminal.

Of the 2,381 deaths before the seventh month of gestation, 1,825 followed abortion. Five hundred and fifty-four did not follow abortion, and for 2 it could not be ascertained whether they did or did not follow an abortion. The 554 women whose deaths before they reached the last trimester did not follow abortion had had ectopic pregnancies or died without a termination of pregnancy; a few (32) gave birth to living, and probably viable, children.

The type of abortion was reported in 1,588 of these 1,825 cases. Of these, 794 (50 percent) were induced (other than therapeutic), 589 (37 percent) were spontaneous, and 205 (13 percent) were therapeutic: that is, were done for medical indications.

Of the 1,825 deaths following abortion 1,324 were attributed, according to the international classification, to puerperal septicemia, 290 to accidents of pregnancy, 163 to puerperal albuminuria and convulsions, 44 to puerperal phlegmasia alba dolens, embolus, and sudden death, and 4 to puerperal hemorrhage.[1]

*Puerperal septicemia was the cause attributed after interview for deaths of 1,324 (73 percent) of the 1,825 women who died following abortion. These 1,324 deaths from sepsis following abortion constituted 45 percent of the total number of deaths from puerperal septicemia in the study.* Ninety-one percent of the deaths following induced abortion, 60 percent of those following spontaneous abortion, and 21 percent of those following therapeutic abortion were due to sepsis. Eighty-six percent of the deaths following abortion for which the type of abortion was not reported were also due to sepsis, this fact suggesting that most of these abortions of unreported type were actually induced abortions.

The period of gestation was reported for 1,461 of the 1,825 cases. In 548 cases it was less than 3 months, in 444 cases 3 months, in 219 cases 4 months, and in 250 cases 5 or 6 months.

[1] According to the 1929 classification 1,324 would be attributed to abortion with septic conditions, about 250 to abortion without mention of septic conditions, and about 200 to other toxemias of pregnancy; the others would remain the same.

A report concerning operations was obtained for 1,777 of the 1,825 cases. Nine hundred and ninety-two (56 percent) had operations of some sort, including 265 of the 583 women who had spontaneous abortions, and 403 of the 778 women who had induced abortions. Of the 205 women who had therapeutic abortions, 38 had other operations as well. The most frequent operation was curettage. Of the women who had spontaneous abortions 212 (36 percent) and of those who had induced abortions 289 (37 percent) had been curetted. Evidently many physicians did not consider fever a contraindication for curettage, for 448 (69 percent) of the 652 women who had had abortions and were curetted were reported to have had fever before the curettage. *Puerperal sepsis caused 94 percent of the deaths of these 448 women*, as compared with 50 percent of the deaths of women who were afebrile before the curettage and 68 percent of the deaths of the women who had no curettage.

CHART VII.—ABORTIONS AMONG WOMEN DYING FROM PUERPERAL CAUSES

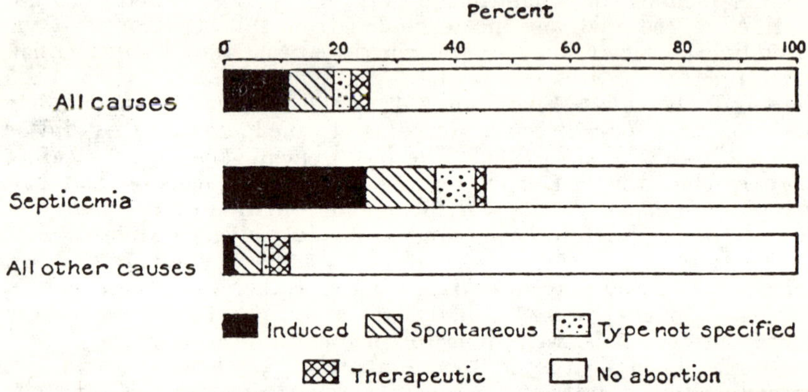


Hemorrhage was reported for 328 of the 652 cases in which there had been a curettage. It was absent in 235 cases, and it was not reported on for 89 cases. Of the 1,086 women who died following abortion and who had not been curetted, 430 were reported as having had hemorrhage and 459 as having had no hemorrhage; there was no report for 197.

Pernicious vomiting was given as the principal indication for 112 of the 205 therapeutic abortions. Other toxemias accounted for 52, hemorrhage, placenta previa, or premature separation of placenta for 14, dead fetus for 12, and various other causes for 15.

Married women made up 90 percent of the women whose deaths followed abortion, but abortion was a more frequent cause of death among unmarried than among married mothers, for abortion preceded the deaths of about one fifth of the married mothers and of more than one third of the 509 unmarried mothers included in the study.

The proportion of maternal deaths that were preceded by abortion increased with the age of the mother up to 30 and then decreased.

The mortality rate for deaths following abortion was higher among the colored than among the white women and among urban women than among rural women. The difference between urban and rural groups was most marked in induced abortions, for which the mortality rate was 11 per 10,000 live births in urban areas as compared with 4 in rural areas.

The proportion of maternal deaths that followed abortion in the various States ranged from 18 percent in Alabama and Wisconsin to 37 percent in Washington. The variation in the per-

CHART VIII.—MORTALITY RATES FOR DEATH FOLLOWING ABORTION AMONG WOMEN DYING FROM PUERPERAL CAUSES

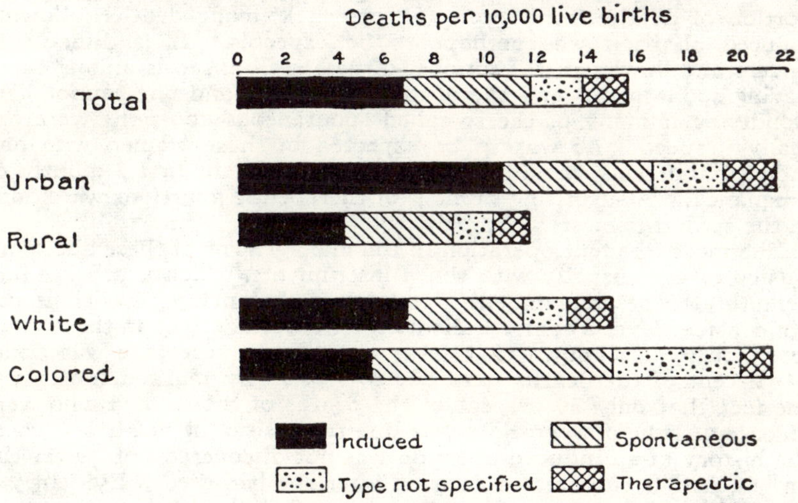


centage of maternal deaths was greatest for induced abortions, which ranged from 3 percent of all maternal deaths in Alabama to 23 percent in Washington.

Three percent of all the maternal deaths followed therapeutic abortion.

---

## COMMENT BY ADVISORY COMMITTEE

In reading the section on abortion it must be carefully kept in mind that the definition of "abortion" as used in this report is different from that of the international list. In this report the term "abortion" is used to mean the termination of a previable uterine pregnancy.

Undoubtedly among this number of deaths were some due to criminal abortions. If the abortions were known to be criminal and death followed, the deaths were assigned by the Bureau of the Census, according to the International List of Causes of Death, as homicides and were not included in the maternal mortality. It was impossible, however, to separate the known self-induced abortions from possible criminal abortions, and therefore they were included in the figures analyzed.

That one quarter of all the maternal deaths in this study followed some type of abortion is probably the most outstanding finding of the study. The further finding that three quarters of the deaths following abortion were due to puerperal septicemia is equally significant. As 1,825 deaths followed abortion out of the total of 7,380 deaths in this series, abortion is evidently one of the greatest problems in lowering the maternal mortality of the country.

The large proportion of induced abortions shows a very serious situation. Fifty percent of abortions of known type were induced and 13 percent of all the abortions were of "type not reported", so that many of these may have been induced. The seriousness of this situation is further shown by the fact that 73 percent of the deaths following abortion were due to puerperal septicemia. The high proportion of deaths from sepsis (91 percent) among deaths following induced abortion was perhaps to be expected. It is difficult to understand, however, the number of deaths from sepsis among those having spontaneous and therapeutic abortions, and one cannot help wondering if many of the so-called spontaneous abortions were not really induced. As was to be expected in those women who had induced abortions, more than half were done in the first 2 months of pregnancy. A surprising number of therapeutic abortions were done in the second trimester of pregnancy.

The most frequent operation in the management of these abortions was curettage (usually with sharp instruments, which is a procedure definitely to be condemned). It is clear that many physicians did not consider fever a contra-indication for curettage; yet in those cases in which it was known that fever existed and curettage was done, 94 percent of the deaths were due to sepsis. In marked contrast is the fact that only 50 percent of the deaths of the women who were afebrile at time of operation were due to sepsis. In not a few cases the history of an induced abortion was not discovered until after the patient had been curetted or even after she had died. Evidently a careful history in many of these cases was not obtained.

Hemorrhage was of frequent occurrence in these abortion cases, but the fact that the patient had had a hemorrhage had very little effect on the proportion of deaths from sepsis after curettage in febrile cases.

As pernicious vomiting was the principal indication given for 112 of the therapeutic abortions, it would seem that the physicians had delayed in doing the abortion or had been called in consultation too late to save the patient's life, or else had improper technique.

Analysis of the figures on illegitimacy brings up the whole problem of abortion in unmarried mothers, for abortions accounted for more than one third of the deaths of unmarried mothers in this series.

This study shows very clearly the seriousness of the problem created by the great number of abortions that are induced each year. It also shows that the practice of curetting every patient who has an abortion is common. Physicians must be made to appreciate the seriousness of curetting these potentially septic cases. The management of an abortion calls for the best medical care that can be given, and in many of the cases in this series it is obvious that such care was not given. The abortion problem is a widespread sociological and economic problem, which the medical profession must have help in solving. However, the physician has one great obligation—to teach the public the dangers entailed by abortion, whether spontaneous or induced.

## PUERPERAL SEPTICEMIA

Puerperal septicemia, as has been shown (p. 5), was the most important cause of death connected with pregnancy or childbirth. It caused 40 percent of the 7,380 deaths included in the study.

Women who have been weakened by hemorrhage, by eclampsia, or by the exhaustion of a long and difficult labor are an easy prey to infection; and infection is the chief cause of death of women for whom an operative delivery is necessary and who survive the shock of the operation itself. It is also the chief cause of death following abortion from any cause.

From death certificates and subsequent queries of indefinite certificates, 2,827 of the 7,537 deaths studied were assigned by the Bureau of the Census to puerperal septicemia. On interview with the attendant, 110 of these were found to be due actually to other causes; 64 of these 110 were not strictly puerperal and therefore were omitted from the study. Interviews also disclosed that 231 deaths assigned to other puerperal causes were really due to puerperal septicemia, and these deaths were so classified in the study. These changes involve only those cases in which the sepsis, although not mentioned on the death certificate, was diagnosed by the attending physician or in which the history of septic temperature, positive blood culture, or autopsy findings made the change in diagnosis inevitable. This gives a total of 2,948 deaths considered due to puerperal septicemia. *The term "puerperal septicemia" as used in this report means obvious and unmistakable sepsis, and the number of deaths here attributed to this cause is the minimum.*

Of these 2,948 deaths 1,324 (45 percent) were preceded by abortion. Ectopic pregnancy was a factor in 65 cases.[1] Placenta previa was present in 53 cases, and 84 women had other puerperal hemorrhage of such severity that it was considered the principal contributory cause of death. One hundred and sixty-nine women who died of sepsis following delivery were reported to have had postpartum hemorrhage as a contributing factor. Eclampsia or severe toxemia of pregnancy was a principal contributory cause in 168 cases.

Operations aimed at delivery were performed on 573 women who died of sepsis at 7 or more months' gestation. Of these operations, 140 were Cesarean sections. Information as to whether there had been any intrauterine manipulation, such as induction of abortion, operative delivery, or curettage, was obtained for 2,549 of the 2,948 cases of deaths from sepsis. There had been some intrauterine manipulation in 1,546 of these cases, or 61 percent.

The time of this manipulation with reference to the appearance of symptoms of sepsis was reported for 1,526 of these cases. In 748 (49 percent) the intrauterine manipulation had occurred only before

[1] Abortion with septic conditions and ectopic gestation with septic conditions are separate titles in the 1929 revision of the International List of Causes of Death.

the onset of sepsis; in 517 (34 percent) it had occurred after the onset of sepsis; and in 261 (17 percent) it had occurred both before and after. In septic cases of less than 7 months' gestation the intrauterine manipulation before the onset of sepsis was usually the induction of abortion; after the onset it was usually curettage. In the last trimester the manipulation before the onset of sepsis was usually an operative delivery, and the manipulation after the onset of sepsis was usually a curettage.

In the last trimester of pregnancy puerperal septicemia caused the deaths of 1,529 women. Most of these (1,386, or 94 percent, of the women for whom a report as to onset was obtained) had a spontaneous onset of labor. Labor terminated spontaneously in 65 percent of the cases in which information concerning termination was obtained; in 34 percent termination was artificial.

Of the 1,474 deaths of women who had reached the last trimester, for whom there was a report on operations aimed at delivery, 573 (39 percent) had had such an operation. Operations in the last trimester other than those for delivery were far more numerous among women who died of sepsis than among those who died of other causes. Blood transfusion was known to have been performed on 64 women who later died of sepsis and who did not have hemorrhage.

The time between delivery and the appearance of the first symptoms of sepsis was reported in 1,303 of the 1,529 cases of women who died from sepsis after reaching the last trimester. Symptoms of sepsis appeared before the actual delivery in 196 cases (15 percent); within 2 days after delivery in 328 cases (25 percent); between 2 days and a week after delivery in 602 cases (46 percent); and a week or more after delivery in 177 cases (14 percent). The 196 cases in which symptoms of sepsis appeared before the actual delivery were carefully studied for the presumable cause of sepsis. Long labor, early rupture of the membranes, or attempts at delivery were apparently responsible in 53 cases; one or more of these, and some other factor, were responsible in 7 cases. Infectious disease, usually respiratory, at the time of labor was the probable source of sepsis in 38 cases. Macerated fetus was associated with sepsis in 18 cases, pyelitis in 15, gonorrhea or pelvic inflammatory disease in 11, and some other cause in 22. In 32 cases no probable reason for the development of sepsis was given.

Symptoms of sepsis developed more quickly among the women who had operative deliveries than among those who had spontaneous deliveries. In general, symptoms of sepsis appeared earlier in women who had longer labors. Attendance at birth, technique at delivery, and nursing and aftercare of the patient are of particular interest in these cases of death from sepsis. A larger proportion of the deaths of women who had been attended by midwives were from sepsis than of the deaths of women who had been attended by physicians. Of the 550 women dying at 7 or more months' gestation who had midwife attendance either alone or with a physician or interne, 239 (43 percent) died of sepsis, while of the 4,065 who died after being attended at delivery by physicians, 1,177 (29 percent) died of sepsis.

The delivery technique of the physician in charge was reported in 1,114 cases of women who died of sepsis after reaching the last trimester. It was said to be aseptic in 445 cases (40 percent). Most of these cases occurred in hospitals. Asepsis was attempted under conditions making its attainment unlikely in 158 cases (14 percent). Ordinary cleanliness was present in 405 cases (36 percent), and in 106 cases (10 percent) ordinary cleanliness was lacking.

More of the women who died of sepsis than of those who died of other puerperal causes had 3 or more vaginal examinations, and a smaller proportion of those who had as many as 3 vaginal examinations had had attendants who used rubber gloves.

Inquiries were made as to the preparation of the patient for operation, and information was obtained as to shaving and scrubbing for 1,348 cases. Of these, 645 (48 percent) had been shaved and scrubbed; 263 (20 percent) were neither shaved nor scrubbed; 428 (32 percent) had been scrubbed only; and 12 (1 percent) had been shaved only. Some antiseptic had been used in 1,094 cases; none had been used in 262 cases. In at least 172 cases women who died of sepsis had been neither scrubbed nor shaved, nor had an antiseptic been used.

Of the 2,948 women who died of puerperal septicemia, 1,950 (66 percent) had had hospital treatment. Only 618 of them, however, were known to have had their delivery or abortion in the hospital. One thousand three hundred and one were known to have had their delivery or abortion outside of the hospital, 25 died undelivered, and for 6 the place of delivery or abortion was not reported. Fatal sepsis developed in the hospital in 420 cases (70 percent) of the 601 women delivered in hospitals for whom the place of development of sepsis was reported, and in 26 cases of women delivered elsewhere. However, at least 69 of these 420 women had had vaginal examinations or other vaginal manipulations before admission to the hospital.

In most cases it was impossible to obtain information whether other septic patients were in the hospital at the same time as were these that died.

There were 898 hospital deaths from sepsis of women who had reached the third trimester; but only 454 of these women were delivered in the hospital, and 105 of the 454 were reported to have had vaginal examinations or attempted operative delivery before admission to the hospital.

The mortality rates from sepsis were higher among the colored than among the white women, and higher in the cities than in the rural areas. This is true of sepsis following delivery as well as of sepsis following abortion.

Deaths from sepsis following abortion make up a large proportion of deaths assigned to puerperal septicemia in the international classification. In the 15 States studied 45 percent of the sepsis deaths followed abortion and 25 percent followed induced abortion. In the separate States the proportion of sepsis deaths following induced abortion varied considerably, being 48 percent in Washington and only 7 percent in Alabama. The mortality rates from septic abortion ranged from 6 deaths per 10,000 live births in New Hampshire to 18 in Washington. The death rates from this condition were low in the New England States of New Hampshire and Rhode Island, and in Wisconsin, Minnesota, and North Dakota, and were highest in Washington, Oregon, and Oklahoma.

## COMMENT BY ADVISORY COMMITTEE

That 40 percent of all the deaths in this study were of women who had such obvious and unmistakable signs of sepsis that there could be no question how they should be classified shows clearly the serious condition presented by this cause of maternal death.

The outstanding findings in regard to abortions followed by septicemia have already been commented on in the section on that subject.

No matter how the figures are analyzed, it is clear that the loss of life from sepsis is enormous. That in the last trimester of pregnancy 1,529 women of this series died of sepsis, 94 percent of whom had a spontaneous onset of labor and 65 percent a spontaneous termination of labor, is nothing short of appalling.

In this series of deaths the midwives had a larger percentage of deaths from sepsis than physicians. This fact, however, does not by any means take the onus of this state of affairs from the physicians. Lack of adequate nursing care at home undoubtedly had something to do with these bad results, but the ultimate responsibility for these deaths rests on the delivery technique of the physician. That technique was classed as aseptic in only 40 percent of the cases in which it was reported upon, and these usually occurred in hospitals. The frequency of vaginal examinations without gloves is to be noted, as well as the relative infrequency of rectal examinations. Preparation of the patient in the majority of the cases was inadequate. It is not surprising to find that under these conditions sepsis developed much earlier in operative cases than in spontaneous deliveries. It is also to be noted that in cases of long labor signs of sepsis appeared earlier.

The deaths of 420 women delivered in hospitals from sepsis that developed in the hospital show clearly that the technique in the hospitals was unsatisfactory.

In many of the septic deaths classified as abortions the physician surely cannot be held responsible. It is admitted that many were induced, and there is no way of telling how many of the so-called spontaneous abortions also were induced. Moreover, infection was present in many of these cases when the physician was called. But the frequency with which curettage was done on these septic cases is not justifiable.

In the cases in the last trimester there is no such excuse for the bad results obtained as may be offered in the abortions. Complications were present in many instances in the last trimester, and operative procedures were necessary, but these facts do not excuse the physicians for the poor technique which they themselves admitted.

What is the reason for the existence of this condition? It is due to lack of proper teaching of obstetrics in some of the medical schools, lack of opportunity to deliver a sufficient number of normal cases, and almost total lack of experience in the simplest obstetric operating, or else it is due to the willful disregard by careless physicians of the fundamentals of asepsis.

The large number of fatal cases of puerperal infection are in the majority of instances due to infection that is introduced from without. Its prevention, therefore, lies in carrying out proper obstetric procedures, consisting chiefly of proper aseptic technique and carrying out only definitely indicated obstetric operations. It must be remembered, however, that there are a certain number of cases of puerperal infection which are endogenous in character; that is, they are due to organisms which the patient harbors chiefly in her birth canal. This type of infection forms another obstetric problem.

## PUERPERAL PHLEGMASIA ALBA DOLENS, EMBOLUS, SUDDEN DEATH [1]

Three hundred and thirty-seven deaths were assigned to puerperal phlegmasia alba dolens, embolus, sudden death, from information given on death certificates. At the interview with the attending physician 48 of these deaths were attributed to other puerperal causes, most of them to puerperal sepsis or puerperal hemorrhage, and 3 to nonpuerperal causes. But 58 deaths were added to these as a result of additional information or as a result of the physician's change of opinion.

Not all deaths for which this cause is given on the certificates are so assigned in the international classification, for certain other causes take precedence over this classification. There were 242 deaths assigned to puerperal causes for which puerperal phlebitis or embolus was given as the principal contributory cause of death. For 123 of these the primary cause of death was puerperal sepsis. An autopsy was performed in only 25 cases.

Of the 344 deaths attributed after interview to phlegmasia alba dolens, embolus, sudden death, 303 were attributed to embolism, 10 to thrombosis, 10 to phlegmasia alba dolens, and 21 to sudden death. Phlebitis was diagnosed either clinically or at autopsy in 52 of the 303 cases in which death was thought due to embolism. Of these 303 deaths, 10 occurred during delivery. The diagnosis can be questioned particularly in these cases, but in one case embolism was proved by autopsy.

Of the 303 women whose deaths were attributed to embolus, 220 were said to have had respiratory distress, 41 were said not to have had it, and for 42 there was no information on this point. Cyanosis was reported present in 197 cases, 53 were reported as not cyanotic, and for 53 there was no report. That the absence of reported cyanosis or respiratory distress does not rule out embolism is shown by a case in which an autopsy was done, and a large embolus was found in the left pulmonary artery.

Abortions preceded 44 of the 53 deaths at less than 7 months' gestation. The abortion was said to have been spontaneous in 25 cases, induced in 13, therapeutic in 4, and of unknown type in 2 cases.

The deaths of 291 women who died after reaching the last trimester were attributed to phlegmasia alba dolens, embolus, sudden death. Of these women, 12 died undelivered. For 7 the termination of labor was not reported. Of the 272 who were delivered, delivery was spontaneous for 203 (75 percent) and artificial for 69 (25 percent). In 40 cases phlegmasia alba dolens, embolus, sudden death was given as the principal contributory cause where the death was attributed to Cesarean section or other operative delivery.

[1] This title, no. 147 in the 1920 revision of the International List, is no. 148 in the 1929 revision, without change of name or content.

Death occurred within the first day after delivery in 33 percent of the 316 cases for which the interval between delivery or abortion and death from phlegmasia alba dolens, embolus, sudden death was reported, and within the first week in 46 percent. Twenty-nine percent of the deaths took place in the second week, 9 percent in the third week, 8 percent in the fourth week, and 9 percent in the fifth week or later.

## COMMENT BY ADVISORY COMMITTEE

Little comment on this section is necessary. This number in the international list may cover many deaths of uncertain cause. A death certificate under this heading is oftentimes accepted without proper understanding of the circumstances of the death.

Twenty-five percent of the women who reached the last trimester died following operative delivery. Some had symptoms clearly suggestive of embolism, but in others the history obtained was of ruptured uterus. Many of the spontaneously delivered patients showed the classical symptoms of embolism with no demonstrable phlebitis. Thrombosis and embolism are the results of infection; and so far as infections are preventable, thrombosis and embolism are preventable.

## TOXEMIAS OF PREGNANCY

Thirty percent (2,221) of all the deaths in the study were preceded by some presumably toxic condition as the chief cause or the chief contributory cause. Most of these deaths—1,900, or 26 percent of the total—were due to puerperal albuminuria and convulsions (no. 148 in the International List of Causes of Death), and 220 that were attributed to other primary causes had albuminuria and convulsions as the principal contributory cause. Sixty-one deaths were attributed to pernicious vomiting of pregnancy, and 40 more that were attributed to causes other than albuminuria and convulsions had pernicious vomiting as the chief contributory cause.[1]

Deaths resulting from the toxemias of pregnancy are assigned in the International List of Causes of Death to various numbers, most of them, as has been noted, to puerperal albuminuria and convulsions. According to the definite rules of classification, some death certificates on which the cause would otherwise be assignable to puerperal albuminuria and convulsions are assigned to puerperal septicemia, puerperal hemorrhage, ectopic gestation, or ruptured uterus, when these conditions accompany the toxemia. For the same reason, because chronic nephritis takes precedence over certain puerperal causes, a number of deaths of pregnant or parturient women from this cause are lost entirely to the puerperal group. Deaths from acute yellow atrophy of the liver are likewise omitted from the puerperal group unless puerperal septicemia appears on the death certificate.

### PUERPERAL ALBUMINURIA AND CONVULSIONS

Puerperal albuminuria and convulsions (no. 148 of the international list) was the cause of the death of 1,900 women—26 percent of all those included in the study. As a puerperal cause of death it was exceeded in importance numerically only by puerperal septicemia. In the last trimester of pregnancy it was of equal importance with puerperal septicemia, each accounting for 31 percent of the deaths at or after 7 months' gestation. Among the rural women, both white and colored, after 7 months' gestation, it was a cause of death of numerically greater importance than sepsis.

The 1,900 deaths were finally attributed to the group albuminuria and convulsions, after interview with the physicians in charge of these patients. Physicians had certified 2,006 deaths as due to this cause, but the interviews showed incomplete or incorrect information for 180, which were therefore not included; 74 deaths, however, were added to this group after interview.

No attempt at pathological classification of these deaths was made. Convulsions were known to have preceded the deaths of 1,305 of the 1,900 women. Five hundred and twenty-one had no convulsions, and in 74 cases information as to convulsions was not obtained. In 130 cases the toxemia was a pernicious vomiting of pregnancy.

[1] In the 1929 revision of the International List the toxemias are divided into puerperal albuminuria and eclampsia (no. 146) and other toxemias of pregnancy (no. 147), which includes pernicious vomiting.

Death occurred in the first or second trimester in 338 cases, and in the third trimester in 1,549 cases; in 13 cases the duration of pregnancy was not known.

A few of these cases seemed to be true cases of fulminating eclampsia, fatal convulsions developing a few days after a thorough examination at which nothing abnormal was found, but *the great majority of toxemic deaths were of women who lacked some or all of the ordinary safeguards.* Approximately one half of the 1,756 women who died of puerperal albuminuria and convulsions after the second month of pregnancy and for whom a report as to prenatal care was obtained had presented themselves for prenatal care, but only 12 percent of the total had received good care.

After the patient was seen by the physician the cooperation of the patient was said to have been good in a little more than one half of the cases in which a report on this point was obtained. It is of interest to note that *about one third of the women who died of albuminuria and convulsions could not have cooperated, because they were in convulsions or in coma when first seen by a physician, or they were not seen by a physician before death.*

CHART IX.—CONDITION WHEN FIRST SEEN BY PHYSICIAN OF WOMEN WHO DIED FROM PUERPERAL ALBUMINURIA AND CONVULSIONS

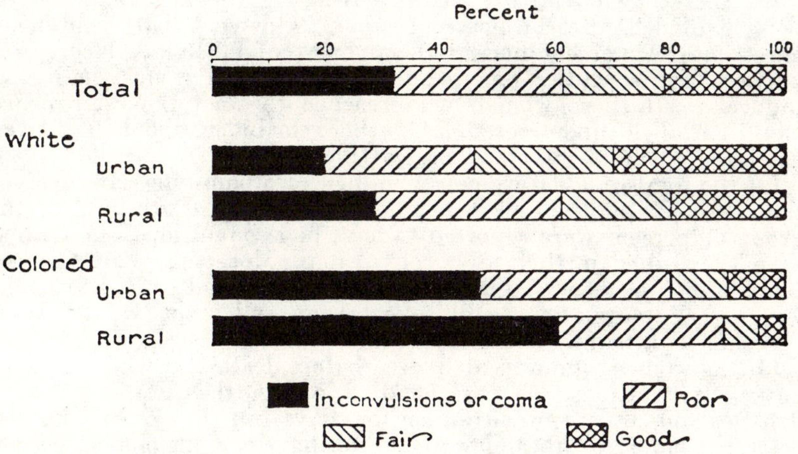


In 1,723 cases the condition of the patient when she was first seen by a physician was known. Of these women, 546 (32 percent) were in coma or were having or had had convulsions; 508 (29 percent) were otherwise in poor condition; 313 (18 percent) were in fair condition; and only 356 (21 percent) were in good condition.

Thirty-six percent of the women who died in the rural areas as compared with 25 percent of those in urban areas were in coma or had had convulsions when first seen. Fifty-six percent of the colored women and 25 percent of the white women were in this condition. It must be noted that only 54 percent of the urban white, 39 percent of the rural white, 20 percent of the urban colored, and 11 percent of the rural colored women who died of albuminuria and convulsions were in good or even fair condition when first seen by a physician.

One thousand and twenty-nine (54 percent) of the 1,900 women whose deaths were attributed to albuminuria and convulsions were hospitalized, 869 (46 percent) were not, and for 2 cases this information was not reported. The great majority of the patients who were sent to the hospital did not reach it until they were in a serious condition. One hundred and thirty-eight were sent to a hospital or were already in a hospital on the first appearance of symptoms. Of the 866 women who were not hospitalized until they were in a serious condition, only 157 were reported to have been put to bed at home at the first appearance of symptoms. More of the white women who died than of the colored had had hospitalization and bed treatment. A number of the women who were sent to the hospital early improved under treatment and were allowed to go home and later returned in convulsions.

Operative delivery comprised part or all of the treatment of many of the women. Twenty-six percent of those who died after reaching the last trimester had an artificial onset of labor. This includes 224 women who had labor induced mechanically, 146 who had Cesarean section when not in labor, 10 who had medical induction, and 3 for whom the exact method was not reported. Fourteen percent died before the onset of labor.

Of the women who died before reaching the last trimester, 47 percent died before the onset of labor, 21 percent had spontaneous onset, and 32 percent had artificial onset of labor. A larger proportion of the white women than of the colored women had labor induced. Of those women who reached the last trimester nearly one fifth died undelivered. Of the remainder about half were delivered spontaneously and half artificially.

Of the total of 1,900 women who died of albuminuria and convulsions 437 (23 percent) were not delivered before death, and of this group 69 percent were reported to have had convulsions. A number of patients died in their first convulsion. More than half (56 percent) of the women who died undelivered and had convulsions died less than 12 hours after the first convulsion, and about two thirds (63 percent) less than 24 hours afterward.

Of the women who were delivered before death and who died after having convulsions, 90 percent died within the first week after delivery and 56 percent within the first day. Of the women who were delivered before death and who did not have convulsions, 63 percent died within the first week and 31 percent within the first day.

Of the women who were delivered in the last trimester 807 gave birth to liveborn and 457 to stillborn children. Eighteen mothers had 1 liveborn and 1 stillborn twin. No data were obtained, however, as to the survival of these children.

Puerperal albuminuria and convulsions caused 36 percent of the deaths of primiparæ and 21 to 24 percent of the deaths of women in subsequent pregnancies. Of primiparæ less than 20 years of age it caused 41 percent of the deaths.

Both the percentage of total deaths due to puerperal albuminuria and convulsions and the rate per 10,000 live births were higher among the colored than among the white women. The highest death rates from this cause among the white women were in Alabama and New Hampshire, the lowest in Wisconsin and Minnesota.

Among the colored women in the States having 2,000 or more colored births annually, the highest rates were in Alabama and Oklahoma, the lowest in California and Maryland.

The death rate from this cause was, in general, higher in the urban than in the rural areas.

### PERNICIOUS VOMITING

Although pernicious vomiting of pregnancy was the primary cause of death given for only 61 of the 7,380 women included in the study, it was a contributing factor in 191 other cases. Nearly all the women whose deaths were associated with pernicious vomiting died before the seventh month, and most of them died before the fifth month.

The duration of the vomiting before the physician was called was given in 164 of the 252 cases. It had lasted less than a week in 49 cases, from 1 to 2 weeks in 24 cases, from 2 to 4 weeks in 28 cases, and 4 weeks or longer in 63 cases. Ninety-three of these cases were said to have been in poor condition when first seen.

The condition that 227 of these 252 women were in when they were first seen by the physician was noted. Twenty-nine women were said to have been in good condition, 62 in fair condition, 136 in poor condition.

Pregnancy was interrupted artificially for 121 women. Labor or abortion took place spontaneously in 47 cases, and 82 women died without labor or abortion. Operation was known to have been refused by 19 of the 127 women dying without operation whose deaths were associated with pernicious vomiting. A few of these women had a spontaneous abortion. There were also other patients who refused interruption of pregnancy for varying periods, and finally consented to operation only when they were in very poor condition.

Of the 112 women with pernicious vomiting who had therapeutic abortions, 16 died of sepsis.

---

## COMMENT BY ADVISORY COMMITTEE

The chief method of attack against the severe toxemias of pregnancy is conceded to be their early detection and control. For this it is necessary to have continuous intelligent medical supervision of the prospective mother from early in pregnancy, early recognition of untoward symptoms, prompt and judicious treatment of symptoms as they appear during pregnancy as well as during and after actual delivery of the patient, and the cooperation of the patient. It is true that a few patients developed toxemias and died who apparently had all these safeguards. A small number of these seemed to be true cases of fulminating eclampsia—fatal convulsions developing a few days after a thorough examination at which nothing abnormal was found. Evidently, in the present state of medical knowledge, death from toxemia cannot be entirely prevented. But the vast majority of toxemic deaths were of women who lacked some or all of the safeguards mentioned.

For many of the toxic deaths studied the physician was not responsible because he saw the patient for the first time when the condition was already acute or because the patient failed to follow his advice. Three fifths of the women were in convulsions or coma or otherwise in poor condition when the physician saw them for the first time. Moreover, some of the women were seen early in pregnancy and advised concerning prenatal care—but the advice was not accepted. Others were seen in the preclamptic stage and induction of labor was advised—and the advice was not accepted. Evidently there is great need for the education of patients and families.

On the other hand, the study reveals serious conditions for which the physicians were responsible. Even though the occurrence of toxemia cannot be entirely prevented, many of the deaths from this cause can and should be prevented by the early recognition of symptoms and prompt and judicious treatment by the physician in charge. Some of the women (12 percent) had had what could be considered as good prenatal care, and the symptoms of approaching toxemia were promptly recognized during the latter part of gestation, but treatment was at fault. Induction of labor (as distinguished from accouchement forcé) was done in surprisingly few of these cases. Prenatal care, so far as the toxemias of pregnancy are concerned, will not save lives unless good clinical judgment and treatment are used.

The number of women who died during the first convulsion was rather surprising. Probably many more women die in this way than is realized.

Probably it is now generally conceded that radical treatment in eclampsia is never indicated except in the best environment and with proper anesthetic. The dire results of teaching radical treatment for eclampsia were manifest—almost universal resort to immediate operative interference in all kinds of cases and by all kinds of practitioners. Cesarean section seemed to be too often regarded as proper treatment for eclampsia. Oftentimes the sections were done without regard to the profound shock from which many of the patients were suffering and without due consideration for the proper anesthetic. Operative interference of all sorts was frequent, even in the cases of multiparous women; a majority of the operations were done under general anesthesia, ether being used commonly and even chloroform occasionally. Epigastric pain, which is a prodromal symptom of eclampsia, was occasionally observed, and was almost always treated as acute indigestion. There were more than occasional instances in which rising blood pressure was noted, but its importance evidently was not realized. In many cases treatment other than vague advice as to diet, or the prescription of a diuretic, was far from prompt. In other cases (202) the treatment was an immediate accouchement forcé, which, though prompt, would be called judicious by no leader in obstetric thought today.

Few of these women were treated along the conservative lines now accepted—with fluids, glucose, magnesium sulphate, and morphine or other sedative and induction of labor. There can be no question that failure to institute prompt treatment and the injudicious treatment they did receive contributed to many of the deaths. It is evident, therefore, that some safe, conservative treatment for eclampsia should be agreed upon and that knowledge of it should be widely disseminated.

## PUERPERAL HEMORRHAGE

Puerperal hemorrhage accounted for 791 deaths (11 percent) of the total deaths of this study. This includes 347 deaths attributed to placenta previa (no. 144*a* of the International List) and 444 deaths attributed to no. 144*b*, which includes postpartum hemorrhage and accidental hemorrhage.[1] Of these 444 deaths 374 were from postpartum hemorrhage and 70 from premature separation of the placenta, adherent placenta, or undefined puerperal hemorrhage.

Puerperal hemorrhage was definitely related to both parity and age. *Among primiparæ this condition caused 7 percent of all deaths as compared with 13 percent among multiparæ.* It caused 5 percent of the deaths of primiparæ under 20 years of age and 15 percent of the deaths from 35 to 39 years. Among the multiparæ 8 percent died from puerperal hemorrhage in the group under 20 years of age, 16 percent in the group from 35 to 39 years. The percentage of deaths from puerperal hemorrhage rose rapidly from 7 for primiparæ to 10 for women in their second pregnancy and to 13 for women in their third pregnancy, and rose again to 17 percent in the seventh pregnancy. 22 percent in the eighth pregnancy, and 24 percent in the ninth pregnancy. It caused 21 percent of the deaths of women having 10 or more pregnancies.

Puerperal hemorrhage caused a slightly larger proportion of the deaths in rural areas (12 percent) than in urban areas (10 percent). It caused a larger percentage of deaths among the white women than among the colored, but the maternal mortality *rate* (deaths per 10,000 live births) from puerperal hemorrhage was higher for the colored than for the white women.

### PLACENTA PREVIA

For 347 of the 408 women who were known to have had placenta previa, it was given as the primary cause of death. Fifty-three of the 408 deaths were attributed to puerperal septicemia and 8 to other causes. Of these 408 women who were known to have had placenta previa, 327 had some bleeding before the onset of labor, 38 had no bleeding then, and for 43 it was not known whether or not there was hemorrhage before the onset of labor. In 310 cases of bleeding before the onset of labor for which the extent of bleeding was ascertained, it was scanty in 44 cases, moderate in 82 cases, and profuse in 184 cases.

The bleeding was said to have begun before the thirteenth week in 7 cases, from the thirteenth to the twenty-fifth week in 31 cases, from the twenty-sixth to the thirty-ninth in 201 cases, and in the fortieth week in 49 cases; in 39 cases the week in which the bleeding began was not reported.

---

[1] Puerperal hemorrhage (no. 144) remains the same in the 1929 revision of the International List.

The first hemorrhage—occurring in some cases before the onset of labor and in others at the beginning of labor—was said to have been dangerously profuse in 107 of the 408 cases, *in 236 cases there had been a warning hemorrhage earlier in pregnancy*, and in 65 cases there was no report as to warning hemorrhage. It was reported that the warning hemorrhage resulted in prompt treatment for the placenta previa in 18 cases, but that *in 216 cases treatment was delayed.* Of the 107 who had no warning, it was reported that 87 had prompt treatment, 14 had delayed treatment, and 3 died at once without time for treatment. In all, 239 women were reported to have had delayed treatment. The delay was apparently due to the physician in 129 cases, and to the patient, her family, or circumstances in 110 cases. At least 9 women died without medical attention. In 46 cases the physician did not arrive until the patient was moribund, but in 351 cases there had been earlier medical care.

Of the 408 women who died following placenta previa, a report concerning operations for delivery was obtained for all but 7. Three hundred and twenty-five (81 percent) were known to have had some operation aimed at delivery. About half (207) of the women were reported to have been delivered by some form of version, in 124 cases preceded by artificial dilatation of the cervix. This was nearly always a version with immediate extraction. In only 2 of these 207 cases was there said to have been a Braxton Hicks version without immediate extraction. Cesarean section was the method of delivery in 41 (10 percent) of the cases. It was done upon at least 7 women who had been packed before admission to the hospital. A forceps operation alone or in combination with some operation other than version was used in 33 cases (8 percent), and dilatation of the cervix—usually manual or bag dilatation—was the only operation for delivery in 17 cases (4 percent). Only 27 of the 408 women were known to have had a blood transfusion.

The uterus was reported packed postpartum in 31 cases. It was apparently done as a routine procedure in only 6 cases. In the other 25 cases the packing was done after the onset of a postpartum hemorrhage.

A ruptured uterus was diagnosed by the attending physician after treatment in 3 cases of death associated with placenta previa.

There was a report on postpartum hemorrhage in the cases of 335 women whose deaths were associated with placenta previa and who had been delivered in the third trimester. Of these women, 156 had a postpartum hemorrhage.

Of the 347 women whose deaths were assigned to placenta previa, 50 women died undelivered, and the rest died soon after delivery.

The interval between delivery and death was reported for 290 women. Of these, 88 percent died less than a day after delivery, and 97 percent died within the first week.

## OTHER PUERPERAL HEMORRHAGE

Puerperal hemorrhage other than placenta previa caused the deaths of 444 women, 443 of whom were known to have reached the last trimester. Of these 443 women the termination of labor was reported for all but 10. It was spontaneous in 249 cases and artificial in 178 cases; the patient was undelivered in 6 cases.

Of the 444 women 374 died from postpartum hemorrhage and the other 70 from adherent placentæ, premature separation of the placenta, or some bleeding during or after labor the exact cause of which was unknown.

**Postpartum hemorrhage**

In addition to the 374 deaths of which postpartum hemorrhage was the primary cause, it was present as a complication in the deaths of 519 other women, so that 893 women, or 21 percent of the 4,188 who died after reaching the last trimester of pregnancy and for whom a report was made on this condition, had postpartum hemorrhage. Of the 374 women dying of postpartum hemorrhage, 50 had no physician at the time of delivery; in 185 cases the physician did not leave the patient until after her death, and in 94 cases the patient's condition was satisfactory when he left; in 28 cases she was in unsatisfactory condition, and in 17 cases a statement as to her condition or as to attendant was not made.

Of the 893 women who had postpartum hemorrhage (including those whose deaths were assigned to other causes), only 78 were known to have had a blood transfusion.

**Premature separation of the placenta**

The diagnosis of premature separation of the placenta was made by the attending physician in 106 cases. In 21 cases the delivery was spontaneous; in 31, there was manual dilatation, usually followed by forceps or version; in 24, forceps or version without manual dilatation; and in 17, Cesarean section. In 8 cases there was some other method of delivery, in 2, the method of delivery was not reported, and in 3, the patient died undelivered.

The uterus was known to have been packed after delivery in only nine cases.

The women whose deaths were associated with premature separation of the placenta were, in general, older and had had more pregnancies than the total group included in the study. Eighteen percent of these deaths were among primiparæ; 69 percent were known to have had three or more pregnancies.

Eighty of the one hundred and six women were delivered operatively, but in 21 cases the deliveries were reported as spontaneous; 3 died undelivered; and for 2 there was no report.

## COMMENT BY ADVISORY COMMITTEE

If the onset of hemorrhage in placenta previa were accompanied by pain, patients would apply for treatment sooner and would not be content with inactivity on the part of the physician. Of 236 cases in which warning bleeding occurred, it was ignored by the patient or by the physician in 216, and in more than half these cases it was the physician who was responsible for the delay. Even among the 107 cases in which the first hemorrhage was profuse, and it could therefore be said that no warning was given, there were a few cases of delayed treatment, for a small number of which the physician was responsible. Placenta previa is not a condition that can safely be treated expectantly.

A Braxton Hicks version, which is of greatest use to control bleeding, was rarely done, but manual dilatation of the cervix with internal podalic version and immediate extraction was done many times. The frequent occurrence of rupture of the uterus, tears, hemorrhage, shock, and immediate death illustrates the seriousness of these procedures and the fact that they are not proper in the treatment of placenta previa. So many of these women died immediately after delivery that relatively few lived long enough to die of sepsis; as it was, 53 died of sepsis.

Treatment for shock in connection with hemorrhage was rarely mentioned in the histories as given in the schedules. Fluids of any sort were infrequently used. That the buttocks of the child could be used to control hemorrhage and that shock could be treated at this time, the labor being terminated by the patient's own efforts, was apparently seldom thought of.

Many women with placenta previa died of hemorrhage after labor. Only 31 of the women were packed after delivery. This would suggest that if proper packing were at hand it would be used more often, and certainly blankets and sheets would not be used as emergency packing, with later death from sepsis.

Unfortunately rupture of the membranes was seldom done in the appropriate cases of lateral placenta previa.

Long distances and bad roads would seem to have contributed to some of the deaths from placenta previa.

It should be emphasized that Cesarean section is contraindicated in the treatment of placenta previa when the patient is suffering from shock or hemorrhage or potential or actual sepsis. If dirty packing had previously been used or if there had been mismanagement of any sort, the delivery should be by vagina whenever possible. But in this study the Cesarean sections for placenta previa were not limited to cases in which the mother and baby were in good condition. The operation was often done after great loss of blood and without coincident blood transfusion, though transfusion would doubtless have been given more frequently if equipment for blood typing and for giving the transfusion had been at hand. The Cesarean sometimes followed dirty packing done before the women were admitted to the hospital. Naturally many women who did not die at once from shock and hemorrhage died from sepsis.

The treatment of placenta previa is to control bleeding and treat shock and acute anemia; it is not to effect the immediate delivery of the fetus, except as a means to this end in properly selected cases.

In the cases diagnosed as placental separation also, shock, even when severe, did not seem to be sufficiently considered in determining treatment. Only one fifth of the women in this group had spontaneous deliveries. About one half the women in the group were delivered immediately.

The frequent use of pituitrin before delivery in cases of women who later died of puerperal hemorrhage other than placenta previa is worthy of comment.

# OTHER ACCIDENTS OF LABOR, INCLUDING RUPTURE OF THE UTERUS

## OTHER ACCIDENTS OF LABOR

Of the 7,380 deaths in the study, 652 were attributed after interview to "other accidents of labor" (no. 145 of the international list). Of these 652, 136 deaths were attributed to Cesarean section (no. 145*a*): these deaths have already been discussed. One hundred and nine deaths were attributed to instrumental delivery and other operative procedures (no. 145*b*). These were not deaths resulting from hemorrhage, sepsis, or toxemia but were thought by the attending physician to be due to shock, exhaustion, or embolism.

The remaining 407 deaths were attributed to "others" under the title "other accidents of labor" (no. 145*c*). Sixty-five of these were attributed to no. 145*c1*, which includes rupture of uterus or bladder during delivery. Sixty-three of these were due to ruptured uterus and will be taken up later. Forty-six were attributed to no. 145*c2*, a group including deaths said to be due to difficult or abnormal labor, faulty presentation, inversion of the uterus, or similar causes. The immediate cause of death in these cases was usually thought to be either shock or exhaustion. There was a group of 296 deaths about which so little was known that it was not possible to attribute them to a more definite cause than "others under this title" (no. 145*c3*). This also includes deaths in which influenza, pneumonia, and certain other diseases complicated an otherwise fairly normal childbirth.[1]

In this latter group there was a report on intercurrent disease for 203. One hundred and thirty-seven (67 percent) of these had some intercurrent disease, and 66 (33 percent) had none. Not only intercurrent disease during pregnancy but various complications after delivery contributed to some of these deaths. Influenza, various types of pneumonia, cardiac disease, cerebral hemorrhage, intestinal obstruction, and anemia were given as nonpuerperal contributory causes of death in 242 of the 296 cases.

## RUPTURE OF THE UTERUS

In addition to the 63 deaths attributed to ruptured uterus (no. 145*c1*) 28 had a diagnosis of ruptured uterus made by the attending physician or at autopsy—a total of 91 out of the 7,380 deaths included in the study. Of these 28 deaths 17 were attributed to puerperal septicemia, 5 to puerperal hemorrhage, and 6 to accidents of pregnancy.

[1] In the 1929 revision of the International List of Causes of Death, other accidents of labor (no. 145) becomes other accidents of childbirth (no. 149), consisting of Cesarean section (no. 149*a*), and others under this title (no. 149*b*). Rupture of uterus or bladder is now no. 149*b1*; the conditions formerly grouped under nos. 145*b*, 145*c2*, and 145*c3* are now included in no 149*b2*.

Ten of these 91 women were primiparæ, and 77 were multiparæ; the parity of 4 was not reported.

Six of these women were not in labor. One had a rupture of a uterine sinus as shown by autopsy; 2 had had previous Cesarean sections; there was no adequate explanation for the other 3. Fifteen of the patients had been in labor less than 6 hours; the others varied to 36 hours or more. In 8 cases a Cesarean section had been done in a previous pregnancy.

The type of presentation was reported for 78 of the 91 cases; it was vertex in 59 cases, face in 6 cases, breech in 6 cases, and transverse in 7 cases.

There was a report as to the use of pituitrin in 75 cases. It was not used in 36 cases and was used for induction in 1 case; in the first stage, in 10 cases; in the second stage, in 13 cases; in the third stage or postpartum only, in 14 cases; and at an unreported stage, in 1 case.

Of the 91 women, 64 had an operation for delivery and 27 did not; 15 of these 27 died undelivered and 12 were delivered spontaneously. As some of the operations were unsuccessful, 6 of the 64 who had operations for delivery died undelivered.

There were many other cases in which the symptoms suggested ruptured uterus, although the attending physician had not made the diagnosis. A careful study of the schedules showed that the history pointed clearly to ruptured uterus in 68 cases and made such a diagnosis probable in 109 other cases.

### INVERSION OF THE UTERUS

Twenty cases of inversion of the uterus were reported. In three of these cases the condition was not discovered until necropsy was done. Whether these cases are a true index of the frequency of this complication cannot be stated, for there were many unexplainable deaths that occurred in severe shock, some of which may have been due to this condition.

The causes of death were as follows: Postpartum hemorrhage, 13; accidents of labor, 5; sepsis, 1; embolism, 1.

---

## COMMENT BY ADVISORY COMMITTEE

A satisfactory analysis of the deaths in this miscellaneous group of 652 cases, "other accidents of labor", is difficult. This is true particularly of the largest subgroup of 296 "other" deaths, although here the nonpuerperal contributory causes of death play an important part.

It is a well-recognized fact that the diagnosis of a rupture of the uterus is not always made in spite of the suggestive history that is often obtained. This statement is supported by the relatively small number in this series of cases so diagnosed and the many probable ruptures not so diagnosed by the attending physician which were revealed by careful study of the schedules. Though spontaneous rupture is uncommon, the possibility of its occurrence, especially when a previous Cesarean section has been performed, must be kept in mind. The relative infrequency of this accident in primiparæ is conclusively shown in this series. Abnormal presentations were common However, many of the ruptures followed apparently needless, and certainly premature, interference with labor.

Study of the case histories of the women whose deaths were caused by rupture of the uterus emphasizes the need for further education of physicians regarding the danger of pituitrin. The use of pituitary extract during labor is still causing maternal deaths from rupture of the uterus.

Although inversion of the uterus was reported as a cause of death in but 20 cases, some of the unexplainable deaths may have been caused by this condition. For, unless the physician in charge is alert and keen, an inversion may be overlooked.

## ECTOPIC GESTATION

Of the 7,380 maternal deaths ectopic gestation was associated with 314 (4 percent). Two hundred and forty-nine of these were attributed to accidents of pregnancy (no. 143 of the International List), 248 to ectopic gestation (no. 143*b*), and 1 (a case of ruptured cornual pregnancy) to "others under this title" (no. 143*c*). The other 65 patients developed sepsis, and their deaths were accordingly attributed to puerperal septicemia.[1]

The deaths reported to be associated with ectopic gestation were more frequent in urban than in rural areas of the States, 194 occurring in urban areas and 120 in rural areas. In every State except Nebraska and North Dakota, the mortality rates from deaths associated with ectopic gestation were higher in urban than in rural areas. The mortality rate for white women was less than for colored women. These rates are probably minimum because the differences in the mortality rates from ectopic gestation in the various States are influenced by the opportunity for exact diagnosis.

Of the 314 women whose deaths were known to be associated with ectopic gestation, 4 had no medical care by a physician, and 44 were seen by a physician only when moribund. Two hundred and sixty-three, however, had been under the care of a physician for a time. For 3 medical care was not reported. Of the 314 women, 253 (81 percent) received hospital care.

The parity was reported for 262 of the 314 women. Of these, 93 were primigravidæ and 169 were multigravidæ.

The period of pregnancy at which symptoms began was reported in 239 of the 314 cases. Symptoms were noted by the third month in all instances in which a report was obtained. In 30 cases symptoms began before the fourth week, from the fourth to the sixth week in 39 cases, from the sixth to the ninth week in 116 cases, from the ninth to the thirteenth week in 38, and at 3 months in 16.

Two hundred and four of the 314 women were operated on for this condition, but 109 died without operation. Twenty-six of the 204 operations were described as elective, 175 as emergency, and there was no report on 3.

Sixteen percent of the women operated on for ectopic gestation for whom duration of symptoms was known had had symptoms for less than a day, 43 percent for less than a week, and 35 percent from 1 to 3 weeks. Twenty-three percent had had symptoms for 4 weeks or more. Of the 26 women who died after elective operations, 17 were known to have had symptoms for more than a week. The duration of the symptoms of the other 9 was not reported. Of the 86 women who died without operation and for whom duration of symptoms was reported 34 percent had had symptoms for less than a day and 60 percent for less than a week.

In all but one case the operation performed was a laparotomy, and in this case there was a puncture of the posterior cul-de-sac only.

[1] The 314 would all be included in ectopic gestation (no. 142) of the 1929 revision, 65 in no. 142*a* "with septic conditions specified" and 249 in no. 142*b* "without mention of septic conditions."

Six women had a hysterectomy done, and three of the women who had an ectopic pregnancy of 7 or more months' gestation had dilatation of the cervix in an attempt to bring on labor.

Eighty-six of the women who died following ectopic gestation had other operations. Only 36 of the 314 women had blood transfusions. Eight of the women who died following ectopic gestation had had attempts at induced abortion in the present pregnancy, and five of them died of sepsis.

In 12 cases the period of viability of the child was reached, the diagnosis being made either at operation or at autopsy in 6 cases. One living child was delivered. The abdominal pregnancy was discovered in the course of an operation that was intended to be a Cesarean section with appendectomy.

---

## COMMENT BY ADVISORY COMMITTEE

Ectopic gestation is more frequently reported as a cause of death in urban than in rural areas. But when one considers the nature of this complication and the fact that it was given as the cause of death for only four women who died without medical care, it is fair to assume that, especially in the rural areas, some of the deaths from this condition are not recognized and the cause of death is not properly assigned. This assumption is further supported by the fact that in those States where hospitalization was more frequent the diagnosis of ectopic gestation was made more frequently.

Of the 314 women whose deaths were known to be associated with ectopic gestation, 4 had no medical care and the condition was discovered at autopsy, and 44 were moribund when first seen. Eighty-one percent of these cases received hospital care. It is interesting also to note the large percentage of these cases that occurred in multigravidae. It is likewise surprising to find that 109 of these women died without operation. As is to be expected, a very large percentage of the others had emergency operations.

The fact that only 36 of these 314 women had blood transfusions shows that this life-saving procedure was not available in many of these cases, for if it had been it undoubtedly would have been used.

That emergency operating was common and that the deaths of 65 of these patients were classified as due to puerperal septicemia makes it very clear that the operative technique must be as perfect as is possible if deaths from sepsis are to be avoided. The removal of the appendix in cases of ruptured ectopic is a dangerous procedure and adds to the deaths from sepsis. (There were 11 such cases.) It has long been recognized that the opening of the gut when there is much blood in the peritoneal cavity should be avoided.

A review of the duration of symptoms suggestive of ectopic pregnancy before the operation was performed shows that only 16 percent of these cases had symptoms less than a day, while 43 percent had symptoms for a week, 35 percent had symptoms for 1 to 3 weeks, and 23 percent had symptoms for 4 weeks or more. These figures show clearly that in many cases the symptoms of the serious condition of ectopic pregnancy were ignored.

## RECOMMENDATIONS BY ADVISORY COMMITTEE

Maternal deaths are due in large part to controllable causes. But how is control of these causes to be established? First, the medical profession and the public must know the facts, and then each group should take appropriate and decisive action. Physicians have the responsibility for leadership in both the medical and the community program for such control. As the facts become more widely known, others will assume this leadership if they do not.

Recommendations for action looking to prevention of maternal deaths are addressed to the medical profession and to the general public.

### *To the Medical Profession*

A. Physicians must assume leadership in the field of maternal care by:

1. Informing the public that the high mortality during pregnancy, delivery, and the postpartum period is due largely to controllable causes.
2. Recognizing that every mother must have adequate prenatal, delivery, and postpartum care. (For definition of adequate see pp. 16, 17.)
3. Instructing the public as to what constitutes adequate maternal care.
4. So organizing the available resources of their communities that every mother can receive adequate maternal care.
5. Warning the public as to the dangers occasioned by abortions, spontaneous or induced.

B. In order that more accurate information may be secured relative to cause and prevention of maternal deaths:

1. Physicians should make a greater effort to study by autopsy and other scientific means every maternal and fetal death, for in many cases this is the only means of ascertaining the true cause of death.
2. Physicians are urged to exercise the greatest possible care in making out maternal and fetal death certificates, so that vital statistics may be more accurate and therefore more valuable.
3. Bureaus of vital statistics are urged to query maternal and fetal death certificates recording an indefinite cause of death; for example, "Cesarean section" alone.
4. Medical societies and departments of health in cooperation should investigate each maternal death within a few weeks of the death.

C. In order that physicians in general may have a better understanding of the fundamentals of obstetric care:

1. There should be larger and better facilities for clinical training in obstetrics.

2. Undergraduate students should have a much wider contact with obstetric patients.

3. The State medical societies, the medical schools, and State departments of health should provide or arrange for postgraduate teaching in the various counties in order to keep the local practitioner in touch with the best obstetric thought and practice.

D. It is recommended that all physicians practicing obstetrics give particular consideration to:

1. The importance of good aseptic technique, including the use of rubber gloves and masks that cover nose and mouth.

2. The danger to mothers from carriers of infection.

3. The dangers of the use of pituitrin during labor.

4. The dangers of multiple, forcible, and radical procedures in obstetrics.

5. The proper indications and contraindications for various obstetric operations, especially (*a*) the dangers of major operations in the presence of shock and hemorrhage and (*b*) the dangers of Cesarean section after vaginal manipulations or long labor.

6. The proper selection of anesthetics.

7. The value of blood transfusions.

8. The dangers of intrauterine manipulation in cases of infected abortion.

9. The dangers of abortion or delivery to women suffering from acute diseases, especially infectious diseases.

10. Knowledge of the symptoms of some of the less common but more serious complications of delivery such as rupture of the uterus.

E. It is recommended that State medical societies working in cooperation with the State departments of health consider the development of some plan by which well-trained regional obstetric consultants may be made available.

### *To the General Public*

There should be widespread education of the public as to the following:

1. That the high maternal death rate is due largely to controllable causes.

2. That it is necessary for all women to have adequate supervision and medical care during pregnancy, labor, and the postpartum period, such supervision and care to begin early in pregnancy and to be continuous through the postpartum period—

*a.* In order to safeguard the health of both mother and child.

*b.* In order especially to control the infections, toxemias, and hemorrhages that this study and others have shown to be real menaces to life.

3. That there is danger of death or serious invalidism following abortions, spontaneous or induced.

4. That the community has a definite responsibility to provide adequate medical and nursing facilities for the care of women during pregnancy, labor, and the postpartum period. This predicates the proper organization of hospitals, outpatient services, and medical and nursing personnel and applies to both home and hospital care. The community should know the standards for hospitals taking obstetric cases that have been drawn up by the American College of Surgeons. (See below.)

5. That judicious selection of the hospital to be used for maternity care is of the greatest importance when hospitalization is planned.

6. That the better education of those caring for women during this period is essential and should have public support. This includes adequate obstetric training for medical students, postgraduate obstetric training for physicians in practice, to keep them abreast of modern developments, the training of nurses in good maternity care, and the training and supervision of midwives in communities where midwives still practice.

7. That it is important to make careful and intelligent selection of the attendant for maternal care.

### STANDARDS OF AMERICAN COLLEGE OF SURGEONS FOR HOSPITALS TAKING OBSTETRIC PATIENTS

[American College of Surgeons; Twentieth Year Book. 1933. Pp. 68–69. Chicago]

(1) Segregation of obstetric patients from all others in the institution.
(2) Special facilities available for immediate segregation and isolation of all cases of infection, temperature, or other conditions inimical to the safety and welfare of patients within the department.
(3) Adequately trained personnel, the entire nursing staff to be chosen specially for work in this department and not permitted to attend other cases during time on obstetric service.
(4) Readily available, adequate laboratory and special-treatment facilities under competent supervision.
(5) Accurate and complete clinical records on all obstetric patients.
(6) Frequent consultations encouraged on obstetric service, a consultation made obligatory in all cases where major operative procedures may be indicated.
(7) Thorough analysis and review of the clinical work of the department each month by the medical staff with particular considerations to deaths, infections, complications, or such conditions as are not conducive to the best end results.
(8) Adequate theoretical instruction and practical experience for student nurses in prenatal, parturient, and postpartum care of the patient, as well as the care of the newborn.

O

UNITED STATES DEPARTMENT OF LABOR
FRANCES PERKINS, Secretary

CHILDREN'S BUREAU KATHARINE F. LENROOT, Chief

# HABIT CLINICS FOR CHILD GUIDANCE

BY

D. A. THOM, M. D.

Bureau Publication No. 135

(Revised 1938)

United States Government Printing Office
Washington : 1939

# CONTENTS

# LETTER OF TRANSMITTAL

UNITED STATES DEPARTMENT OF LABOR,
CHILDREN'S BUREAU,
*Washington, November 23, 1938.*

MADAM: There is transmitted herewith a revised edition of Habit Clinics for Child Guidance, first published in 1923 as Habit Clinics for the Child of Preschool Age, by Dr. D. A. Thom, director of the habit clinics of the Community Health Association of Boston and director of the division of mental hygiene in the Department of Mental Diseases of Massachusetts.

The revision is an enlargement of the original edition, based on Dr. Thom's experience in the habit clinics over the past 15 years. It is believed that the method developed by Dr. Thom and here set forth will be of interest to all concerned with the physical and mental health of children.

Respectfully submitted.

KATHARINE F. LENROOT, *Chief.*

HON. FRANCES PERKINS,
*Secretary of Labor.*

# HABIT CLINICS FOR CHILD GUIDANCE

## INTRODUCTION

Fifteen years have elapsed since the Children's Bureau published a report entitled, "Habit Clinics for the Child of Preschool Age; their organization and practical value." This report was the first of its kind and embodied what at that time represented a fairly comprehensive review of the organization and development of the first clinic in this country to deal specifically with the mental health of the preschool child.

Since the preschool period is the habit-forming period, this clinic was called a habit clinic. It was felt that there was a real need for this subject of the mental health of the child to be presented to parents, teachers, nurses, and general practitioners in a way that could be utilized by these various groups in their everyday contact with children. It was therefore not considered within the scope of the publication to discuss the psychological mechanisms which motivated the type of conduct that brought children into conflict with the group or rendered them unhappy and inefficient. The author has repeatedly stressed the need of reducing mental hygiene to terms that would have a practical value to those individuals making daily contact with children. The last 10 years have borne witness to the fact that those mental-health clinics which have rendered a real service to the community—that is, to the home, the school, the hospital, the medical clinic, and organizations concerned with child welfare—have survived. They have created for themselves a place of importance in the fields of parent education, pedagogy, and medicine.

It has now seemed wise to revise the report in order that it may be more useful to those interested in this field.

In the revision the name habit clinic has again been used rather than child-guidance clinic, as the publication is concerned primarily with preschool children and many of the problems of older children, dealt with in most child-guidance clinics, are not discussed. The following discussion will be open to the criticism of being rather superficial and lacking the precise technique necessary for the solution of many of the more complex problems with which parents are confronted. It may be said, however, that in dealing with these obviously more involved situations, parents must necessarily seek help from those who have had training and experience in this particular field. Parents do not treat fractures or serious infections, nor do they attempt surgical procedures; neither are they equipped to solve the more serious problems pertaining to the mental health of the child. Experience, however, has led us to believe that the parent, the teacher, the nurse, and the general practitioner are in a position to render valuable first aid. They can prevent the development of many serious mental problems if they are equipped with such knowledge of mental hygiene as falls well within their grasp.

From a practical point of view there is a large group of cases which will benefit from the understanding and guidance that can be given directly in the home, where the problem originates. It is recognized that there are exceptional cases so complicated and involved that they will tax the skill and ingenuity of the specialist. The outstanding question is how the clinic can best serve the community in which it is located, the health agency with which it may be affiliated, and the school and social agencies which are dependent upon it for advice and treatment. Its function is not limited to the treatment of individual cases but should include, for educational purposes, the dissemination of such knowledge as has been acquired by experience.

In the organization and development of clinics it is necessary to be practical, and this requires that one evaluate the total situation. A physician, a social worker, or a nurse may complicate a home situation instead of helping it unless the family rather than the individual is kept in mind as the unit. For example, it may be much easier for the mother of five children to wash extra sheets three or four times a week than to bring a youngster afflicted with enuresis to the clinic the same number of times. On the other hand, much may be accomplished with only the minimum of inconvenience to the mother if a weekly clinic visit is made. Without minimizing the value of intensive work or implying that one method will be applicable to every case, it may be pointed out that many of the problems presented at the habit clinics have been treated successfully by merely directing attention to something that was obviously wrong in the environment. In other words, there was no need to use a pick and shovel when a rake would do the work. An important causative factor may easily be overlooked by parents, a nurse, or even the family physician, and yet be quite apparent to a well-trained psychiatrist.

Inasmuch as the behavior of the child represents the response which that particular individual makes to his environment, the clinic must have first-hand knowledge of this environment. An irreducible minimum for an investigation should be outlined and carefully followed in every case in order that important environmental situations directly affecting the conduct of the child may not be overlooked. This part of the clinic program should be carried out by a well-trained social worker, who, by virtue of her training, is in a position not only to describe environmental situations but also to interpret to the psychiatrist how these particular situations are affecting the child. She must be in a position to evaluate the social, economic, cultural, and intellectual level of the child's home and the surrounding conditions, the personalities with whom the child has to deal, and the adjustment of these personalities to one another. She must bring to the attention of the clinic the facilities in the community that can be utilized in helping the child to make a better social adjustment.

In order to understand the behavior of the child, an appreciation of the intellectual differences in children is also necessary. This part of the program is in the hands of the *psychologist*, who obtains the information relative to the child's mental equipment, his attitude toward work, his ability to concentrate, and his particular interests and aptitudes. The *psychiatrist* must take all the available information, together with the material gathered from his direct personal contact with the child and the parents, interpret this information, and utilize it in making a plan. This plan must take into consideration not only the particular problem for which the child was brought to the clinic but the child's adjustment to life in general.

Although a clinic for child guidance is concerned with the child, the family must be considered as a unit. Where there is a problem child, not infrequently the mother, father, brother, sister, or some other relative represents the offending aspect of the environment. It is likely that certain parental attitudes need to be altered. Perhaps the behavior of a problem brother or sister must be treated. A change in schools may be necessary. Foster parents may have to be introduced as a temporary expedient. Possibly help must be sought from social agencies interested in relief, placement, and observation of children under supervision. It is not unusual to find that the child who has been brought to the clinic is not the one who is most in need of treatment. The shy, diffident, well-mannered child in grave need of help may have been left at home while his much better-adjusted, tempestuous brother who causes his parents annoyance has been brought for help. It frequently happens that two or three members of the same family receive clinic treatment at the same time or that several members of the same family benefit by the treatment which one maladjusted member receives at the clinic.

Mental hygiene has made great strides during the last 10 years, and the general public is very much better informed about the importance and value of mental health. The time has already arrived when the larger social agencies are finding it necessary to have upon their staffs someone well trained in child-guidance work. Already such agencies have clinics for both children and adults. It has become an absolute necessity for all organizations dealing with the problems of human beings, whether it is with reference to disease, poverty, or delinquency, to have some knowledge of mental hygiene. The necessity of recognizing the importance of mental health has been stressed by the leaders in the fields of sociology, penology, industry, and education.

There is still a long way to go, however, before parents in general will be as deeply concerned over defects in personality and over undesirable habits as they are over physical ailments. There are advantages in small, informal clinics wherever they can be established in the community as an adjunct to highly organized mental-health clinics which are always available for service. The ideal place for one of these clinics concerned with the mental health of preschool children is in association with other services for children, especially general health clinics. A clinic serving preschool children and some older children can be assimilated easily by a health center and it can operate as part of the medical routine. There must be some more highly organized mental-health centers here and there, with opportunities for research work and training. A medical background is absolutely essential to clinics interested in mental health. Every child must have a careful physical examination, and all abnormal conditions having a physical basis should be corrected before any attempt is made to interpret the symptoms on a psychogenic basis. There is no branch of medicine in which greater care is needed to prevent the introduction of all sorts of quacks and charlatans than psychiatry. The association of a mental-health clinic with a recognized medical organization stamps its work as part of a well-rounded and well-qualified medical program.

The simplicity of such an organization has much to recommend it. It has the advantage of offering to a community a service that is as vital to its welfare as the school or the hospital. It offers to the parent, the nurse, and the teacher valuable aid in developing a happier and more efficient group of children. It permits the individual child who is momentarily out of adjustment with life the opportunity of understanding himself as well as being understood by those upon whom he is dependent for his rehabilitation.

## HABIT-CLINIC PERSONNEL AND PROCEDURE

In the routine clinical procedure of the habit clinic the close cooperation between the psychiatrist, the psychologist, and the social worker will be stressed repeatedly. Although each has a specific job in which he excels, there is no sharp line of demarcation. In fact, an occasional invasion of one into the territory of the other is to be desired.

It is the function of the clinic and the purpose of the combined groups to make a careful investigation and study of the child's behavior, his mental attitudes, and his personality deviations, and to evaluate his assets as well as his liabilities. It is the purpose of such an approach to understand and eventually to straighten out asocial and undesirable tendencies before they become a fixed part of the child's personality make-up. If this is done many children will approach adolescent and adult life unhampered by the crippling influences of their early training and unhappy experiences. There is reason to believe that a relationship exists between the emotional instabilities and conduct disorders of early life and the problems of delinquency and neurotic disturbances later on.

### THE PSYCHIATRIST

The psychiatrist is the logical person to act as the director of any clinic whose function is to study and treat behavior problems. He is a medically trained person who has specialized in mental health. Hence, he not only is concerned with behavior as it affects the individual's conduct in relation to the community but is also seeking the motivating forces which lie behind those inner conflicts leading to unhappiness and inefficiency. Only a medically trained person who has also had training in psychiatry is qualified to decide which cases need physical treatment and which cases can be helped only by psychotherapy. He must also see that cases needing both types of treatment are adequately cared for.

The psychiatrist is dependent upon others of the clinic group for complete understanding of the child. He needs information from them in order to outline treatment and see that the child is properly supervised. Details of therapy may be carried on to advantage by the psychologist, the social worker, or the speech worker, but the final decision should rest with the psychiatrist. A well-organized clinic group will have no difficulty in determining just where each individual fits in best if the prevailing spirit is one of cooperation.

The psychiatric interview must be so conducted that the parent feels at ease. (See case presented in section on Habit Clinic Procedure—Interview With Psychiatrist, p. 17.) The psychiatrist should try to win the confidence of the parent. This can be done only if the parent is convinced that the doctor is interested in understanding the problems confronting the child and those of the parents as well. It is fair to assume that if the parents are making mistakes in the training of their children, they are not doing so willfully and viciously. They are without doubt anxious to discover what mistakes they are making and why they are prone to make these particular errors. It tends to build up a parent's self-esteem and make him feel capable of carrying out the details of treatment if the psychiatrist and the other clinic workers treat him as a responsible being. There is danger, at times, that the psychiatrist will take advantage of his position as the one in authority. By a critical, unsympathetic attitude he will humiliate parents with all the obvious mistakes which they have made. He will send them away from the clinic more discouraged and less able to cope with their problem than when they came. It is a very delicate piece of work to deal with a mother who has been a failure with her child (for this is often the problem), especially if one has to point out the seriousness of the difficulty as well as the difficulty itself. It is in this respect that the habit clinic differs from most agencies. Hospitals, schools, and many other organizations have the law behind them, or if not the law, the fear of death or destitution, or an actual and conscious want, and they afford concrete and tangible assistance. The habit clinic has no definite authority but has to depend for its cooperation upon the parental instinct and a friendly contact, and its assistance is at times very subtle and intangible.

The psychiatrist examines all the information which he himself has collected from his interviews with parent and child, together with that obtained by the social worker and the psychologist and from medical reports. He then attempts to interpret the child's behavior in terms of his personality make-up and his environment. Here is where the psychiatrist tries to apply to this child his knowledge about children in general. He is seeking to determine the hopes, interests, ambitions, love attachments, grudges, fears, and disappointments which have created conflicts within the child himself. He seeks to discover just how these conflicts have affected the child and his relationship with the world in which he lives. He is concerned with what can be done with those environmental situations which create emotional turmoil in the child. Parents are by far the most important influence in the child's environment, and so it is their attitudes that cause the psychiatrist the greatest concern. The conditions and relationships in the school and the neighborhood are likewise important, as is the social, economic, and moral status of the family in their particular community.

The relationship between the psychiatrist and the child is one that requires time, patience, judgment, and understanding. The psychiatrist has no instruments with which to measure resentment, humiliation, fear, jealousy, and other less well-defined attitudes which the child may be experiencing. We know that the child who is in conflict with himself and his environment is usually unhappy. He is not satisfied with his lying, stealing, or truancy. Rarely is it an end in itself; it is merely a means of escape from some situation which is felt to be intolerable. It is with these intangible problems that the psychiatrist has to deal, using such understanding as his experience, education, and training permit. Perhaps his success is due more to his inherent wisdom and ability to understand the motives that actuate human behavior than to his psychiatric knowledge. Both are essential if one is to succeed in being helpful to the child in trouble and to his worried, harassed parents.

In the majority of cases the results are good. In some the improvement is quick and very marked—in the mother's eyes a miracle. In others the progress is slow and the condition is complicated and not fully appreciated by the mother, who takes the attitude either that it is useless to come to the clinic as the child is not improving, or that the problem is too unimportant to bother with. In either case there must be frequent calls at the home in order to educate the mother and insure the proper following out of the treatment. Sooner or later these children show the effect of the work done upon them, and the mothers express their gratitude. It is in these cases that the social services are most important, as the results depend upon careful, persistent, tactful work that means not merely a series of calls but a program of education.

It is essential that the psychiatrist who deals with the behavior disorders of childhood should be optimistic as well as patient. All too frequently many of the problems which are brought to the clinic have been in the making for a long time. These habits have become firmly fixed, and they are very much a part of the individual. Attitudes built up as the result of long-continued, unhappy experiences are not eradicated easily. The psychiatrist must devote weeks, months, and sometimes years to the treatment of a single case. At times he must even acknowledge failure. Yet he must always think in terms of the future and in terms of success.

## THE PSYCHOLOGIST

The duties of a psychologist in a clinic devoted mainly to the problems of preschool children are many and varied. What they are will depend upon the problems of the individual children seeking clinical help. At one time his function may be to determine the level of memtal development that the child has reached; at another, to throw some light upon the reason for slow language development; or yet again, to give advice upon some school problem, of which there are many. Since the contact of the psychologist with the child usually covers a long period, he is in a position to observe any special handicap that the child may have. Loss of hearing, defective eyesight, inarticulate speech is sometimes discovered; even a peculiar mannerism may sometimes serve as a clue to some more obscure difficulty which leads to the child's being directed to the right sources for care and treatment.

When one seeks to reconstruct the behavior of a child by the formation of correct habits, much depends upon the child himself. One of the first questions that confronts a worker is the native ability of the child, or in other words, how much may be expected of him in the reeducational process. It is to the psychologist with his specialized training that one looks for an answer to this question.

The various studies made in recent years upon the development of child life indicate that mental development proceeds in an orderly, continuous way. A child must attain the lower mental levels before going on to the higher. By administering and interpreting many standardized tests now available it is possible to determine different age levels. Has the child reached a level that one of his age usually reaches, or has his mental growth failed to keep pace with his chronological years? On the other hand, has his mental age gone beyond his chronological years? It is essential that these fundamental questions be answered first, for many problems arise through ignorance of these facts alone. To expect a child to function on a level of which he is not intellectually capable only brings strain and stress to both child and parent. On the other hand, many problems are often created by failure to recognize that a child's mental development is beyond his chronological age. A few cases will illustrate this.

Sylvia is a child whose mental development has not kept pace with her years of living. At 6 years 8 months she was brought to a clinic primarily for her many fears. Fears of animals, of strangers, and of school were among them. There were other problems of stubbornness, temper tantrums, and too much dependence upon her mother. She had entered the first grade in the public school but was soon excluded because of her peculiar behavior. She gave no attention to the subjects presented but wandered around aimlessly, talking to herself.

Careful study of Sylvia showed a high degree of mental retardation. In most respects she was capable of doing no more than the average 4-year-old child is able to do. Expecting her to hold her place with children some 2 years in advance of her mentally, necessarily led to difficulties. Furthermore, in the treatment of any of Sylvia's problems one will have to keep in mind the immaturity of the child and expect no more of her than she can attain.

---

Jean represents a child whose difficulties were due in part to advanced mental development. Poor adjustment to kindergarten, a strong desire to dominate, and resistance to authority were some of the problems for which her parents sought clinical guidance. Although Jean's chronological age was only 5 years 8 months, tests indicated that she was over 8 years in her mental development. She wa recognized by both parents and teachers as a bright child, but at no time had her true ability been recognized. It can readily be seen why Jean did not find school work on a kindergarten level interesting.

Slow speech development is a problem which usually gives a parent much concern. Many children are brought to a clinic for this reason alone. With such a case, the role of the psychologist is very important. It may even be that the problem is solved by the psychological study alone, for tests may determine that the child has not reached the mental age at which speech develops. The speech retardation may prove to be only a part of the child's general retardation.

The services of the clinic were consulted in regard to Celia's slow speech development. She was 6 years 3 months of age and had begun her first-grade work in school. From this she was soon dropped. Two older sisters were spending much time trying to teach her but with little success. In spite of their effort Celia had only a few words at her command. Her problem was soon solved, for all tests showed that Celia had not reached the mental age at which speech develops. Her slowness in talking could be explained by a mental retardation below the age at which a child begins to use language.

There may be other reasons why a child is not learning to talk. Chief of these is deafness or loss of hearing.

Grace represents such a case. At 4 years of age she had acquired scarcely any vocabulary. Several tantrums at times made it difficult for the parents to discipline her. In the tests that could be given her at the clinic she responded like a child of average intelligence. However, her behavior suggested deafness, and a hearing test was recommended. Audiograms showed that the child suffered from marked impairment of hearing. In this case slowness in learning to talk was due to deafness and called for very different treatment from that of a child whose poor speech is due to mental retardation.

Proper school placement is of great importance for the mental health of the child. School failure should be avoided whenever possible. Formerly little attention was paid to a child until he had failed two or three times. Attempts are now in progress to make such adjustments much earlier, with the result that the clinic services are often consulted when it looks as if the child will not make the grade during the first year. In this way, failure, with its emotional effects, is often averted. More enlightened mothers are even bringing their children to the clinic to determine their readiness and fitness for school. For these problems the services of the psychologist are very necessary.

Robert was a little chap whose age allowed him to enter the first grade. His mother questioned his readiness and came to the clinic seeking advice. All tests confirmed the mother's suspicions. Robert was slow in his development and was in every respect a much younger child than his chronological years. His poor ability in some special things gave every reason to believe that Robert would fail if he began his first-grade work at that time.

---

Proper school placement was a matter of concern to Richard's mother also. She was aware that he read well for a child only 6 years 3 months of age, but she questioned his ability to do second-grade work without spending the first year in school. The clinic was consulted. Richard's advanced mental development, together with the fact that educational tests showed his preparedness for second-grade work, justified his going into that grade. He was advanced to the second grade, where he adjusted himself easily and happily.

These cases represent only a few of the many problems coming to the clinic in which the services of a psychologist are essential. Furthermore, because the work is varied and demanding, it is important that only those who have had adequate training and experience should assume the responsibility of doing the work. The qualifications of a clinical psychologist should comprise more than a mere knowledge of the technique of administering the tests and the ability to compute the intelligence quotient. Determining the intelligence quotient is but a small part of the psychological study and means little unless interpreted in relation to good developmental, medical, and social history of the child. Personality traits, handicaps, if any, and special abilities or disabilities also come in for study. Only one who is familiar with these various aspects of a child's development can ever hope to do justice to the child in such a study.

After the intelligence quotient has been determined, a question which one may reasonably ask is whether the intelligence quotient remains constant or relatively the same throughout life. Though the constancy of the intelligence quotient has been studied extensively, the question is not definitely settled at the present time. The age at which the psychological study is made will influence somewhat the intelligence rating. To a clinical psychologist who has worked with a young child before his language has developed to any extent it is not surprising to find that the child has raised his rating perceptibly at a later date. Also, a child from a poor environment may change his scoring when placed for a while under better circumstances.

However, an experienced worker will recognize the potentialities of development and differentiate between what may be a permanent retardation and an underdevelopment due to poor environment.

The whole subject of a psychological study might be best understood by pointing out some of the many interesting facts that may come to light during an examination. The first requirements are proper rapport between the psychologist and the child and establishment of a proper attitude toward the tests in general. The psychologist gets his first knowledge of the child from the way in which the situation is met. With one child rapport is quickly established. He comes readily and alone with the examiner to the examining room. He may be a little shy at the beginning but he soon learns that the examiner is a friend and not someone to be feared. In a short time he is very much at ease and complies with all requests. He works with effort and persistence and meets the most difficult test even though his efforts may not be crowned with success. His attitude is one of independence and of meeting new situations alone and unaided.

With another child the very opposite may be true. His mother may have to accompany him to the examining room; he remains fearful of the examiner throughout the examination; he is never at ease; he responds to tests largely under protest; his effort is poor; and when he meets the slightest difficulty he appeals for help. In fact, his attitude is one of dependence and a constant seeking for assistance. At no time does he meet the new situation independently and unaided. In truth, the response to the test situation may often be an indication of the way the child is meeting life in general.

When the child's cooperation has been obtained, the more formal tests are given. The object of the standardized test is to determine how the child's development compares with that of other children of his age. If he has not come up to the standard, what are some of the factors that may possibly affect his future development? One must allow for the premature child to catch up to his actual age; for the child whose physical activities have been curtailed because of many illnesses; for the child with a birth injury; and for children with other handicaps. Handedness also may be observed at this time. At an early age the child begins to show a preference for the use of one hand. Interference in the development of the use of the hands may work out disadvantageously to the child. The little child who has been forcibly changed from the use of the preferred left hand to that of the right is all too frequently recognized by other signs of difficulty.

Further insight into the child's mental development is had by the use of language tests. There is no phase of development that requires more careful observation and study. To distinguish between good all-round language development and mere superficial verbalistic fluency is possible only to one who has a knowledge of language tests and experience with children who show various phases of speech acceleration or retardation. It may be said that this phase of development can be most misleading. The child who speaks a great deal and at an early age is generally regarded as intellectually superior, but this impression may or may not be correct. On the other hand, the child with poor enunciation and little facility in the use of words is often considered retarded. These deductions may or may not be true, depending upon the nature of the language development.

The type of child who has only a parrotlike speech development is well known to the clinical psychologist. He enunciates clearly and has several language patterns. When using these freely and spontaneously, and in the manner in which he has learned them, he seems quite like the average child. He fails, however, when he is asked to use these words in a new way or to show that he knows what they mean.

Daniel's history illustrates such a development. He articulates fairly well and uses rather long sentences. His comments are usually built around some personal incident or some object in the immediate situation. When Daniel is asked to indicate the meaning of some word he has used, he is unable to do so. All that a word seems to do is to elicit a response that has been learned and associated with it. He apparently has no grasp of its meaning. He also fails when it is necessary to comprehend simple questions. He has learned to repeat words in a parrotlike way, but he can do little in using them intelligently. In truth, his acquisition and use of words are comparable to the learning of the defective, who gets the repetitive learning but can do little with his material in new situations. Daniel's intelligence quotient falls into the feeble-minded grouping.

Another phase of development often recognized in a young child is that in which his information is much in advance of his ability to reason independently. This is often seen in an only child or one who has been under the tutorship of an adult a great deal. Such a child may know colors and coins, may have a number concept beyond his years, and may use pencil and paper with ease. In fact, he is much at home with things that may be learned by individual help and attention. It is when such a child is faced with a problem which draws upon his own initiative and ability to reason independently that he fails. His whole attitude is one of waiting to be shown rather than of puzzling the problem out for himself. While the ability to learn readily from others is a measurement of intelligence, it does not constitute the sum total of intelligence. Neither does much learning make one particularly intelligent. It is not so much the amount that the individual learns as his ability to use what he has learned that is essential. It is in this respect that the overambitious parent is often deceived. The mother, in her zeal to hasten the mental development of her child, sets about teaching him all he is capable of acquiring, often to the disadvantage of the child. When the latter has reached the saturation point, he gives the impression of being overstimulated and confused and of possessing knowledge much in advance of his years but having little meaning to him. He has learned facts, but his intellectual immaturity does not allow him to use them well. This is the type of child who may have a very high intelligence quotient at an early age, but whose intelligence quotient drops perceptibly at some later examination. This child may experience difficulty in adjustment to his early school work, the reason often being that, through having much direction and supervision by a second person, he has built up such dependence that he is inadequate when this support is withdrawn and he is obliged to fit into the methods of teaching by group instruction.

78985°—39——2

A similar mistake is often made with the dull, slow child and the feeble-minded. Refusing to accept consciously the fact of the child's mental inadequacy, the parent attempts to compensate for his deficiency by forcing the rote learning. But the learning is not assimilated, and this becomes very evident when the child is called upon to apply it in some simple reasoning problem. Instead of finding it aptly applied, one gets a regurgitation of incidents and facts, a talking about something, as it were, without any proper relation to what the child is saying. In other words, he talks all around a question without in the end answering it. This type of child, too, is well known to the clinical psychologist and often has accompanying behavior problems.

Within recent years considerable study has been made of the so-called verbal, abstract, ideational type of child as compared with the practical, concrete type. While little is known psychologically concerning these differences, it is well recognized that such a difference exists. One child has no difficulty in mastering the symbols required for academic progress and has no trouble in reasoning out a situation not in the immediate present. In contrast to this child is the one for whom all forms of symbolic education are acquired with effort or are not acquired at all. In the immediate situation and in working with concrete material he is intelligent, but he fails miserably in his attempts to meet academic requirements. In other words, he has a type of intelligence which may adjust well in a program that calls for the practical everyday duties of life, but will be very much out of step in a bookish, academic environment. Again, this type may be recognized at a very early age and profitable advice given with reference to educational plans, if the parent will accept it. Too often this is not what happens. The plans and ambitions of the parents for the child will not allow this. They tutor, they drill, they nag, and they force, and all their efforts have only a very detrimental effect upon the child.

One cannot hope to portray all the types seen in a clinical service, and it is not the purpose of this writing to do so. Rather, the aim has been simply to indicate the nature and variety of problems that a clinical psychologist may meet and to emphasize the importance of adequate training and experience. This work requires the ability not only to administer the tests but also to interpret the results and to recognize the various phases of development with their possible relation to the problem for which the child is seeking clinical help.

## THE SOCIAL WORKER

The social work in the habit clinic is complex and varied. All types of problems are referred from many different sources. The visiting nurse who finds a physically well child refusing to eat; a family-welfare worker who sees a mother so overwhelmed with the difficult behavior of one child that her agency's help is of little value to the family; the social worker from a child-welfare agency who seeks help for a child with the problems of defective speech or continued bed-wetting; parents worried and harassed by the ordinary, everyday problems of life as they are related to the child—all turn to the clinic for assistance. Many of the children come to the clinic directly from a nursery school or a kindergarten. In these groups the teachers often note the child who finds difficulty in making adjustment to other children, who is obviously the victim of unwise training; and they will guide the mother to the clinic. Probably the most satisfactory referral is the one made directly by the mother who realizes that her child has a problem with which she needs help, for cooperation is then assured.

It is the social worker in her role as clinic manager who makes the important first contact with individuals or agencies wishing clinic help. She selects the cases which the clinic is best equipped to handle, makes the appointments for attendance, and when the mother and child arrive steers them through the routine clinical examinations and interviews.

The social worker is a member of the team consisting of psychiatrist, psychologist, and social worker, which makes a threefold study of the child. She investigates and studies the environment in which he is living, including the home and the neighborhood, and especially that most important part of the child's environment, the adults with whom he comes in contact. She learns from the parents, the teacher, and the nurse what has been observed of the child's personality, his reactions to punishment, his choice of playmates, his affections, moods, impulses—whatever will help to make up a picture of the child as he really is. She is, moreover, in a position to obtain much valuable information through visiting and observing the child informally in the nursery, the nursery school, the school, the home, the settlement house, the playground, or the community center. For in this way the child may be observed at his play or occupation, quite at ease and unperturbed, free from the fear and anxiety that are frequently associated with the more formal clinic contacts.

To this cross section the social worker adds a longitudinal view—she learns something about the family stock from which the child comes, the conditions under which he was born and reared, his development, the accidents and sicknesses he has had, and his reactions to them—everything that will help to explain the child to the psychiatrist when he comes to the clinic.

When the child has been studied at the clinic and a plan of treatment has been made, the social worker assists in carrying it out. The direct treatment of the child is carried on by the psychiatrist. However, the success of the program for the child of habit-clinic age depends largely on the cooperation of the grown-ups responsible for his training. The father's and the mother's attitude toward masturbation, the method of handling a temper tantrum, the teacher's persistence in correcting a speech defect, may all have to be changed if the child is to be helped. It is often necessary for the social worker to explain to parents again and again the clinic findings, to show them the important role each step plays in carrying out the plan of treatment satisfactorily. Reassurance and encouragement are often necessary, since the task of supplanting poor habits with good ones may prove a long and tedious process.

Frequently the plan for the child's treatment involves some service which the clinic is not prepared to give. For this reason the social worker must be familiar with all possible resources in her community and must know the type of case that each organization can best serve.

A more complete physical examination may be necessary. Deafness, for example, may cause temper tantrums or give an appearance of general retardation and must be ruled out before any plan can be made by the clinic. Enuresis (incontinence of urine) cannot be considered a habit problem unless no physical basis for it can be found. Intensive neurological studies and an intensive investigation of the endocrine glands may be essential. Only those most experienced in these particular fields of medicine can be of real help to the child.

Camps or schools give a temporary change of environment which is very helpful in determining the effect such a change makes in the child's problem. Even with a group of children of the preschool age, the only possible solution sometimes seems to be long-time placement in a foster home. In such an event the child-placing agency gives invaluable assistance. If, as often happens, the mother is so preoccupied with some worry, financial or other, that she fails to recognize the necessity of help for her child or if her own worry is adding to the child's difficulties, the cooperation of a family agency that can work out a budget and give supplementary relief or steer the mother to a relief-giving organization is the first step in treatment. The social worker must know the clinic or agency that can best help the child, considering his age, his problem, and the family finances.

Although the most important part of her work is the service to the child who comes to the clinic, the social worker in the habit clinic has other duties, among which the supervision of students who may come to the clinic for practical training is important. The students will acquaint themselves with the clinic methods by the study of records and through staff conferences at which the psychiatrist, the psychologist, and the social worker present their parts of the investigation and treatment. Study of the contacts other agencies have had with new clinic cases gives the students the opportunity to learn of the community resources at first hand. Follow-up visits test out their ability to make satisfactory interviews and personal contacts. Finally, a few cases are turned over to the students, always under careful supervision.

The material which is gradually collected in the form of records is particularly valuable for research purposes, as it deals with young children whose problems may be projected into the future and who as a group lend themselves to follow-up studies and research. The collecting and analyzing of such data as may be obtained should be useful in showing various trends and in evaluating results of treatment at the clinic when compared with carefully controlled untreated problems of a similar nature.

The amount of educational work which the habit-clinic social worker can do seems to be limited only by the time which she can give to it. That the child's early years are important in his future adjustment to life's problems is still not widely appreciated. Talks to mothers' clubs, to groups of teachers, and to others interested in child training, on the importance of mental health and the value of the services of a child-guidance clinic, especially to preschool children, are time-consuming but unquestionably another important part of the job.

With so broad a scope of activities it is most important that the social worker not only fulfill the usual requirements of education, training, and experience but also have a sufficient reserve of strength and energy to enable her to meet numerous and varied demands with skill and resourcefulness, to be ready to tackle a new situation with initiative, and to be able to see the old problems with a fresh point of view.

## HABIT-CLINIC PROCEDURE

Parental education may be said to be the backbone of habit-clinic procedure, supplemented by a direct psychiatric approach to the mental health of the child in an attempt to understand his particular difficulties in making the necessary adjustments to life. The sources of habit-clinic cases are varied. Social agencies, nursery schools, kindergartens, private physicians, hospitals, nurses, and parents all refer cases for study. As education in mental hygiene has become more general and parents have become more concerned over evidences of maladjustment or inadequacy in their children, and more enlightened concerning the environmental factors affecting conduct, an increasing number of cases have been referred by the parents themselves. Whether the child is referred by a nurse, a teacher, a social worker, or the parents, the procedure is the same.

A visiting nurse entering the home of Mrs. S found the mother very much upset, nervous, and agitated on account of having been worried all day by her little daughter Mary, aged 2 years 2 months. Casual inquiry at this time revealed the following facts: The child was extremely disobedient, almost to the point of being negativistic. She absolutely refused to respond to a direct command and could be managed only by constant coaxing. Although Mary had been weaned months before, the mother had resorted to the use of the bottle in order to comfort her before her nap and before her bedtime, and as a help in getting sufficient nourishment into the child to keep her from losing weight. At every meal the mother was put through the typical ordeal of feeding the child herself, often being rewarded for her efforts by having the child spit the food out on the floor. It was also mentioned quite incidentally that the child wet the bed every night and had done so ever since the mother had resorted to bottle feeding.

With this information at hand, the nurse reported the situation to the supervisor in charge of the settlement house where a clinic was being held, having first interested the mother in the habit clinic and what it is trying to do for this type of case. The supervisor then referred the family to the social worker of the habit clinic, who within the next 2 or 3 days made a careful social investigation of the home. The following is a brief summary of her report:

### SUMMARY OF SOCIAL WORKER'S REPORT

Case of MARY SMITH

The family live in a very poor and crowded district. The street is narrow, unpaved, and cluttered with papers like an alley. There are three-story brick tenement houses on each side, and one has the feeling that it is a congested neighborhood, as the street is crowded with children, there is a great deal of noise, and many people are hanging out of the windows.

The patient's family, consisting of father and mother, Mary, and a little girl of 6 months, occupy a four-room tenement with bath, on the third floor, for which they pay $20 a month. The house is very clean and is neatly and prosperously furnished. It has a living room, a dining room, a kitchen, and a bedroom. All members of family sleep in one room. The patient has a crib by herself.

The mother is a slight, delicate young woman of 20, who enjoys housekeeping and is very much interested in her home. She went 2 years to high school, then worked as a clerk before marriage, and has been married 3½ years. She has a bad temper and is easily excited. She told the worker that when the patient does not mind her immediately she becomes impatient and "feels all stirred up inside."

The father is a short, well-built man of 24, who drives a garbage truck for the city, earning $24 a week. He is in good health, is interested in his home, and plays with his children. He and his wife differ in regard to discipline, he often telling the child that she can do things which her mother has forbidden.

The patient was born full term, instrumental; one eye was black and blue. Development was quicker than that of the average child. First tooth: Four months. Walking and talking: Under a year. The patient has had no diseases or convulsions. The only evidence of illness is that 3 weeks ago she had a fever of 103 and was nauseated.

*Habits.*—Sleeps from 6:30 p. m. to 6 a. m. Is restless and occasionally cries out for mother in her dreams, awakens, but goes back to sleep again. No night terrors. Has a 2-hour nap in daytime.

*Feeding.*—She is not finicky but has a capricious appetite. At different times refuses different foods. Always has to be coaxed and occasionally spits out her food. Will not drink milk except from a bottle. Is always given one when put to bed.

*Enuresis.*—Wets bed every night.

*Disposition.*—Affectionate; demonstrative; generous; not jealous, pugnacious, nor domineering; very stubborn and inclined to be negativistic. Always has to be coaxed to do things; is very disobedient.

*Play life.*—Enjoys playing with other children but can amuse herself if left alone. Likes dolls.

*Summary.*—There is no evidence of nervous or mental disease in the family. The chief problems are refusal of food, enuresis, and disobedience. The mother is excitable and easily loses patience with the child. The father seems sensible, but the parents disagree in regard to discipline.

The mother was asked to report with the child at the clinic the following week, at which time the child was immediately taken in charge by the psychologist, whose report is here summarized.

### SUMMARY OF PSYCHOLOGIST'S REPORT

Some 15 or 20 minutes before the psychological examination was begun, friendly relations were established. The child, after an initial hesitancy and shyness, quickly became interested in playing and enjoyed especially the drawings of a cat with long whiskers. As she is of that age where best examination results are obtained with the mother present, provided she uses discretion, the mother was given the usual instructions as to how she could help in the examination. The mother was quite interested, and excellent cooperation was secured. She smiled encouragement from time to time and did not let Mary know when a failure had occurred. She wisely refrained from distracting her by urging her to do better.

Mary showed but slight hesitancy about entering the examination room. As soon as she saw the pictures and the colors her self-consciousness disappeared. The tests given her were presented as games and she quickly caught the play spirit and very willingly tried to do everything that was asked of her. The mother, too, was pleased and incidentally quite surprised that the youngster did things which she had never tried before.

Mary is 2 years and 2 months old. She developed rather more quickly than the average child. Her first two teeth came in at 4 months. She said such things as "mama" and "papa" at 6 months and a large number of words plainly at 9 months.

As far as formal tests are concerned, this child made a very good showing. With one exception she did satisfactorily all tests that the average child of 2 does. Pictures took her eye, and she interestedly pointed to objects in the pictures and named one or two in each. She quickly imitated such movements as raising arms and clapping hands and quickly carried out simple requests such as "Bring me that ball," "Now throw it to me," and "Go over there and sit on that chair." Before eating a piece of candy, she removed the paper in which it had been wrapped. Her one failure in the 2-year test was that of copying a circle with a pencil. As her mother has never allowed her to use a pencil lest she mark up the house, this failure is insignificant. She passed four of the 3-year tests. She knew her full name and her sex and she took delight in pointing out her eyes, nose, mouth, and hair. She pointed to shoes, stockings, and dress, and was familiar with the names of common objects, such as penny, a knife, a key, a watch, and a pencil. In all informational questions she did exceptionally well.

Summing up results, we find that Mary has a mental age of 2 years and 6 months, as against an actual age of 2 years and 2 months, which gives her an intelligence quotient of 116. Her developmental history, her general alertness and interest in things about her, her quickness in learning, and her rating on formal tests show a child above the average in intellectual equipment.

### INTERVIEW WITH PSYCHIATRIST

Shortly afterwards the mother was interviewed by the psychiatrist, and although the following conversation was not taken verbatim, it represents what was said as nearly as can be remembered from the notes dictated a few hours later:

DOCTOR. I understand from Miss W, who visited you the other day, that Mary is becoming quite a problem.

MRS. S. She is, indeed. I hardly know what to do with her. She refuses to eat anything, and she gets me so worked up and so tense inside that I go into hysterics.

DOCTOR. Then perhaps you are not feeling very well yourself.

MRS. S. I am feeling all right now, but at times I get nervous.

DOCTOR. Under what conditions are you most apt to get worked up, Mrs. S?

MRS. S. Usually when I have had arguments with my husband regarding Mary—how to make her mind and what I should do. When I am trying to make her mind or take her food, he butts in and says, "Let her alone. Don't keep bothering the child." And on other occasions when she is doing things that he doesn't like, he asks me why I don't make her mind.

DOCTOR. One may assume from the report which Miss W brought to me that you and your husband get along very well, that you are both fond of and very much interested in Mary, and that you want to do everything possible to have her overcome these undesirable habits.

MRS. S. Yes, sir. Mary's behavior is the only thing over which we have any arguments at all, and we both want to do all we can to help her.

DOCTOR. You know, Mrs. S, that a child of Mary's age, especially a child of Mary's intelligence, has a very much better understanding of the ordinary things going on about the household than you give her credit for. It is surprising how early a child learns that there is some doubt in the minds of her parents about just what is right and what is wrong, and, quite naturally, when there is any doubt in the child's mind about what course he is to follow, he is very apt to take the easiest one. So it is extremely important that you and Mr. S have a definite understanding about what you are to expect of Mary. You know, too, that not infrequently parents are apt to discipline children in a rather erratic way. By that I mean that much depends upon how the parent happens to be feeling at the time the child needs discipline. If the mother is in a cheerful state of mind and not tired out by the household duties, some breach of discipline may be looked upon as quite amusing, the parents may speak of it as "cute," and the mother may laugh at the child instead of reprimanding her. On the other hand, if the same thing happens at the end of a hard day when the mother is worried and annoyed and somewhat out of temper herself, the child may be punished, sometimes severely and out of all proportion to what she deserves. Of course, you understand that I don't mean that is the method used in your home, but it is a method used in most homes more or less. I just mention it so that you will understand better what I mean by the importance of getting together with your husband and talking these matters over.

Mrs. S. Yes; I know lots of mothers who do just that—laugh at the baby as "smart" one day and slap him for the same thing the next.

Doctor. I would also call your attention at this time to something that you probably know already, and that is, that it is very bad to have the parents question each other's methods of discipline before the child. It is much better to have the mother or father carry out his or her own method, even if the other parent is not in full agreement with what is being said or done, and then discuss the whole thing in private after the child has gone to bed. It is only in this way that the child learns that the parents are united in their efforts to bring about the desired manners and habits. I think it is of the greatest importance that you talk these things over with your husband and have an agreement that will prevent any discussion of authority before the child.

Mrs. S. Yes, sir; I see exactly what you mean.

Doctor. Now we will discuss the feeding problem. I understand that Mary has not as yet given up the bottle.

Mrs. S. I had her weaned from the bottle, but she absolutely refuses to take milk from the cup. It was only when I put a little water with it that I could get her to drink it. I took her to the doctor, and he said if she wouldn't take milk from the cup, to let her have it from the bottle, and that is what I have been doing the last few months. She gets the bottle every morning at 10 o'clock when she takes her nap and every night when she goes to bed.

Doctor. Of course, you appreciate the fact that Mary is old enough to give up this bottle and that her clinging to these habits so strongly simply represents a desire on her part to stick to those infantile methods which she should be gradually giving up. The feeding problem, and the bed-wetting as well, represent habits that are quite normal for infants but that she should have outgrown some months ago, and it is going to be a great deal easier to break her of these habits at 2 years of age than it will be at 4 or 5. There is no better time to begin than the present.

Mrs. S. I realize all that and am willing to do whatever you say.

Doctor. Tell me a little about other difficulties with her feeding.

Mrs. S. She absolutely refuses to take any food unless I feed her.

Doctor. You mean that you have to sit down beside her at each meal and actually take the food from her plate and put it into her mouth?

Mrs. S. Yes; and she even spits it out.

Doctor. Then mealtime must be a very trying experience for you.

Mrs. S. Yes; it is the worst time I have.

Doctor. Then let me tell you what I have learned from my experience regarding children who cause so much difficulty by refusing food. In the first place, we must remember that it is a very natural thing for all human beings to crave attention, and this is particularly true of children. The refusal of food is frequently a method that children use to get the time and attention of the parents. At that time they become the center of attention, and it is a battle of wits between the mother and child to see which one will win. The mother frequently puts the food on the table with serious doubts and misgivings in her own mind as to whether the child will eat it, and perhaps her first remark is, "You have got to eat this. You are not going to get up from the table until you do eat it. You didn't eat any breakfast and you cannot go out to play until you have eaten your lunch." This immediately puts the child in a rather defiant mood. Even if it had not occurred to the child to refuse his food, this in itself acts as a challenge. It is just as though there were a little play going on, in which the child is taking the leading part—a situation in which both children and adults like to find themselves. We know that the child knows that invariably, if he does not eat his meals at the regular time, the anxiety of the mother will make her only too willing to provide food between meal hours. So in this way the child is not only able to defy the parent and attract attention and win his battle, but he is also able to get the amount of food which his system requires. It may be that he doesn't get the best type of food and the kind best suited to nourish him, but he gets the food which pleases him most and satisfies his hunger, and that is about all the child wants.

Mrs. S. But, Doctor, if I let her go without her meals she will get so thin.

Doctor. It will be hard at first, I know, but I would suggest that from now on, or at least during the next week, you and your husband agree to the following plan: Place on the table a smaller amount of food than you would naturally want the child to eat. This should include milk, cereal, fruit, and whatever else you may wish her to have, and absolutely nothing should be said regarding the food itself or the child's eating it. If the child is eating with you and your husband, pay no attention whatever to her eating. After you have finished and sufficient time has been given the child to eat her food, remove the dishes and say nothing at all regarding the amount of food the child has eaten. If Mary has not been in the habit of having milk between meals, under no circumstances give it to her.

Mrs. S. She has been having the bottle at 10 o'clock, just before she takes her nap.

Doctor. Then, under those conditions, I should give her an equal amount of milk in a cup. On the way home, I should drop into the drug store and get some straws and let her use those during the coming week. It will be a step away from the bottle and will interest her in taking the milk from the cup.

But to continue regarding the more general statements as to her feeding habits: Do not be concerned if she does not eat much for the first few days. It will take a day or so for her to learn from your apparent lack of interest in her eating that no one is very much concerned whether she eats or not. In other words, try to get away from romance at her feeding periods. Mary will soon find that she no longer occupies the center of the stage during the meal hour. I appreciate that you will be just as concerned, but the important thing is not to let Mary know it. The task I have outlined is a difficult one, I know, but it is not nearly so difficult to manage now as it is going to be a year or two from now; and although the results may be discouraging at first, you may be assured that in the end it will work out not only to Mary's advantage but to your own.

Mrs. S. Well, I'll try this week and see if I can stand it.

Doctor. I don't want you to look for improvement today or tomorrow or the next day, but I want you to think ahead 3 or 4 months and then picture Mary eating in a perfectly normal, healthy way without causing you or the rest of the family any disturbance. The only way to do this successfully, that I know of, is to follow the plan that I have just outlined.

It is absolutely essential that you and Mr. S work together on this matter, because if you do not cooperate the whole plan is doomed to failure, and this first victory for Mary may work out to her disadvantage in later life. I am sure you know many people your own age who are terribly finicky about what they eat, having all sorts of digestive upsets, refusing to accept any suggestion made by others—the type of person who is generally disliked and hard to get along with. It is just such people that children with all sorts of finicky habits are quite likely to develop into.

Mrs. S. I certainly wouldn't like Mary to grow up like an old woman who lives near us. She's just like that, and nobody can stand her.

Doctor. Do you think you will be able to carry out the plan I have outlined? I mean by that, do you feel that you will have the courage to let Mary go for a few days without what you feel is a sufficient amount of food in order to make her appreciate the fact that whether she eats or not is a thing which primarily concerns herself, and that going without food is not going to develop a tremendous upset in the home?

Mrs. S. I think I see what you mean, and I surely will make every effort to carry out your instructions and get my husband to also.

Doctor. Now, let us consider the problem of enuresis. I understand that Mary wets the bed practically every night.

Mrs. S. Yes, Doctor; every night. It has been much worse since she has been getting the bottle just before she goes to sleep.

Doctor. Now, since the time is getting short I want to outline a plan for that with less explanation than for the feeding problem, as I think this is a much more mechanical thing and will respond to treatment more easily.

Mrs. S. I have whipped and whipped her, and as it does no good I have given it up as useless.

Doctor. You were wise in giving up whipping her for this habit because she is undoubtedly in no way to blame for it, and it is quite an injustice to whip children for things over which they have no control.

Mrs. S. I agree with that.

Doctor. Now, at what time does Mary usually go to bed?

Mrs. S. At 6:30.

Doctor. And at what time does she have supper?

Mrs. S. At 4.

DOCTOR. Then I would suggest that you follow out in detail this plan. Let Mary have her supper at 4 o'clock, with such liquids as she is in the habit of taking, bearing in mind that she is to take the milk from the cup and not the bottle. Between 4 and 6:30 she is to have no fluids whatever. Before going to bed she is to be taken to the toilet, and you must see that she passes her urine. When she is put to bed make her understand that she is to be taken up later on in order to prevent her from wetting the bed. What time do you go to bed yourself, Mrs. S?

MRS. S. At 12 o'clock.

DOCTOR. Do you mean that you go to bed every night at 12 o'clock?

MRS. S. Yes.

DOCTOR. Isn't that rather late?

MRS. S. Well, after supper my husband listens to the radio until about 10:30. Then I make tea, and we have a little lunch, and by the time I get the dishes cleared away it is about 12.

DOCTOR. Then I would suggest that you make a tour of inspection every hour in order to determine at just what time Mary wets the bed, and that at 10 o'clock, 3½ hours after she has gone to bed, you get her up, thoroughly awaken her, and take her to the toilet. Make sure that she realizes why she has been wakened; that is, that it is in order to prevent her from wetting the bed. It is important that you do not pick Mary up in a semidrowsy state and simply place her on the toilet; she must be awakened thoroughly and given to understand exactly why you have wakened her. Then you can put her back to bed and allow her to remain until you get up in the morning, which I presume is about 6 o'clock.

MRS. S. Yes, sir.

DOCTOR. I am sure that if you follow out the instructions I have outlined regarding the feeding and bed-wetting, you will be able to report considerable improvement when you return next week.

MRS. S. I hope so, for it makes me so much extra work to have her go on this way.

DOCTOR. Before you go, I want to remind you again of the most important and fundamental thing that I have said this morning, and that is that you and your husband discuss this matter of discipline openly and frankly and decide upon a plan that will insure cooperation. It seems only natural, inasmuch as you see more of the child than your husband does, that the discipline should be in your hands and that he should support you and help you follow out the plan that you agree upon. Under no condition allow Mary to feel that there is any disagreement between you two as to what is best for her to do. As soon as she finds out that the household is divided against itself the battle, so far as you and your husband are concerned, is lost, and a great injustice is done to Mary.

I see by the tests that have been worked out this morning that Mary is a keen, bright little girl of unusual intellectual equipment, which means that she will be all the more capable of taking advantage of any failures which you and your husband make.

You may be assured we will do everything possible to help you during the next few weeks, and there is every reason to believe that by Christmas time Mary's difficulties will be well overcome. Can you arrange to come back a week from today?

MRS. S. Yes.

DOCTOR. Then that will be all this morning. But the problem of correcting her undesirable habits will have to be solved very largely by you rather than by Mary. I should like to get just a bit acquainted with Mary before you go.

The mother brought the child into the examining room, but no effort was made on the first visit other than to make friendly contact with her. She appeared to be a bright, keen little girl, well developed and fairly well nourished. She seemed interested in everything in her environment. In running about she fell down and knocked against a chair hard enough to hurt herself considerably. She immediately began to cry, but it was not difficult to attract her attention to something else, and the tears did not last long. Her attitude in the clinic during the short period of observation revealed nothing that had not been brought out by the reports of the social worker and the psychologist.

Had this child been a year older, with her rather superior intelligence, an attempt would have been made to interest her in keeping a record of her success regarding both feeding habits and enuresis. She would have been given a chart such as the accompanying one, and every effort would have been made to arouse her interest in obtaining as many stars as possible on her chart, which she would bring to the clinic the following week. Not only can the chart system be made a matter of great interest to the child, but it also serves as a detailed record of what has been done during the clinic intervals. That is, instead of having the parents report that the child has done pretty well or poorly regarding such problems as feeding, enuresis, and temper tantrums, we have a very definite quantitative record of exactly what success has been attained.

The chart system has been criticized by some as savoring of bribery, but there is no reason why the child should be denied some visible evidence of approbation of his efforts. Neither is there any reason why such efforts should not be rewarded if conditions permit. The incentive for most efforts, in either children or adults, usually resolves itself into a striving for approbation or reward and it is rather unreasonable to deny children the same approbation that most adults are seeking.

The following chart shows how the record is kept:

NAME: *Sally Jones* OCT 5 to OCT. 12.

EVERY STAR MEANS SUCCESS IN EATING MY MEALS.

| | *Breakfast* | *Dinner* | *Supper* |
|---|---|---|---|
| Monday | | | |
| Tuesday | | | |
| Wednesday | | | |
| Thursday | | | |
| Friday | | | |
| Saturday | | | |
| Sunday | | | |

However, it was not feasible to utilize the charts for Mary, as they were beyond the comprehension of a child 2 years old; but if the parents, who were keenly interested and who had at least average intelligence, cooperated, there was every reason to believe that the child's problem would not be particularly difficult to solve.

An effort has been made in the foregoing paragraphs to give the reader a fairly good idea of exactly what takes place during the first visit in the case of every child coming to the habit clinic. Whether the problem is one of enuresis, feeding, or masturbation, or whether it is one of the more difficult personality defects—such as jealousy, shyness, cruelty, or abnormal fears—extreme tact and diplomacy are needed, in order, on the one hand, not to offend the parents, and, on the other hand, to impress them with the importance of the mental side of the child's life. They invariably feel that they have used all the patience and good judgment that might be expected of any one handling the problem with which they are confronted. Thus it is necessary to generalize and speak in a more abstract way on the first visit than is necessary after working relations have been established and the parents have developed confidence in the clinic. It is essential in conversing with parents to explain the points made by examples that are well within their comprehension. Care must be exercised not to criticize harshly or unjustly, and it must always be borne in mind that the interest of physicians is primarily therapy and not science or morals.

## COOPERATION WITH OTHER COMMUNITY AGENCIES

It must be kept in mind that if children as a group are to benefit by the available knowledge regarding mental health, every resource of the community must be utilized to its fullest extent. It is of paramount importance that every organization interested in the welfare of children should make a careful survey of what other organizations with similar interests are doing and of which activities have been most successful. The value of the resources which such agencies have for supplementing the work carried on by a child-guidance clinic cannot be overemphasized.

The available facilities which can operate independently or in cooperation with the clinic vary according to the size of the community and the interest and progress that have been shown in the field of child guidance. In urban communities there are usually many organizations which are directly or indirectly concerned with some aspects of this problem. Some social agencies providing service for children or families are equipped to do child-guidance work and others have psychiatric social workers on the staff able to give the treatment indicated by the study of the child made by a child-guidance clinic. Public agencies such as the schools or the juvenile court also may be equipped to provide child-guidance service to some of the children needing such service. In addition, there are usually a great variety of agencies that can assist the clinics. Any well-organized clinic should use all the facilities in the neighborhood that are of value in the treatment of the problem and that would help the future development of the child.

In the treatment of preschool children health centers and nursery schools and kindergartens can render significant service to the child. These important centers of training should be recognized by child-guidance clinics for their educational value in helping parents to understand that a child's emotional life is as important as his intellectual equipment and his physical endowment. These centers should also assume the responsibility of studying behavior problems in order to treat the child with wisdom at a time when wise treatment means so much to all concerned.

The public-health nurse, for example, is in a most strategic position not only to recognize undesirable habits and personality traits, but in many instances to institute simple methods which will correct these tendencies before they become firmly fixed as a part of the child's personality. Every nurse should have some training in mental hygiene. This is particularly true of those engaged in community health work. Many of the simpler problems of eating, sleeping, and toilet habits are matters of training which the nurse should manage efficiently.

Teachers in nursery schools and kindergartens should look upon the development of personality as an educational problem. They, too, are in a unique situation and should render valuable service to the parents and the public by detecting deviations from normal conduct, whether it is in rate of achievement in school work or whether it has to do with the child's ability to get along with his playmates. They usually enjoy a friendly and cooperative relationship with the parents of children under their charge and are often in a position to know intimately the home conditions under which the child is being reared. Herein lies the opportunity for much valuable work in the field of parent education.

Older children and some preschool children may need service from other types of organizations. Important among these are case-work agencies which provide service to children in their own homes and assist parents to understand their needs, such as family agencies, children's agencies, and visiting teachers in the schools. Some of these agencies provide the financial assistance that is essential to the dependent family. Others place the child in an environment best suited to his need, whether this is a foster home, a special institution or hospital, a nursery school, or a vacation camp. Clinics and hospitals carry out the examinations and treatments that are essential to health as well as the follow-up service for the child who is in need of medical care. Other agencies giving service to children are those providing organized activities for boys and girls or opportunities for recreation such as Boy and Girl Scout or Campfire groups, Big Brother or Big Sister Associations, organizations for young men or young women, recreational centers, organized playgrounds, settlements, and churches. Some children may need the special service of the school for social counseling, school placement, or vocational guidance.

The work of a child-guidance clinic should be that of a community center. Only by intelligent pooling of all community service can we be sure that the child is receiving all the advantages which the community has to offer.

## THE CHILD AND HIS PERSONALITY

Almost every discussion of the child and his personality carries with it a long dissertation on heredity which is likely to leave one either in a state of increased perplexity or with some very dogmatic ideas, depending on the author. Some writers maintain a consistently noncommittal attitude, and others state their views for or against the importance of heredity with great conviction. Thus, for example, John Stuart Mill made the statement, "Of all the vulgar modes of escaping from the consideration of the effects of social and moral influences on the human mind, the most vulgar is that of attributing diversities of conduct and character to inherent natural differences"; whereas Frederick Adams stated just as emphatically that in his opinion both "experimentally and statistically, there is not a grain of proof that ordinary environment can alter the salient mental and moral traits in any measurable degree from what they were predetermined to be through innate influences."

The consensus of opinion of physicians dealing with the practical problems connected with the subject of heredity is well expressed by Kirkpatrick in the following paragraph:

> From the individual standpoint, heredity should neither be ignored as of no importance nor yielded to as inevitably fixing one's destiny. Instinctive and hereditary tendencies are the roots from which the physical, mental, and moral life develops. Some individuals develop more readily and to a greater degree than others. All are of the same human characteristics, but each may make the most of his environment. Some cannot go as far as others in certain directions nor as easily, but no one has exhausted his possibilities of development. The practical problem is to expend our efforts upon the useful characteristics which we possess in the greatest degrees.[1]

It seems only reasonable at this time when so much disparity exists in the opinions of various writers on heredity that a conservative point of view, such as that presented by Kirkpatrick, should be tentatively accepted. Such a hypothesis makes it possible to get away from the pessimistic attitude to which the fatalist clings with undying tenacity. Doing this is not seeking a fool's paradise and becoming oblivious to the biological facts of life. Whatever may be the relation between the germ plasm and the color of eyes or the size of foot, and whatever research may determine in regard to defective germ plasm—how it affects the number, size, and distribution of brain cells, evidently resulting in variations in inherent mental equipment and setting definite limitations on brain development—no one, as yet, is ready to say that personality and all its component parts are not molded and colored by social heritage to a great degree. After all, social maladjustments are more frequently due to emotional instability than to intellectual defects. More is to be gained by concentrating upon the study of environment and its effects on the de-

[1] Kirkpatrick, Edwin A.: Fundamentals of Child Study, p. 29. Macmillan Co., New York, 1917.

velopment of personality than by accepting a hopeless, fatalistic theory of heredity.

In the attempt to understand the child it must not be forgotten that just as he has ears, eyes, a brain, and a heart, so he has instincts and emotions. He has, for example, an instinctive fear of falling and is afraid of loud noises. He has an inherent hunger for self-expression that is constantly infringing upon a code of laws and customs of which he has, as yet, no understanding. We must remember that the child has plans, hopes, and ambitions; he has doubts, fears, and misgivings; he has joys and sorrows, some very slight and fanciful, others very deep and real. This emotional life is thwarted and gratified in much the same way at the age of 3 that it is going to be at 30.

With all these instinctive and emotional drives, which have much in common with those of the adult, there is necessarily lacking the stabilizing factor of experience which can come only with years. The child is confronted with many new situations to which there is a definitely unpleasant emotional tone. For example, many of the primary experiences of children with animals are accompanied by fear. Jealousy is often aroused when the child first appreciates that the mother is giving some of her attention to other members of the family. Anger is aroused repeatedly until the child appreciates the reason for the acts which give rise to these emotions, and then suddenly and unexpectedly the emotional reaction changes. The child, therefore, must be considered as an individual with all the equipment necessary for registering joy and sorrow, pleasure and pain, but with little experience for properly evaluating the details of the situation so that the quantity and quality of the emotion will be adequately expressed. Regrettable as it may be, adults all too frequently stimulate some of the child's most undesirable emotional reactions for their own amusement, leaving permanent scars on his personality.

Childhood is not only the opportune time but the only time to initiate a program of mental health. Seeds of pugnacity, selfishness, and feelings of inferiority are sown early. They may not bear fruit until later—perhaps never; but if one expects to develop an adequate, well-rounded, self-sufficient personality, one must plant the seeds for it during the child's earliest years and carefully nurture them. The mental life of the child is characterized by his tendency to imitate, his suggestibility, his love of approbation, and his marked plasticity. These qualities, in association with his lack of experience, training, and education, render an interpretation of his mental activity less difficult at this time than in later years. All these factors may be utilized to great advantage in our efforts to stimulate, inhibit, or alter his reactions to the problems of everyday life. In the effort to understand human behavior the thoughts and feelings of the child must be taken into account. His daydreams become matters of importance. More intimate knowledge of his mental life is needed. It is necessary to take time to find out why he is queer, quiet, or reserved, why he is worried or sad. The situation demands the utmost ingenuity and patience in assisting the child to solve his own problems and at the same time appreciation of the fact that it would be of little value to solve them for him.

The infant at birth has no habits, and the habitual reactions which he acquires in the process of growing up are dependent upon his experience, training, and education. He seems, however, to have certain inherent tendencies which manifest themselves at an early age. Thus one child reaches out and embraces the world in a happy manner and another withdraws and rejects all attention. Such tendencies seem to be present at birth. Yet these so-called instinctive reactions are all modified, either to the advantage or to the disadvantage of the individual, through the effect of environment. Habits represent the child's responses to the innumerable, ordinary, everyday-life situations. Knowledge of an individual's habits makes possible a fairly accurate guess as to what may be expected of him in ordinary situations. As Doctor Dewey has pointed out, habits are not like a garment to be put on and taken off as the occasion demands, or as it pleases us. They are very much a part of us; we are the habit.

We begin to acquire habits at birth and continue to acquire them to a greater or less degree, depending upon our plasticity, until the end of life. The functions of eating, sleeping, and elimination become habitual. We develop habits of conduct toward those in authority. In some situations we acquiesce; in others we rebel. We have habits of conduct which include morals and manners. Our mental attitudes toward life are but habits of thought, and such traits as selfishness, shyness, cruelty, and fearfulness are merely emotional responses that have become habitual through repetition. Lying, stealing, and a disregard for the rights of others are likewise responses to certain situations, which through repetition become a part of the life pattern; in other words, they are habits.

It therefore becomes obvious that habits considered in their broadest sense are nothing more nor less than the individual himself, his happiness and efficiency being largely dependent upon the habits which he acquires in the process of growing up.

Almost from the moment the child is born he is confronted with all the varied life situations evoking what we think of as adult emotional responses. The child does not advance very far in life before he knows what it is to be jealous, to be fearful, to be angry, to love, to hate, to feel inadequate, and to experience sorrow and disappointment. He is continually subjected to environmental situations and personalities which stimulate these varied responses and lay the foundation for mental attitudes which eventually become habitual.

The child is recognized as being amoral (without morals) at birth. His responses to life are those that are essential to the preservation of self. He reaches out for that which brings him pleasure, smiling upon those who cater to his appetites, provide him with food, drink, and creature comforts, and stimulate pleasant bodily sensations by fondling and kissing him; and he rejects things and people not serving his immediate needs. His demands for attention must be recognized; his attempts to exhibit an influence over his environment must not be thwarted or there will be evidence of resentment. He is, indeed, a self-centered, egotistical individual who feels no responsibility toward life except that of trying to satisfy his own needs. All that he acquires in the way of ideals, altruistic tendencies, cooperation with his environment, and desire to please must come from his experiences with life, and during his early years these experiences are to a very large extent closely tied up with his parents.

It is therefore important that parents appreciate the raw material with which they have to deal, that they know something about these inherent strivings of children, their emotional stability, and their intellectual equipment. As time goes on parents should be intimately acquainted with the personality make-up of the immature individual whose future life is so dependent upon their interest and wisdom. They cannot afford through ignorance to twist and distort the personality make-up of the developing child through a domineering intolerance or humiliation, or by teasing, ridiculing, and cheating him, and destroying his sense of security. The child subjected to personalities that are egotistical, domineering, unstable, quick-tempered, and ill-mannered, has a right to become rebellious. It must be kept in mind that the child is not satisfied with being simply a passive part of his environment. He is persistently reaching out and struggling to make the environment satisfy his emotional needs. The parents' duty is to see that the emotional needs of the child are satisfied in a way that is compatible with the requirements of society.

In any effort to understand the behavior of children and to recognize the importance of the part environmental factors play in their conduct, it is essential to keep in mind the personality make-up of the individual child. No two children are subjected to the same environmental influences. The material situations may appear to be not very different, but the personalities of parents and others who are responsible for the training of the child vary widely, and these personalities are the most important aspect of the child's environment. To a very large extent the habits and the mental attitudes which become incorporated into the child's personality make-up are dependent upon the wisdom of the parents. They are the ones who must prepare children to live in a world outside the home. They must see to it that children are both ready and willing to make the necessary adjustments to life as it really exists. In this outside world the environment will not be altered to suit the child, as it frequently is in the home. Parents themselves must keep in mind, and must help the child to grasp the idea, that the individual and not the world makes most of the compromises and concessions when conflicts arise.

78985°—39——3

## THE PARENT AND THE HOME

The home must be considered the workshop in which the personality of the child is being developed; and the personalities of the parents will make up, to a very large extent, the mental atmosphere in which the child has to live. This mental atmosphere may easily become contaminated and can be quite as dangerous to the mental life of the child as scarlet fever or diphtheria would be to his physical well-being. Faulty habits are not infrequently due to the imitation of bad examples. Yet one is quite safe in saying that the mere imitation of the bad example is not nearly so dangerous to the child's mental health as may be the way in which the indiscretion is treated by the parent. In any study of environment, therefore, it is absolutely essential to have the fullest details possible regarding the personalities of the individuals with whom the child comes into intimate contact.

Parents who are largely responsible for the inadequate development of their children's personalities may be divided into well-defined groups. There is first of all the mother who, although worn and wearied by her routine household duties, tries to supplement the family income by putting in several hours a day sewing, washing, baking, or scrubbing when she should be in bed. She has little energy, either physical or mental, to give to any consideration of the welfare of her children. In striking contrast to her is the work-avoiding, duty-shirking, pleasure-loving mother who feels that her duty is ended at the birth of the child and turns over her responsibilities to a nursemaid. Again, there is the mother with excellent intentions, whose unintelligent interest is apt to defeat its very purpose. Usually she is oversolicitous and caters to every whim and desire of the child. All too frequently she is emotionally unstable and the child soon finds out that she has no definite rules and regulations about discipline. What is condoned today is punished tomorrow; and in spite of his ability to make rapid adjustments, the child finds it difficult or impossible to follow a consistent line of conduct. More pathetic than any of these situations, however, is that of the mentally defective mother who does the very best she can with her limited endowment and yet fails and recognizes her own failure.

So far only the mother has been considered but it must not be forgotten that the father's influence also must be considered. He may spread peace and harmony where chaos was wont to prevail, or he may disrupt and render chaotic that which was peaceful. The stern, righteous, rigid father who dominates the household by fear, is, from a mental point of view, perhaps the most undesirable. Yet there is no reason to envy the child who has a quick-tempered, impulsive father always ready with a sharp word and a blow. Lucky is the child who does not have his discipline handed out in an erratic manner by an emotionally unstable father.

Needless to say, the foregoing types fail to furnish the child with the very companionship which he needs most. Cheerfulness, affection, and kindly consideration; frankness and honesty in answering questions, so that speech and action may be free and uninhibited by fear of punishment or silent contempt; manners and speech that are not forbidding—all these tend to play a part that cannot be overestimated in the development of the child's personality.

To evaluate parental personalities requires more than a study of the personality make-up of isolated individuals; it entails a study of a complex relationship between two human beings endeavoring to carry out a very difficult task, usually without training or experience and sometimes without interest or desire. One need not be surprised that two such individuals do not always create a quiet, peaceful, happy home in which the child will find everything necessary for a healthy outlook upon life. Sometimes even an intelligent, well-educated man and woman with common interests will not make for efficiency when operating together as parents.

Much sentiment has rightly been lavished on the home—the place where the disheartened and the troubled find understanding and comfort, the fortress where those in need may find safety and security from a critical, demanding, competitive world. Unfortunately not all homes serve this ideal purpose. All too frequently the average person—man, woman, or child—makes less effort to keep up his morale in the home than in the shop, office, school, and place of recreation. Too frequently the home becomes the reservoir into which are poured all the resentment, disappointment, grief, and frustration associated with the unhappy experiences of the day. A tired, harassed mother finds in the family circle the only audience that cannot run out on her when she recites her trials and tribulations. A father at the close of a trying business day settles down at home with no feeling but indifference as his contribution to the family circle because he is preoccupied with expressing his grievances against those in authority, his irritation with his fellow workers, his feeling of failure, his anxiety about economic security. It is not surprising that the children in such a home soon regard it as the dumping ground of all unhappy and unhealthy adult emotions—a place used by all its inmates in their efforts to air the grievances against a world that has cheated them of something vital to their well-being. Such a home finds it difficult to compete with commercialized amusements—the dance hall, the night club, and motion-picture theaters.

Much good may come of talking over personal dissatisfactions in an orderly, intellectual way, but an unintelligent outpouring of grievances by a group of unhappy individuals seeking self-pity serves no useful purpose. Children who see in their parents unhappy, defeated, critical individuals do not want to be like them, nor are they inclined to find in their own home an ideal pattern for the future.

Unfortunately there are parents who have to live on such a low economic level that the problem of bare subsistence is confronting them at all times. When the clinic is faced with such a situation a relief agency must lay the foundation for any improvement involving mental hygiene. There are also parents whose intellectual equipment is so low that it would be beyond their comprehension to carry out even a common-sense program. For the problem child of such parents placement is absolutely essential. More numerous than any of these are, however, the parents whose own lives are so unstable emotionally that little or nothing constructive can be done for the child or for the family until the parents have recovered from their own mental difficulties. For this they need help, which may be provided either by referring them to some adult psychiatric clinic, or, if time permits and it seems wise, by treating the parents as well as the child at the habit clinic.

The child looks to his parents for his sense of security. In his parents he meets authority for the first time and his love relationship with them is constantly being endangered. He has to recognize that many of his desires are unattainable. In fact, it must seem to him at times that many of the goals which he is pursuing belong in the realm of the forbidden. He must learn to postpone the desire of the moment for that which his parents teach him is more worth while in the future. The habitual reactions with which the child meets these situations depend upon the wisdom with which his parents meet them. Parents who are still trying to meet the problems of adult life with the same emotional responses they used as children will obviously fail. Those who have had experiences deeply laden with emotion which are incompatible with their own ideals and supposed adult maturity, are suffering from a state of mind which necessarily affects their conduct toward their children. When the child's behavior sets off these potential emotional bombs, the task of developing adequate habits in the child is indeed a problem. The wise parent will make an effort to understand his own emotional life as well as that of the child.

The following case is a good example of a mother who brought a child to the clinic when the child should have brought the mother.

A woman about 40 years of age brought her little girl, 7 years old, to the clinic for examination, stating that she acted like a child 4 years old. The mother was unable to give any concrete examples of the child's immature acts. As far as could be discovered the child had no bad habits. She slept and ate well and was frank and honest. She would have liked to be affectionate if her mother had permitted her to be. She showed no cruel tendencies, and about the worst the mother could say was: "She takes up with any child she can find, regardless of creed, color, or nationality. I will not stand that." The mother stated that she would not permit her child to associate with the Catholic children in the neighborhood and that the Protestant children were not good enough.

The patient appeared to be a bright, keen, alert little girl, who answered all questions quickly and accurately. She manifested an interest in the examination and in her surroundings. She had an intelligence quotient of 98. As far as the history obtained from the mother and the examination of the child were concerned, there seemed to be little evidence to indicate that the child was either abnormal or unusual.

The mother was interviewed again, and it was ascertained that the child was not wanted, that the mother and father had been quite happy until her birth, and that she was looked upon as a stumbling-block to their happiness and economic success. The father's attitude toward the child was one of indifference. He rarely gave her any attention. The mother stated that she was not fond of her because the child was hateful and always made the mother regret being kind to her. When the mother and father were together they both ignored the child, and she was sent off by herself and not permitted to play with other children.

Further investigation of the case by the social-service department of the clinic revealed the following facts: The mother was looked upon in neighborhood as being "different." Although she was very affectionate toward her husband, the neighbors stated that it was not unusual for her to tell the child that she hated her. It was later ascertained that until a year before the patient was born the mother was looked upon as a very desirable neighbor. About that time she went away to live with a man who had been a boarder in the house and returned to her husband only after the authorities made complaints. Shortly after her return the patient was born. Since that time the whole situation had changed.

One of the most pernicious influences to which a child is subjected is that of persistently interfering members of the family group. Grandparents are perhaps the worst offenders in this respect, although other relatives may complicate the problem of bringing up children quite as much, if they are so inclined. This is particularly true, of course, if these individuals are living in the same household, but not infrequently their influence is felt even when they reside at some distance. Too much stress cannot be laid on the necessity of having the right to discipline the child vested entirely in the parents. Nothing does more to lessen parental authority than to have some line of action which the parent has decided to carry out questioned in the presence of the child.

Another situation frequently arising with reference to the problem of discipline is that brought about by the divided household; that is, the inability of the parents to agree upon any plan of action for training the child, each one forming as the occasion arises a spontaneous judgment entirely on an emotional basis. Much of the difficulty arising because of divided opinion regarding some particular act of the child might be avoided if parents themselves could get some clearer idea of the relative importance of so-called misconduct in children. For example, all too frequently the same punishment is meted out for some quite accidental offense, such as breaking a window with a baseball, as would be given for some obviously voluntary, malicious act involving cruelty.

For the child who has the misfortune to have a physically handicapped parent—especially a mother—it is very important, on the one hand, that too much stress should not be laid upon her incapacities, and, on the other, that the child should appreciate at the earliest possible age the burden which the parent is carrying and the consideration to which she is entitled. One frequently sees problems of delinquency arising under these conditions because the parent has been physically unable to "make the children mind." Much can be done by appealing to the child's spirit of fair play, especially when the object of his sympathy is always before him.

All too often adults are prone to utilize what appears to be the most potent means of obtaining obedience from the child; namely, fear. As this is one of the most primitive and easily stimulated emotions it is used more freely perhaps than any other. "If you don't stop crying, I'll go back to the hospital again," is a threat of a convalescent parent. "Don't touch the telephone," a mother remarks. "It will bite you." "The policeman will get you if you are not good." "The doctor will put the stick down your throat if you don't answer his questions." Fortunately for the child's peace of mind he soon finds that such promises and threats are not to be taken seriously, but unfortunately he is unable to distinguish between the persons whom he can trust and believe and those whose advice and warnings are simply idle prattle. Consequently he is likely to develop an absolute disregard and disrespect for the opinions of others, and later in his life he will be insensitive to praise or blame.

Cheating the child by making promises which the parents know they cannot keep or which they have no intention of carrying out is perhaps the origin of the absolute disregard for truth and the exaggerated suspicion seen in many children at an early age.

"The doctor has a lot of nice things in his bag which he will give you if you stop crying," one mother was overheard to say. She followed this up with the statement that "Mother is going to buy you heaps of pretty things as soon as the doctor is through," and made other promises which obviously she had no intention of carrying out.

The parents who take time to understand their child, who know his responses to praise, blame, rewards, and punishments, and who are affectionate and tolerant without being unduly sentimental and spineless, are the ones who will have the most to offer their children. The child imitates the habits and attitudes of his parents. They are a constant source of suggestion to him at a period in life when he is most plastic.

## HABIT PROBLEMS ASSOCIATED WITH EATING, SLEEPING, AND ELIMINATION

The physical well-being of the child is largely dependent on the efficiency of three fundamental organic functions; namely, eating, sleeping, and elimination. These functions become controlled and regulated by habit, and therefore habits of eating, sleeping, and elimination are the first to receive attention. The mother of the newborn infant is confronted with the dual responsibility of supplying proper nourishment and helping the infant to develop desirable habits for taking this nourishment at such times and in such ways as will best serve his physical needs. Almost at once she must also teach him to sleep at regular hours and without special attention; and, a little later, she tries to establish regular toilet habits. When these habits are properly established at a reasonable time, the child has been provided with a lasting foundation for both mental and physical health.

It is in connection with these simple physiological processes, however, that many of the initial mistakes in child training are made, either because parents ignore their importance entirely or because they become unduly worried and anxious over the difficulties encountered. The consequences of ignoring an undesirable habit are not always apparent. The immediate effect may be trivial compared with the ultimate results. On the other hand, oversolicitude on the part of parents introduces into their relationship with the child an indefinable something that the child assumes to be doubt, misgiving, or weakness, and that prevents him from looking to them for guidance, an essential factor in child training.

The methods recommended for establishing satisfactory habits in infancy are discussed elsewhere.[2] The discussion here is rather based on the fact that mistakes are made and undesirable habits formed. Inasmuch as these undesirable habits cause parents much concern and interfere with normal personality development, the habit clinics can be of valuable service to the community.

### EATING HABITS

No problem causes parents more concern than that of the child who has difficulty in taking and digesting his food. The more common feeding problems are refusal of food, sucking of food after taking it into the mouth, regurgitation, and vomiting. The fact that parents develop a marked anxiety with reference to these difficulties makes them oversolicitous, and this, in itself, is a most important factor in perpetuating the difficulty. A part of the body which is easily affected by emotion is the gastrointestinal tract. Physiological research has established the fact that emotions of various sorts, such as fear, anger, and excitement, directly influence the flow of digestive secretions. It is therefore not surprising to find that an organism so

---

[2] See Infant Care (Children's Bureau Publication No. 8, 1938), pp. 44–49.

highly developed, yet so unstable, as that of the nervous system of the child may very clearly reveal the relation between psychogenic and physiological processes.

It is usually not difficult to pick out those children whose loss of appetite and inability to digest and assimilate food are due to psychogenic rather than physiological causes. Nevertheless, it is essential to have these cases clearly differentiated by careful physical examinations. Many children who come to the clinic because of difficulty in feeding are not poorly nourished, anemic individuals. On the contrary, their physical condition is frequently such that one sees little cause for anxiety until the history of the case is presented. In such cases it is found that although the child's intake of food is fairly good, the food is of such a quality and taken under such emotional stress that it fails to serve the child's needs. The mother states that the child absolutely refuses to take food unless she sits down by his side and actually carries out all the necessary motor processes to get the food from the plate to the child's mouth, and even then she may have to tease, coax, threaten, and sometimes punish the child in order to make him swallow the food. After satisfying herself that the proper amount of food has been taken by the child, the mother is naturally quite dismayed to have the food vomited before the child leaves the table. When one considers the effects of emotion upon the process of digestion, it is not surprising to find that under emotional strain the stomach rejects the food.

A somewhat different problem is presented by the child who becomes antagonistic toward certain types of food—as, for example, soups, cereals, or vegetables of a special color. Such antagonisms persisting over a long period of time may have been aroused by injudicious methods utilized the first time the food was presented to the child. There is no doubt that parents sometimes make a great mistake in forcing a child to eat some new food which they consider absolutely essential to his well-being, the parents themselves being dominated by the idea that unless they are successful at the first attempt the battle is lost. Under such conditions there is apt to be a very unpleasant emotional scene which will linger in the mind of the child and be recalled the next time the food is presented. It therefore seems wise to guard against making an event of introducing a new article of diet into the child's menu. The food should be presented without comment and without any evidence of doubt in the mind of the parent or nurse that it will be eaten. But if, for some reason known or unknown, it is not taken at that particular meal, an unpleasant scene should be avoided and it should be presented at a later date without comment or show of indecision.

A certain amount of manual dexterity is required before children are able to feed themselves, and all too often parents find it easier to feed the child than to teach him to feed himself. Feeding is one of the first complex acts which the child is called upon to do for himself, and it is not surprising that he accepts this new responsibility with a certain amount of reluctance. Usually, however, success brings with it a kind of satisfaction which stimulates the child to make further efforts toward accomplishing the task.

It is of paramount importance to avoid discussing the child's feeding habits in his presence. Such discussion tends to fix the event in the mind of the child and make him cognizant of the fact that he is the center of attraction during the meal hour. Many children find that a negativistic attitude, not only toward feeding but toward sleeping, playing, and general obedience, is one way of attracting the attention which they desire.

Once the physiological causes of loss of appetite and malnutrition have been eliminated, it invariably works out well to serve the child only a small quantity of food, first making sure that it is well prepared and then allowing a sufficient period of time in which to eat it slowly. If it is not eaten, the food is removed at the end of that period without any ceremony, this procedure being repeated for a series of meals. Under those conditions much of the drama in which the child delights is eliminated, and much of the unpleasant emotional reaction produced by creating an antagonistic attitude in the youngster is avoided.

Some of the cases illustrating the difficulties associated with feeding will give more detail regarding the importance of neither directing the child's attention nor arousing his antagonistic attitude toward his food and the necessity of allaying the doubts and fears in the minds of parents so that they may at least appear less concerned.

Allen was brought to the clinic at the age of 3 years with the following history: Birth was difficult, necessitating the use of instruments; birth weight, 10 pounds; breast-fed; normal development; no illnesses or diseases. At the age of 2 he was treated with radium for a persistent thymus; at the time of the clinic visit he had enlarged adenoids and tonsils.

According to the mother this child never slept restfully but tossed and twisted about in his crib, often talking and crying out. He was extremely finicky about food and had marked likes and dislikes. He did not care for milk and refused vegetables, but he would sometimes eat seven apples a day. He was fond of meat, which was given to him occasionally. He never wanted the food set before him at mealtime.

He was considered somewhat shy and diffident, especially with strangers and adults. He played fairly well with other children on the street—usually with girls about 2 or 3 years older, but also with boys when he had the opportunity. He was fond of throwing a ball and wanted to be doing just what others were doing in games. He was very active. He was very fond of his mother and was often called "mother's boy." He was chummy with his father and most considerate toward his sister, 2 years younger than he. He was very selfish and most reluctant to divide things with others, always keeping the "lion's share" for himself. His mother stated that he was very stubborn and would not do as he was told, being, in fact, more likely to do the opposite. She punished him at times, but she believed that a more effective method of discipline was the threat to leave him.

At the clinic the child was keen and responsive. He answered all questions quickly and in detail, cooperated well, and was interested in the tests. He enjoyed being the center of attention and was very pleasant and kindly about it all. He paid much attention to his mother and little sister. His intelligence quotient was 130, and his mental capacity 1 year ahead of his chronological age.

There seemed to be nothing unusual or significant in the home situation. Both parents were fairly intelligent, very friendly, and cooperative. Although the father was an occasional drinker, he never came home drunk, nor was he a man of dissipated habits. The parents were working together for the good of their children. The father's salary was adequate. The family occupied a four-room apartment which was in good condition and well kept. The furnishings were of the average type.

*Summary.*—It appeared that this child, 3 years 4 months of age, was of rather superior intellectual endowment. His environment presented nothing outstanding in the way of a social problem at the time of the examination. The principal anxiety of the parents was the feeding problem, the child being poorly nourished and underweight, extremely finicky about food, showing strong likes and dislikes for various articles of food. The child was stubborn and very negativistic. He rebelled against authority whenever he was thwarted and whined a great deal.

The first and most important step in the treatment of this case appeared to be the regulation of the sleeping hours, it being perfectly obvious that a child of 3 years should retire before 10 p. m. The mother was instructed that before any improvement could be expected the child must be trained to go to bed at 7 o'clock and have at least 12 hours of sleep. She was warned of the initial difficulty in trying to put this new program into operation and was given a careful explanation of how much easier it would be to institute such a program at this time than 2 or 3 years later. Her cooperation was thus assured.

The next step necessitated a rather long, detailed explanation to the mother of the means and methods which children use at an early age to obtain their own way. The futility of trying to get the child established on a proper diet while giving him apples and candy whenever he refused to take milk and vegetables was pointed out to her. She was also advised that just so long as stubbornness served the child as a means of obtaining what he desired just so long would he utilize that method; and that it was extremely important for him at this age to learn that whining and rebelling would not serve as a method of gaining his own ends. A diet was carefully prescribed, and the mother was instructed to place only moderate portions of food before the child at each meal. She agreed that the food should be left before him for a period sufficiently long to permit him to eat slowly, yet not long enough to permit him to play with it, and that it was then to be removed. She also promised that he would receive nothing between meals except the extra milk which was prescribed in the diet because of his being underweight. The parents were in no way to concern themselves with what the child was eating. A careful record of the success or failure of the treatment was to be kept on a chart. The entire plan was explained to the child as simply and concisely as possible.

The results in this case alternated between success and failure for 5 months. Cooperation of the mother during the first part of the treatment was not all that had been hoped, but each time she returned to the clinic, regardless of whether success or failure had been reported, renewed efforts were made to have her carry out in detail the plan outlined.

At the end of 6 months the following report was made: "The child is doing remarkably well; eats all vegetables including carrots, spinach, and string beans; still has a strong dislike for milk but takes one glass per day." A month later the report read: "Patient continues to take his food without difficulty; has shown marked physical improvement; takes great interest in presenting his chart, which shows a perfect record for the last 2 weeks; is much less negativistic; is no longer shy; and takes great pride in telling the physician of his improvement."

With the establishment of proper sleeping hours and feeding habits, the child became more obedient and less selfish and lost many minor neurotic manifestations, such as nail biting, whining, and restlessness at night.

*Comment.*—This case is particularly interesting because success in treatment came only after a period of 5 months, during which time the outlook seemed rather discouraging. It emphasizes the importance of persistent and continued education of the parents in a certain group of cases where cooperation is not of the best and where suggestion is not accepted readily by the child. The results, however, justified the efforts.

---

Barbara, aged 6 years 9 months, was brought to the clinic by her mother because of persistent vomiting and enuresis.

The child's history was as follows: Normal birth, full term. Development retarded; walking delayed until child was over 2 years of age; speech still quite indistinct; teething delayed. Illness included pneumonia at 2 months, whooping cough at 2 years, influenza, and chickenpox. Child subject to coughs and colds.

The child slept and ate well and had no history of any undesirable habits with the exception of enuresis both day and night and persistent vomiting after meals, a habit which began about 4 weeks before the first clinic contact.

The child was described as shy and unwilling to speak unless spoken to, even at school. She frequently hung her head when spoken to by her teacher and refused to answer. She was extremely selfish and was jealous of the other children. At home she was quarrelsome, but outside the home she got along without difficulty. She seemed to have a normal interest in other members of the family with the exception of the younger sister, Susan, toward whom she was very antagonistic.

At the clinic she seemed to be a dull, apathetic child who hung her head and refused to look at the examiner. She was lacking in self-confidence and displayed absolutely no interest in her surroundings. One felt at once that there was a problem of mental deficiency. This impression was borne out by subsequent tests and psychometric examination, her intelligence quotient being 64, which seemed a fair indication of her mental equipment.

The home environment was poor. The family lived in a very narrow tenement street. They had an apartment of three rooms which were very untidy, with dirty clothing lying about on the floor. The hand towels and dish towels were very much soiled. A pail in one corner of the kitchen was used as a toilet. The mother and the youngest child, aged 2 years, shared a double bed, and the father, the patient, and Susan slept in another double bed. They had lived in this place for 5 years. Although conditions were extremely poor, they had shown considerable improvement during the last few years. Previously the family had lived in one room and was very much in debt. The father had been drinking; the mother had taken no interest whatever in the children. At the time of the clinic visit the father had stopped drinking, the mother was taking more interest in the children, and they were no longer in debt.

The patient was brought to the clinic because of persistent vomiting, which began about 4 weeks prior to the visit, and for enuresis, which had been almost continuous since birth. No attempt had ever been made to establish a routine that would break up the latter habit.

It was not difficult to determine how the vomiting had its origin. The mother was pregnant and had been vomiting during the preceding months, frequently in the presence of the child. How much of the behavior of the child was imitation and how much was stimulated by the physiological reaction of seeing another vomit was difficult to say. However, as soon as the mother was instructed about the necessity of seeking privacy during these vomiting periods, and after it was explained to the child (although she was mentally deficient) how unnecessary it was to persist in this habit and how foolish it would be for her to continue to take food if she persisted in throwing it up immediately, the problem seemed to be solved, for within 2 weeks the vomiting ceased completely.

Further investigation showed that Susan, 2 years younger and of higher intelligence, was also troubled with bed-wetting at night. The routine corrective measures were at once instituted for both children. A chart system was introduced and rivalry was stimulated between them. The results in both cases were extremely satisfactory.

Another youngster was subsequently added to the household, making four children in all. When the oldest was just over 7 the mother found it necessary to go out to work and took a job cleaning a theater at night. She left the house at 10:30 p. m. and worked for 8 hours, sleeping most of the day. She well represents the type of mother who is worn and wearied by toil and who has little to contribute to the welfare of the home. She was, however, extremely grateful to have her burdens lightened as much as they were. Both children continued to visit the clinic at frequent intervals, the mother feeling that they were more easily disciplined when they had to make a report to the clinic occasionally.

*Comment.*—The interesting point in this case is that it shows how important imitation is in the mental development of children and also that feeble-minded children do respond well to the simple training method.

---

Carrie came to the clinic at the age of 5½ years. Birth and development were quite normal. There was nothing of significance in her history nor in the physical examination made at the time of the first visit to the clinic.

The patient was brought to the clinic by her aunt, who stated that she would not eat unless fed, that she held her food in her mouth, and that she persisted in regurgitating it. When left alone at her meals and told to eat she invariably hid the food and told fanciful tales about what had become of it. On one occasion when she was told to eat her breakfast, she hid the food on the attic stairs and said she had eaten it. When taken to her uncle's store and given crackers she secreted them on her person and then threw them away, sometimes hiding them behind barrels in the store but always insisting that she had consumed them. She was said to be able to play all day without food. There was, however, no difficulty in getting her to eat ice cream and candy.

The child's father and mother had both died during an influenza epidemic, when she was 2 years of age. At that time the patient had been taken by the aunt and uncle, with whom she had continued to live. These relatives were apparently devoted to her and were as seriously interested in her welfare as in that of their own child. At the time of her parents' death she had not learned to feed herself, and the struggle to teach her had persisted ever since. She had formed the habit of not eating unless her aunt sat down and fed her, which meant cutting up the food and conveying the morsels from the plate to her mouth. More recently the child had begun simply to hold the food in her mouth, refusing to swallow it. The aunt reported that breakfast was a daily ordeal, as she felt that the child must be forced to eat before going to school. She further stated that Carrie had gone beyond all limits of the normal hunger period for the ordinary child. Except for her capriciousness regarding food, there seemed to be no undesirable habits. She slept well, was ordinarily obedient, had well-established toilet habits, and seemed to have no particular defects in her personality make-up.

At the clinic Carrie did not appear at all undernourished and seemed to be happy and cheerful. Her only comment regarding not eating was as follows: "I dream of a beautiful fairy in yellow who told me that I should not drink milk." After having a careful physical examination, however, the child did drink a glass of milk and eat a half slice of stale bread without any hesitation.

The aunt was instructed not to be so solicitous over the child's meals. She was told to prepare the food and place small quantities of it before the child, telling her that she would have 15 or 20 minutes to eat her meal and that it would then be taken away and she would have nothing else until the next meal. She was strongly urged to carry out these instructions faithfully until she came to the clinic the following week.

The problem was also discussed with the child, an effort being made to impress her with the importance of taking her food at regular intervals and also of eating it without assistance from her aunt. The following week the aunt reported to the clinic that the patient got along well for the first 4 days after their visit but that since then "has been carrying on pretty much the same way as she always has." She found it more difficult to discipline the patient than her own child and clung tenaciously to the idea that she wanted to do for the child what the child's mother would have had her do. One could see that she was activated by the idea that she wished to avoid showing any partiality toward her own child.

The family lived in a comfortable, sunny apartment, which, however, was kept in an extremely untidy state. When the social worker visited the home, the table was piled with dirty dishes and half-eaten food, and such food as could be seen in various pans looked most unattractive and poorly cooked. The floor was unswept, and there were large pails full of unwashed clothes standing about. The aunt's clothing and person were dirty, as were those of the children. At this time the aunt felt that she was at the end of her resources with regard to the patient and said, "I wouldn't mind trying to feed her if she would only eat what I feed her." Yet she seemed glad to have the child as a member of the family, in spite of her difficulties. She felt that the child had been spoiled by her own parents, who had lost an older child as the result of an accident when the patient was 1 year of age. This had undoubtedly made the patient's mother very solicitous and anxious, and the child had been permitted to have her own way. The aunt stated that she felt the child's difficulties with eating were getting worse, rather than better.

It seemed impossible in this particular case to organize the child's routines in a satisfactory way in her own environment, and an effort was therefore made to remove her from her surroundings until normal eating habits could be established. This was accomplished by sending the patient to live with another aunt in one of the nearby suburbs when the aunt with whom she had lived went to the hospital to be confined. While living in the new environment she did extremely well and no eating problem was evident. Shortly after returning home, however, she resumed her old habits. Attempts were made to persuade both the aunt and the uncle to have the child go to the study home of a local child-welfare agency for an extended period, but their attachment to the girl and their inability to appreciate the gravity of the situation made such attempts futile.

## HABITS OF ELIMINATION

The function of elimination frequently becomes the center of undesirable behavior, ranging in seriousness from simple delay in establishing toilet habits to serious neurotic manifestations and perversions. The most common problem concerned with elimination is enuresis, and as this is the type of behavior for which habit training is particularly important and with which it is very successful, the discussion will be largely limited to this.

Enuresis may occur both day and night. It occurs in both sexes with about the same frequency. It may begin in infancy and last until the sixth or seventh year, or it may cease at the end of the first year with the condition returning at indefinite periods and lasting from a few days to a few months at a time. Doctors Holt and Howland state, "Probably the most important cause is habit, resulting from poor training. Habit is often a potent factor in continuing the incontinence, even after the primary cause has disappeared."[3] It is with this group of cases that the habit clinics are concerned.

Before starting to treat enuresis as an undesirable habit, it is, of course, necessary to eliminate, so far as possible, every organic cause for the condition. Conditions affecting the bladder, acute inflammations, and calculi are the most common causes. An adherent prepuce (phimosis), a narrow urethral meatus, or local irritations from worms or fissures in the rectum may be the cause. Enuresis may be associated with a highly concentrated acid urine when the fluid intake has been insufficient, or it may be brought about by increasing the fluid intake, which naturally increases the amount of fluid to be excreted. The more general conditions, anemia, malnutrition, and an unstable nervous system (of which enuresis is only a symptom), should receive proper consideration.

After all organic conditions have been excluded as causes of the enuresis there still remains a large group of cases which are dependent upon faulty habit formation for their cause and persistence. Even in those cases where definite physical causes have been found and cured, the condition may persist from habit.

There are certain general principles that may be applied in every case of enuresis. The child should so far as possible be following a regime that is free from any excessive mental strain. He should have a simple, bland diet and definite hours of sleep. Routine measures should be instituted to avoid constipation and to stimulate free elimination through other sources than the kidneys. One of the first and most important steps in the treatment of enuresis is to interest the child in making an effort to overcome the habit. This should be brought about by appealing to the child's love of approbation rather than through punishment or humiliation. The chart system has been utilized with success in this connection. Not only does a chart serve to keep a definite record of the child's achievement during the interval that he is away from the clinic, but in a way it serves as a motive for

[3] Holt, L. Emmett, M. D., and John Howland, M. D.: The Diseases of Infancy and Childhood, p. 647. Tenth Edition. D. Appleton & Co., New York [1933].

the effort needed to overcome the habit. The child keeps his own chart, makes a mark for each day and night of success, and over each mark a star is placed. In a certain group of cases, suggestion, when the child is going to sleep at night, has worked well. The mother sits down by the bedside of the child and just as he is about to fall asleep she has him repeat over and over again, "I am not going to wet the bed." This suggestive treatment is similar to hypnotism, which has been used successfully in many adult cases and which lends itself quite easily to home treatment.

Not infrequently one finds that parents for one reason or another have taken for granted that a particular child will continue his habit of bed-wetting long after the time when he should have been trained to the dry habit. One mother stated that she herself had wet the bed until after she reached of age of puberty and for this reason she had ignored the problem in her 7-year-old daughter. Another mother explained that the child had inherited weak kidneys from the father's side of the family, the patient's grandfather and father having both been troubled in this way. A third mother reported that none of her four children was "dry" before reaching the age of 5 years and that she just assumed that the patient, who had come to the clinic because of night terrors, should also be wetting the bed at 4½ years of age. Such an attitude in parents invariably prevents them from starting on any intelligent plan of training; indeed, they often seem to get a feeling of satisfaction when their half-hearted attempts at training fail.

It is not unusual to find children reverting to the habit of enuresis despite adequate training. A little girl, 4 years old, who became intensely jealous of the newborn baby, began wetting her bed and her clothes again after having overcome this habit more than a year before. Another little girl who was devoted to her nurse began wetting the bed when the nurse left her to care for a younger child. Peter, aged 6, found that the bed-wetting of his younger sister, aged 4, got so much attention that he began the same performance after having been perfectly trained for 3½ years.

One must keep in mind that there are many emotional and environmental situations which are related to enuresis, especially in those cases in which the child has been "dry" for a long period. Notwithstanding the fact that punishment and humiliation are not usually successful as methods of treatment, it is perfectly fair and just to impose upon the child a certain amount of care and responsibility which go with looking after the soiled linen. Such tasks as putting the clothes to soak, airing the bed, and washing off the rubber sheet, should be handed out, not as punishment, but rather as aids to correct a difficult situation. It may, however, provide the essential motive if the child is to take the problem seriously enough to make it worth his while to get over the habit.

It is also wise to point out to children the disadvantages associated with the habit of bed-wetting. It prevents overnight visits to friends and relatives and perhaps riding on trains. It is frequently an obstacle to the child's privilege of having overnight guests or of going away to camp. These disadvantages should be presented as reasons why every effort should be made to overcome the habit and not as threats against its continuance.

Daniel, first seen at the age of 5 years 2 months. Born at full term; birth weight, 7 pounds; breast-fed; development normal.

He was in the habit of going to bed at 6 p. m.; slept alone; was restless only on rare occasions, when he would talk during sleep. He was not finicky about food; had a good appetite and no history of constipation or indigestion.

His mother stated that trouble began when he was 2 years of age. At that time he was very ill with pneumonia. Following this illness he began to soil himself and wet his clothes and his bed. This condition persisted for 2 years, but for the last year and a half he had been troubled with enuresis only at night. This occurred about 5 nights out of 7. The mother stated that she had spanked him, rubbed his nose in the urine, and deprived him of things, and at the time of her clinic visit she was refusing to give him clean pajamas over long periods of time, trying to impress him with the fact that he must learn not to wet his bed.

The child was generous and friendly, liked other people, played with other children, and was not jealous. He was inclined to be obstinate and could not be driven, but could be easily disciplined if coaxed. The child had no particular fears and enjoyed playing outdoors with other children. On the other hand he spent much of his time playing dolls with his little sister.

In his psychological examination he received an intelligence quotient of 92. He was fairly cooperative but inclined to be boastful, constantly saying, "I can do this," "I can draw that." He was particularly interested in drawing. In fact, it was difficult to hold his attention because of his interest in making pictures. He was attending kindergarten and preferred going to school to staying at home.

The home environment was quite satisfactory, the family occupying a small house consisting of five rooms. The home was clean, tidy, and attractive; each child had a room to himself. The mother was interested in her children and ambitious for them, looking forward to getting a larger house and a yard for them to play in, where they would be away from the dangers of automobiles. She was, however, of a neurotic make-up, having had two nervous break-downs. The father was in a successful business with his brother, earning an adequate salary. The two children were both in good health and enjoyed each other's company. The mother was in fairly good health at the time of the visit to the clinic.

*Summary.*—Child, 5½ years of age, with an average intellectual equipment, coming from a good home, troubled with enuresis 5 nights out of 7, with no other undesirable habits. The treatment, to date, had consisted of cruel humiliation and severe punishment.

The fact that the patient had been treated at numerous clinics led the mother to believe that the case was hopeless. She maintained that she had carried out all the directions given her by the physicians, but in spite of this the enuresis continued.

The boy, as seen at the clinic, was attractive and bright, interested in his environment, and anxious to demonstrate his ability in printing and drawing. He discussed his problem openly and frankly, without any apparent embarrassment, and expressed willingness to cooperate. Physical examination and laboratory examination of urine were both negative.

The routine treatment for enuresis was outlined as follows: The patient's diet was to be simple, free from spices and sweets, with only a moderate amount of meat; his evening meal was to be served at 5 p. m., after which he was to have no fluids. He was to retire at 7 p. m. He was to be taken up, thoroughly awakened, and sent to the toilet at 8:30 and again at 10, and then permitted to sleep until morning, when he was to be awakened at 6 o'clock. Stress was laid on the fact that the child must be thoroughly awakened and made to realize why he was being aroused. The mother was warned to be sure that the child voided when he was taken up. A chart was then brought out and given to the boy, and the method of keeping the record was carefully explained.

The child responded to his part of the program with much enthusiasm, but the mother showed considerable skepticism about the routine outlined. They returned to the clinic 1 week later, and at that time it was apparent that she had not carried out the directions, in spite of her statements to the contrary. She had instituted her own treatment with kidney pills. She was, however, prevailed upon to continue the prescribed routine for a month and was requested to visit the clinic each week. The report of the next visit to the clinic read: "She is much pleased with the change that has taken place in the patient, feeling that the chart brought it about. She is anxious that the younger child, aged 2½ years, be admitted to the clinic for the same trouble. She states that she did not continue to experiment with a patent medicine but decided to follow the advice given."

The next time she brought both children. She reported that the bed-wetting had completely ceased and that she was greatly relieved.

*Comment.*—The only comments that need be made on the above case are in reference to the tactfulness necessary in getting cooperation from the parents and in making them feel that, although they have tried various remedies at different times, they have perhaps never put into operation any plan that took into consideration all the aspects of the individual case.

This case of enuresis was uncomplicated by any other nervous symptoms or undesirable habits, and it is worthy of note that the enthusiasm which the child showed in keeping the chart was, in itself, favorable from a prognostic point of view.

---

Another case of this type was that of Ellen, aged 3 years 9 months when first seen at the clinic. The patient was born at full term; birth and development were normal; she was breast-fed to the age of 11 months.

The child's hours in bed were from 7:30 p. m. to 6 a. m. Sometime previous to the clinic visit she began waking up during the night; she seemed frightened, cried out, and talked about soldiers. She had always been finicky about food. She would not take milk until she started attending nursery school, but she had since developed a liking for milk and ate everything except meat. She did not eat between meals.

The patient was very shy and said nothing in the presence of strangers but clung to her mother. She was very quiet, and her mother stated that she was capable of entertaining herself. When younger, she had had a very bad temper and had frequently gone into tantrums. She was extremely jealous of her younger brother. This jealousy was carried so far that when her mother had first begun to nurse him the patient had not lost an opportunity to slap or otherwise bother him. She did not care to play with other children and was self-centered and retiring. She was obedient and rarely had to be disciplined. Her play life was occupied largely with her dolls, occasionally with her brother, and rarely with other children.

The patient had an intelligence quotient of 84. She attended kindergarten, where she was getting on fairly well.

The home consisted of a five-room tenement on the second floor of a three-story brick building. The family had lived there for 8 years. It was clean, and although in poor condition, well furnished. The patient had a room to herself. She was more attached to her father than to her mother and lacked normal interest in her brother.

The problem as described by the mother was enuresis, which occurred both day and night. This condition had persisted since birth. For a long time there had been difficulty in sleeping. The child was put to bed at 7:30 p. m. and usually went to sleep within half an hour. She woke up at 1 or 2 a. m. and then every hour thereafter until 6 o'clock, when she insisted on getting up. This wakefulness, accompanied by crying, had become a very disturbing factor in the household. For the 3 preceding weeks the child had developed an unusual fear of soldiers and upon waking cried out in fear, saying, "Don't let the soldiers get me!" The story was that she had been taken by her mother to see some soldiers drilling. This had alarmed her for some unknown reason, and since that time she had talked constantly about soldiers, saying that they were going to take her away. When she awoke at night she cried out to her mother, "Close the door, the soldiers are coming!" She refused to go into any room alone since this event and wanted her mother constantly by her side. She had become much afraid of the dark.

At her first visit to the clinic she was extremely shy and would have nothing to do with the examiner, speaking only to her mother in whispers. She resented any attempt of the doctor to become friendly, and because of this timidity the first clinic visit was unsatisfactory.

Routine measures for the enuresis were instituted, however, as described in the preceding case, except that the child was permitted to go to bed at the usual hour of 7:30, was awakened at 10, and was permitted to sleep until morning.

The mother was instructed to take the child again to see the soldiers drilling and allow her to observe them as closely as her fear would permit. The mother was told to assure her and to instruct her about soldiers.

At the end of the month the mother reported that the child had shown considerable improvement and had not wet the bed for 2 weeks, had slept better, and was no longer afraid of soldiers. The fact that the mother had taken her to see the soldiers drill every day seemed to dissipate her fears. The child was more friendly toward the doctor but was still shy and bashful.

Improvement continued during the summer months, and in September the child entered kindergarten. The teacher reported that she got along well, showed normal interest, and adapted herself to the school work. She enjoyed the association with other children, was quite unselfish, well-mannered, and obedient. The mother reported that the patient was getting along very well—that she did not wet the bed and that she had no difficulty about her eating. She no longer entertained any fear that disturbed her either day or night.

*Comment.*—It was interesting in this case to note the degree to which this child was able to make satisfactory adjustment to both home and school conditions. She became relatively independent of her mother and interested and affectionate toward her little brother. She was sleeping well, her appetite was good, she had no difficulty with enuresis, nor was she any longer disturbed by fears and terrifying dreams.

Although it was impossible in this particular case to determine the underlying cause of the terrifying wakeful periods, it is of interest to note that many favorable changes took place subsequent to, if not simultaneously with, the treatment of the enuresis. This happens so frequently in the treatment of this disorder that it leads one to believe that the feeling of inferiority and shame associated with enuresis in many cases colors the entire mental life of the patient. It is of practical importance in the treatment of mental problems where enuresis happens to be one of the symptoms (inasmuch as enuresis is one of the most trying problems to the parent, although one of the most easily curable) to institute treatment for the enuresis at the earliest possible date.

## HABITS OF SLEEP

Most of the problems that arise in relation to sleep are brought about by poor training or lack of training on the part of parents. Children frequently get the idea that bed is a place to be avoided, because it has been used as a means of punishment. When Mary is naughty, she is threatened with being sent to bed. Tommy, on the other hand, is told that if he is good he may stay up a half hour later. Both attitudes imply that bed is a place to be avoided.

A sleep routine should be established to which parents and child will conform, for there is no demand made upon the physical well-being of the child in which sleep and relief from physical fatigue do not play important parts. The tired child is usually an unhappy child. Tantrums, enuresis, stammering, various mannerisms, and numerous other physical and emotional problems are frequently caused by fatigue due to insufficient sleep.

The importance of sleep should be taken for granted, neither featured nor ignored, and the parents' attitude should be precisely as it is toward the meal hours. The hour for retiring should not be permitted to be a time for "putting on a show" and getting attention. The child will soon learn that after he has been adequately prepared for bed, comfortably tucked in, and had his parting "good night" said, the ceremony is over and a belated request for a story, a trip to the bathroom, or another drink of water is just a way of trying to get attention or exert a little influence over the solicitous mother. Yielding to such requests is the beginning of an indulgence on the

78985°—39——4

part of parents that may cause them much trouble later and create in the child a feeling of dependency that will prove a real handicap.

The overtired child or the child who is said to be suffering from growing pains may exhibit considerable restlessness—tossing, turning, twisting about, and complaining of not feeling rested the next day. These periods of physical unrest need not cause parents undue anxiety. They are indications that there is need for more rest, less violent physical exercise, and perhaps a warm relaxing bath before retiring. Night terrors, so called, are a matter of deeper concern because they are invariably related to some disturbance in the psychic life of the child. There is no doubt that many fears are planted during the early life of the child, are awakened by subsequent experiences, and eventually play an important part in producing night terrors. Children should not be threatened with violence of one kind or another for indiscretions, because the anticipation of punishment, like threats from other children, may lead to serious disturbance of sleep.

Not infrequently intelligent parents create sleeping difficulties for the child by reciting to him, just before he retires, stories that are tinged with the mysterious and the unexpected. They often leave him in suspense in some very exciting part of the story in order that a happy experience may be anticipated the following evening. It is obvious that such a proceeding is unwise for the imaginative child. The mental activities created in this way often prevent the child from going to sleep and frequently create both motor and mental unrest. Many programs presented over the radio at the present time are of this nature and lay the foundation for a bad night, which is followed by fatigue and irritability the next day. Many children have strange, vague, ill-defined worries and anxieties over death, sickness, school, and parental relationships. Strong emotional tension is associated with these worries and they assume undue proportions in the mind of the child after he has withdrawn from the day's activities which have been demanding his attention. Threats of punishment, fear of being deserted by parents, or of being subjected to bullying and teasing by other children, and many other everyday environmental situations which threaten the child's security are subjects that are worthy of investigation when one is endeavoring to solve a problem related to sleep.

As the child advances to the age when he is able to read and comprehend sensational newspaper headings relating to lurid tales of murder, suicide, robbery, immorality, and other topics that excite curiosity, a new factor is introduced which often disturbs his mental life and results in sleepless nights. Fortunately, much of the material derived from radios, newspapers, and other contacts which the child must make in his everyday existence, does not register on his mind before his fifth or sixth year. All these new avenues of enlightenment make a valuable contribution to mankind in general, but they are a menace to a certain group of highly sensitive, imaginative children. It hardly seems necessary to mention that fear stimulated by putting children in dark closets and down in the cellar, by threatening them with unusual punishments, and by scaring them with weird tales, is cruel and vicious and leaves scars upon their mental life that are rarely completely healed and that may lead to the most violent type of night terrors. Some children are extremely sensitive and sympathetic to the worries and anxieties of parents, and during periods of extreme economic depression, when the security of the entire family is threatened, when there is grave illness in the home, or when undue emotional tension exists between parents, a state of mind is created in the child that frequently prevents normal sleep.

Besides creating a happy, carefree, unperturbed state of mind for the child before retiring, it is also important to provide proper sleeping arrangements. The bed itself should be neat, clean, and orderly in appearance, with clothing suitable to the season. In other words, it should have an inviting appearance. The room should be well ventilated but not necessarily cold or drafty. The shades should be drawn so as to avoid bright early-morning light. Some of the minor details such as the type of night clothes, placement of bed, and arrangement of furniture can be left to the child when feasible. The act of retiring should be taken for granted, featured neither as one of the crosses that children have to bear nor as an unusual privilege, but as one of the events that take place in the routine of a happy day. The matter of adequate sleep is a subject that cannot be ignored in any consideration of the mental and physical welfare of the child, especially during the first few years when habits are being established. Sleep is nature's way of conserving the child's energy against the demands made upon it by rapid physical and mental growth.

John, a 2-year-old boy, was referred to the clinic because of irregular sleeping habits, enuresis, soiling, irregular and finicky feeding habits, and disobedience. His birth and development were normal, and his intellectual equipment was average. His parents were young and unintelligent. He had developed into an undisciplined and untrained child. The mother had never made any attempt to train the child to toilet habits, and the irregularity of his eating had been taken for granted. In other words, the child ate when he felt hungry rather than when food was served to the other members of the family. His mother could not remember that the child had ever slept well. She stated that he was put to bed at 7 o'clock but rarely went to sleep before 2 or 3 in the morning. He insisted on getting out of bed and going into the living room to join his parents. In spite of their efforts, which were undoubtedly feeble and misdirected, he would stay up until 12 or 1 o'clock. He rarely slept later than 6:30 in the morning, at which time he would get up to have breakfast with his father. He then returned to bed and slept until 12.

The child was irritable, demanding, and extremely difficult to get along with. Whenever he was crossed or an effort was made to get his cooperation in doing something that did not please him, he would cry; and at the age of 2 he had already found that tears were apt to get him out of many difficult situations.

The mother was a weak, negative sort of individual, entirely lacking in imagination, who took little care of her own health or personal appearance, and who was a poor housekeeper and a bad manager. She was inconsistent in her discipline, so that in one mood she tried to control the child by cuffing and slapping him and in another mood she would indulge him in everything. When she slapped him, he slapped back; when she was resentful, he, too, was resentful. In other words the mother had settled down to a rather childish, infantile, emotional level, as was shown in her efforts to control the child with threats of the doctor, the nurse, "the cop," and anything else that might for the moment have affected the child's conduct. The problem was obviously one of parental education and of getting the child into a nursery school where he could live in a well-organized environment for at least part of the day.

---

Sarah was a tall, undernourished girl just under 5 years of age. She was brought to the clinic by her mother because of night terrors which had existed since infancy. For the first 6 months she had been difficult to feed, became much undernourished, and had suffered from constipation; otherwise her development was normal. The feeding difficulty had, however, continued to manifest itself in indifference to food. She apparently enjoyed the attention that was associated with being fed by her mother, who indulged her in this respect.

This child, only 5 years of age, was frequently allowed to stay up in the summertime until 9:30, although she did go to bed somewhat earlier in the winter. Retiring was usually accompanied by a good deal of talking and laughing with her brother, who slept in the same room. The mother stated, "Nearly every night Sarah has night terrors. After a half hour to an hour of sleep she starts screaming and will yell out, 'I won't do it,' 'I don't like you,' or some other similar expression." The mother found it difficult to awaken her during these times. There was usually a short crying spell, and then the child would finally settle down and go to sleep. These episodes would be repeated several times during the night, but the child would have no recollection of terrifying dreams nor could she remember much about what had happened during the night. These night terrors were invariably worse when she was sick, but the mother had been unable to associate them with any actual experiences.

The mother described Sarah as "a high-strung, nervous child." At the clinic the psychological examination showed that she had a superior intelligence, rating 2 years above her chronological age. Her cooperation was excellent and her general behavior indicated excellent training and manners. The home from which the child came was above the average economically and culturally, and the parents were rather superior intellectually—in fact, the mother was "an amateur student of psychology and child training." It appeared, however, that the parents' influence on their child had been counteracted by that of the grandmother, who was said to be psychotic and who insisted upon "smothering" the patient with her affections and attentions, which the patient resented. The relationship with her grandmother was of such a nature that this ordinarily quiet, well-behaved, sensitive child resented it and made every effort to repel the grandmother's advances by assuming a domineering attitude herself. The mother was advised to regulate the patient's routine so that she would have adequate sleep, more rest, and regular meals; to eliminate so far as possible the contact between the patient and her grandmother; to see that the child was kept interested and occupied; and to secure the cooperation of her maid in this plan. The child was placed in a kindergarten in an effort to provide a routine suited to her needs, and to bring her in contact with intelligent and unemotional adults as well as a normal group of children of her own age. The mother reported at the end of 2 months that the night terrors had disappeared.

## RESENTMENT TOWARD FRUSTRATION EXPRESSED IN AGGRESSIVE ACTS

The ways in which the behavior of children brings them into conflict with their constantly changing environment are many and varied. Equally numerous and varied are the causes of this behavior. For example, a child may present a picture of restlessness, destructiveness, pugnacity, and marked impulsiveness, with other evidences that he lacks normal inhibitions. Such behavior may have its basis in certain organic defects either inherited or acquired at an early age, mental deficiency being a classic example of this group; or it may be a reaction to physical limitations associated with diabetes, infantile paralysis, or cardiac conditions. Not infrequently acute inflammatory conditions of the brain or its coverings resulting in meningitis and encephalitis (commonly known as sleeping sickness) are followed by such disturbances in the child's behavior, due to impairment of the normal processes leading to inhibition. Very often, however, these difficult behavior problems are not due to any of the causes mentioned, but are the result of poor training or lack of training. In this case one sees an undisciplined child who undoubtedly has the ability but has never learned the necessity of exerting what are commonly known as will power and self-control.

Nor is the behavior of the child always constant. For a period, at least, offensive attitudes may alternate with defensive, and the child may put up a good fight against personalities and situations that are too strong. There may be vague, intangible situations which are overpowering to him. Rebellion may be of no avail against the subtleties of a persistently oversolicitous parent. The child will finally succumb to defeat and accept a plan of life ill suited to his needs and necessitating much in the way of fantasy to make it tolerable. What appears to be simply an undesirable habit such as enuresis may have its roots deeply seated in jealousy. Cruelty may be regarded by the parent as "just ordinary meanness" when actually it is an unconscious protest of the child against his own inadequacies. The sullen, unhappy child, apparently lacking in affection for anyone, may be crying aloud for someone who will take time to find out what his emotional needs really are and to see that some effort is made to satisfy them.

The varied responses which human beings make to life do not lend themselves well to any rigid classification. Because there is wide diversity in the constitutional make-up of individuals, and because these individuals are called upon to adjust themselves to environments that are varied and constantly changing, situations are created which are necessarily extremely variable and complex. It is with great difficulty and always with more or less danger that broad generalizations are set forth to be applied to the individual case. Every child must be considered as a living organism struggling to make such adjustments to his environment as will permit him to survive and enjoy natural growth and development and to accept and conform to the restrictions which society imposes upon his behavior. Acquisition of the personality traits that lead to conformity is insisted upon by those who are responsible for the orderly growth and development of the child. It is the function of child training, so far as the wisdom and ability of parents permit, to see that the child is mentally and physically equipped to meet the world outside the home. Society deals harshly with those who fail to recognize the necessity of subordinating self to the social group. Unfortunately, force rather than understanding is too frequently exerted in efforts to make children conform. Fear is often in the foreground of most parental and social doctrines. The child is taught at an early age that the way of the transgressor is hard, and yet in spite of all this pressure exerted from without, the world is full of unhappy, inadequate, poorly adjusted individuals who have not profited by their early training. The question arises whether education should not be substituted for fear.

From the clinical point of view there are three distinct groups of problems of this kind: (1) There is the group represented by the child who because of certain limitations of intellect, physical defects, or emotional instability will be a problem regardless of his environment. (2) There is the child who, in the process of growing up, goes through phases involving certain changes in behavior which cause concern to his parents. These situations are not so much the problems of the particular child as problems of a particular stage of development, and, if handled wisely, they need cause but little anxiety. (3) There is a type of child behavior that is only a symptom of a problem environment. Many of the cases referred to clinics fortunately belong to this last group. Constructive effort to change the environment and give the child a better understanding of his difficulties is invariably helpful in these cases. Examples will be included in the following discussion.

## ANGER AND TEMPER TANTRUMS

In considering such aspects of conduct as temper tantrums it is necessary to appreciate fully the different planes upon which moral conduct is enacted in relation to the age of the individual and the stage of social development.[4] Those who deal with children are concerned very largely with conduct carried out on a low moral plane.

During the early years of life no moral judgments are formed and the child does not think of himself in relation to others. The child is fundamentally selfish and consequently interprets everything in terms of self, his own acts as well as those of others being evaluated by the amount of pleasure or pain they bring to him. He must learn by experience that a certain line of conduct is a paying proposition, so to speak, and that another line of conduct is not; and by "paying" one implies a gain to the child in pleasure and comfort. With proper training and in the proper environment the average child soon learns that conduct carried out in consideration of those

[4] No more practical exposition of this subject has been presented than that of Prof. William MacDougall in his Social Psychology.

with whom he comes in contact in his everyday experiences brings him more pleasure and less pain than he would otherwise have. He does not take long to learn that certain experiences are associated with definite pain—for example, touching the hot stove—and ordinarily he can learn in the same way that little or nothing is to be gained by what is commonly called a temper tantrum. Such a tantrum has been described by a parent as follows: "The child lies down on the floor, yells, kicks his heels, and throws his arms about with the intention of inflicting bodily harm on those who come near him."

The tantrum is, of course, purely instinctive and must be met on its first appearance in such a way as to impress on the child not only that nothing will be gained but that such action is positively painful in its results—painful in the sense of bringing a definite loss or of being similar to the experience of putting his hand on the hot stove. This crude and more or less undesirable method of directing and inhibiting conduct during the early years of life should be discarded as soon as possible in favor of appealing to the child's love of approbation, which manifests itself early. Here the attempt is directed toward influencing the child's conduct by appealing to his desire for praise, on the one hand, and his desire to avoid blame, on the other. With children who have reached this stage of development it has been possible to utilize in the clinics a chart system to give the child tangible evidence of the approbation of the doctor, the parents, and others whose praise he most desires.

Temper tantrums, as was said before, are usually physical manifestations of the emotion of anger, which may be stimulated when any of the varied instinctive reactions are thwarted. It is important to know this when attempting to understand the tantrums of the child, because it is necessary to determine the cause of the anger, which many parents say they are unable to account for. It is only after the child, through training and experience, has developed various means of meeting and overcoming his difficulties, that the emotion of anger ceases to be one of the most dangerous stumbling blocks. The instinct of pugnacity, of which anger is the associated emotion, is essential in the development of most successful individuals. It is the driving force to which much of the success in human affairs is due, and it should be controlled rather than stifled, if it is to work to the advantage of the individual.

In every case that involves outbursts of temper it is absolutely essential to study the environment in which the child is being reared, in order to know under what conditions, in what places, and with whom these tantrums are most common. It is of equal importance to make a careful personality study of the child in order to understand as fully as possible the conflicts that he has and the purpose that these emotional upsets serve. It is futile to treat each outbreak by punishing the child or by permitting him to gain some undesirable end. Either method is doomed to failure. Such conduct must be interpreted in terms of the child's experience, if his personality is to be molded so that he will be capable of making a satisfactory social adjustment in later life.

Harriet was first seen in the clinic at the age of 2 years 5 months. The birth had been normal. The patient was breast-fed until 23 months of age.

The mother stated that it was very difficult to wean the patient; she cried so much and went into such temper tantrums that the mother nursed her until 3 months before her next child was born. Teething, walking, and talking all developed normally. She had had none of the children's diseases and had had no injuries or operations.

She refused to go to bed unless accompanied by either her father or her mother. She retired at 8 or 9 p. m. and slept until 8 or 9 a. m. Two or three times during the night she would wake up and scream. Her mother said, "She is probably having temper tantrums in her sleep and is dreaming that she cannot have what she wants." There was no feeding difficulty—she ate everything that was given to her—but there were some indiscretions in diet, such as tea for lunch. Enuresis occurred occasionally. The child had been known to masturbate. Her mother said that the child had a "terrific" temper; that she would lie on the floor and kick and scream on the slightest provocation. When she did not get what she wanted to eat or was crossed at play she developed one of these tantrums. Sometimes they occurred when the mother had no idea what the exciting cause might be. They occurred frequently when she was playing with other children. Following one of these tantrums the child had had "peculiar attacks," getting blue in the face, the mouth remaining partially open, the body becoming stiffened. These spells lasted about 10 minutes. During the 2 weeks preceding the clinic visit she had had seven such attacks.

The policy pursued by the family at that time was one of acquiescence. The patient was said to be generous "when she wants to be"; was jealous; did not want others to have things she could not have; did not get along with other children because she was pugnacious and fought them; was "always very bossy and domineering and always makes other children playing with her do what she wants even if they are twice her size." She was afraid of the dark, would not go to bed without a light; was afraid of animals, especially cats and dogs. At times she had shown marked affection for her father. Her father took no part in disciplining her, and her mother had found that corporal punishment was of little avail.

The father was Italian and the mother was Irish-American. The mother said that the father considered her an idiot and had been brutal to her. She did not know how much he earned. He was very close with his money and gave a dollar a day on which to run the house. He spent little time at home. The mother felt intellectually superior to the father and was always conscious of the racial difference. She said that the father hated their older daughter, Mary, but was devoted to Harriet, whom he fondled and petted. He was also quite indifferent to the baby. They lived on a short, paved street in a three-story brick tenement house. They had a two-room apartment on the first floor. Father, mother, and Harriet slept in a double bed, and Mary slept on the davenport. The mother had furnished the rooms with her own money, and they were fairly comfortable and well kept.

Prior to their marriage the father and mother had lived in Boston as man and wife. At the same time, he was keeping company with another woman. Even at that period he was extremely cruel and abusive to the mother and was very irritable. He would throw cups at her when things he desired were missing at the table. He was arrested in 1918 and was sentenced to jail for 3 months. After his release quarrels were frequent, and in self-defense the mother had scalded and bitten him. Although he was still very rough, showed temper, and drank a great deal, he had not used physical violence of late. The mother knew that he was not true to her and questioned his relations with the patient. There was a story of his having infected the older daughter with gonorrhea when she was 4 years old. His sexual demands were excessive and he masturbated frequently.

At the clinic the patient appeared to be a quiet, demure, neatly dressed little girl, who sat quietly by her mother until she left to enter the examining room. The child then went into a violent tantrum, lying on the floor, kicking her heels, and yelling at the top of her voice. This behavior continued during the half-hour interval while the mother was talking to the physician, but it was not followed by one of her spells. The mother verified the history as given by the social worker and said that the child had been "cranky since the day she was born, always crying and whining." She said, "I could not do a thing with her—she has never slept soundly. I always have to lie down with her and sing her to sleep." Sometimes the patient stayed up until 10 p. m.

and she never had a nap. When the patient got jealous of other children she tried to inflict pain upon them. Whenever her mother paid special attention to other children in the neighborhood or to the patient's sister, she went into a violent temper, bit her sister, pulled her clothes, and tried to bite her mother. Her mother repeated that she was afraid the patient had learned to masturbate from her father.

*Treatment.*—The problems of enuresis and of establishing routine hours of sleep were attacked first. The mother was instructed to see that the child was put to bed at 6 o'clock and that she remained in bed at least 12 hours. She was warned against all the difficulties that would arise in starting out on this program, but she was told that they would be only temporary and slight compared with the trouble that would occur if the child was not taught to appreciate that tempers could not be used successfully to get her own way. The routine method as described for enuresis was to be followed, and a chart was given to the mother for the purpose of keeping a record rather than to interest the child.

At the end of 2 weeks the mother returned to the clinic, stating that she had instituted the 12-hour sleeping regime but found it impossible to carry out the measures suggested for breaking the habit of enuresis.

The situation was particularly difficult because the child cried violently, the tenant downstairs threatened to have the family put out, and other neighbors became irritated. The father told the mother that she had no brains—what could she expect of the child? He said that he thought coming to the clinic was a waste of time. Under such conditions it was too much to expect the cooperation necessary for improvement. Jealousy and pugnacity continued, and the patient, on one occasion after her last visit, had had a violent temper tantrum on the street. The mother stated that to her knowledge the child had not masturbated since the last visit, and she was encouraged by the improvement which followed the routine hours of sleep.

*Comment.*—This case illustrates one of the difficulties of instituting treatment that may cause more or less temporary annoyance, not only to the family but to the neighbors. It is not to be expected that a mother will get up two or three times a night to awaken a child, if she knows that such a disturbance of the child's sleep will be followed by a violent temper tantrum and by threats and insults from her husband and the neighbors.

It is hoped that the time is not far distant when facilities will be afforded for taking such children out of the home and training them, temporarily at least, under more favorable conditions.

---

Isabel, aged 2 years 8 months; birth and development history negative. She had always enjoyed good health; slept well; had well-established toilet habits; had a poor appetite and was very finicky about food. Her mother always had to supervise her feeding, and she refused to eat cereal, eggs, or oatmeal, but was very fond of meat.

The child spent much time sucking her fingers, especially when moody. She was active and interested in outdoor activities. She enjoyed being with other children in spite of the fact that it was difficult for her to get along with them. Only on unusual occasions did she have an opportunity to play with children other than her younger sister. When the opportunity arose to play with other children during vacation periods in the summer months, she met every unpleasant situation by developing a violent temper tantrum. She was domineering and always wanted to be the boss. She was considered a fighter and was rough and pugnacious toward smaller children. She whined constantly, and it was frequently difficult to determine just what she wanted. She would lie on the floor and kick and yell, and was extremely irritable and impatient. After getting the object for which she had tenaciously fought, she would throw it away immediately. She was very destructive. Her fear of the dark developed after the following incident. While her father was playing with her she ran into a dark closet, and her father stood outside the door making a noise like a cat. She seemed to enjoy it at the time and asked him to continue. Since this incident, however, she had refused to go to bed unless the door was left open. In spite of her apparent lack of affection, she made heavy demands upon her mother's time and wanted to be constantly by her side. She rarely showed any affection for either parent and utilized kisses only to get out of some situation that was apt to be followed by punishment. She was rough with animals but not cruel. She was ordinarily kind and generous toward the baby in the household but at times was rough and pushed and slapped her. Her mother admitted that she did not give much time or affection to the child and said, "I am not naturally affectionate, and my husband is more interested in the children." The mother was of average intelligence and appeared interested, but one felt that this interest was rather superficial and that one of her fundamental characteristics was to take the path of least resistance. For example, she met the finger-sucking problem by giving the child a bottle.

*Comment.*—The outstanding features in the foregoing case were the unaffectionate attitude of the mother toward the child and the indifference the child showed for the parents. The child's negativistic attitude toward life stood out very prominently. She was always on the opposite side. In other words, she belonged to a group of children who, between the ages of 3 and 5, develop what may be termed "contrasuggestibility."

This condition in children usually lasts but a short time and passes without leaving any undesirable effects upon the personality. On the other hand, there are many individuals in adult life who are chronically negativistic, who are immediately prompted by any suggestion from an outside source to take the opposite side of the question presented. Many of these individuals develop unusual ways. Their habits of living, of dress, and of eating are all such as openly to defy custom and tradition. In children this negativistic attitude toward sleep and general conduct is often difficult to explain, but frequently it represents an effort to attract attention and to keep themselves in the limelight and hear themselves discussed. Invariably these negativistic children are pointed out by the parents as "simply impossible youngsters."

It seems wise, when this negativistic attitude is first recognized, to minimize it so far as possible, to see that the child gains nothing by such reactions but rather t t they work out to his loss. Above all, the apparent peculiarity of the child should never be discussed in his presence. This is one of the situations in which the child must be led and not pushed.

This case brings out the importance of allowing children to associate with others of their own age. One of the most fundamental and important instinctive forces is that which is commonly termed the herd instinct. Very early in life the child is capable of benefiting greatly by association wth other children. He thus has an opportunity of seeing his own acts mirrored in the reactions of those of his own age and is able to get a better understanding and develop a more sympathetic attitude toward others by virtue of this understanding. It is, therefore, not surprising to find that the child who has been confined to his own household 9 or 10 months in the year, making contacts only with those in the family, experiences great difficulty in understanding and getting along with others when the opportunity arises. In these days, when the hazard of automobile accidents in crowded, congested districts cannot be ignored but must be considered by every interested parent, the nursery and the nursery school afford the desirable opportunities for youngsters to get together. In the performance of their simple tasks, in their play life, and in the educational training received, they will learn much concerning the problems of everyday life as they are related to the group rather than to the individual.

Although not yet 3 years of age, this child was rapidly developing into a cold, calculating, unaffectionate individual who utilized pretense of affection toward others only to gain her own ends. This attitude, of course, only reflected that of the parents toward the child, and it is not surprising that she utilized such asocial reactions as temper tantrums and negativism to keep from being obliterated from the family horizon.

The treatment in this case dealt primarily with the mother. She manifested more interest than the foregoing history would indicate that she was capable of; and as she was of an intelligence above the average, the situation seemed quite hopeful. The treatment of such a case must continue over a period of several months. Much can be expected when this child enters the nursery school in the fall and makes daily contacts with other children. Much has already been accomplished by presenting to the mother the program to be followed, and by changing her attitude toward the patient as much as possible.

Anger is the child's emotional response to a situation in which his demands are not satisfied and he is being thwarted in his efforts to attain some particular end. It is an expression of resentment toward barriers and restraints set up by his environment. It is evidence of dissatisfaction and may be of value in leading to greater effort to attain the goal, if it does not confuse and dominate him. Anger is not an emotion to be eradicated by drastic methods but one which the child should learn to control. Any normal child or adult will be confronted with many situations in life in which any other emotion than anger would be entirely inappropriate. Indignation is a controlled form of anger and has been the driving force behind many a movement that has benefited mankind.

The child must learn, as he develops, that uncontrolled anger is invariably a handicap in that it results in confusion of thought and action, thus defeating the ends for which he is striving. Rigid discipline which depends upon force and fear for its success may prevent for the moment any expression of anger on the part of the subdued child, but external influences are of little use in teaching the child control of a normal and often useful emotion.

It is the expression of anger resulting from the constant conflict between the child and his environment which should cause concern. This is an indication that for one reason or another the emotional needs of the child are not finding adequate outlets and that he is not capable of making the compromises which are essential under such conditions. Such a child is unhappy, critical, and intolerant, and his pugnacious tendencies get him into all kinds of social difficulties.

There is no better way of teaching a child self-control than by example. Parents who are habitually quick-tempered, who lose control of themselves on the slightest provocation and are always shouting at their children, are obviously setting a bad example. Even if the child, through fear, is submissive in the home, he is likely to compensate for his pent-up resentment in his contacts with other children, especially those whom he can dominate through fear and bullying.

John, 2½ years old, was sent to the clinic from the nursery school with the following statement: "He has a bad temper, is always fighting, strikes and slaps other children without provocation, and always wants what his brother has and fights for it."

In the attempt to determine the cause of this exaggerated pugnacity, rather contradictory statements were encountered regarding the patient's older brother, Henry, aged 4. The home life of the two youngsters was said to be very unhappy and chaotic. The mother and father were always fighting, and both were said to be impulsive and quick-tempered. The father had been arrested for assault and battery, and on her first visit to the clinic the mother bore evidences of his cruelty in the shape of scars.

It appeared that John had always been "mother's boy" and his older brother, Henry, had been the father's favorite. From the nursery school it was learned that the older brother was very sensitive and extremely quiet, that he was absolutely obedient and more polite than other children. At times he was troubled with enuresis and stammering. The mother's story, however, was quite different. She claimed that Henry was bossy and domineering, always wanted his own way, was jealous of the younger brother, had a violent temper, and sometimes bit other children when he was angry. She further stated that he had an intense fear of her, that when she "exploded in anger" or threatened to punish him "his legs actually shook."

When the mother's attention was drawn to the discrepancy in the descriptions of Henry's personality she said that the picture which she had given the previous week "was only true when he was having ill turns" and that usually he was extremely timid and never asserted his own rights, that John would "knock him down and walk all over him and Henry never made any resistance whatever." He was extremely affectionate and liked to be petted and he was afraid of the dark, where he "saw things and people."

In the examining room the child seemed very quiet. He had a marked flush and breathed through his mouth because of a profuse discharge of mucus from both nostrils. The cervical glands were enlarged, especially on the left side; and the adenoids and tonsils were enlarged. The lad was underdeveloped and poorly nourished. He was immediately referred to the medical clinic, and the mother was requested to return to the habit clinic at the end of 10 days.

Careful social investigation revealed the following facts: The father and mother were "always scrapping," and on several occasions the father had been arrested for assault and battery. They were living with the maternal grandmother because the father did not support or provide for the mother. The grandmother reported that there were two distinct factions in the household. The younger child, pugnacious John, was lined up with the mother against the father and timid Henry. Because of the father's work during the day and his pursuit of pleasure at night he spent little time at home. Consequently Henry was left alone pretty much to fight his own battles. The mother had at all times been the protector of John, who had learned from experience that he could tease and torment his older brother without fear of retaliation when his mother was about. Henry undoubtedly had learned that it was the better part of valor to submit to tormenting by his brother rather than to raise his mother's wrath. So day by day the younger lad had become more domineering and pugnacious while the older boy had become more subdued and submissive, only occasionally turning upon his brother and biting and scratching in a crude, instinctive way at such times. This was not mere speculation but was borne out by the fact that John had improved rapidly since entering the school, where he had less opportunity of manifesting his arrogant, domineering ways without punishment. Henry, on the other hand, had retained his shy and diffident manner.

*Comment.*—The two important points brought out in this case are: (1) The effect of environment on the development of personality and (2) the importance of certain types of symptoms in making a prognosis. A question that is constantly brought up is: If environment is such a tremendous factor in the development of personality, why is it that two individuals coming from the same environment should be so diametrically opposite in character and disposition? This case seems to bring out the fact that it is not the physical environment that counts but the mental atmosphere of the environment. Here were two boys who were born of the same father and mother and reared in the same home, but for whom the mental atmosphere of the home was entirely different. One lived an absolutely sheltered life, basking in the affection of an oversolicitous mother, and the other was living a life of torture, being subjected to the torments of the younger brother and to the persistent reproaches of the mother. It is not difficult to understand why these two children should have developed entirely different personalities, one characterized by a domineering pugnacity and the other by submission and a feeling of inferiority.

With reference to the second point, the prognosis is always discouraging when the individual's personality defect has caused his retreat from contact with humanity. Such a personality defect deprives the individual of the opportunity to develop new interests outside himself. It takes away the necessity of his making an effort at social adjustment and gives him time in which to build, in fancy, life as he would have it. The individual who remains active, keeping in contact with the herd, has ever before him the opportunity of learning life's lessons by experience and by the necessity of adjusting himself to the demands of society.

---

Katherine was a Negro girl who was brought to the clinic at the age of 2 years 9 months. Birth and developmental history were quite normal. She had always had good health except for measles and bronchitis when she was 2 years old.

Her habits regarding food had given considerable trouble. Until the beginning of the second year she always had to be coaxed; had to be forced to eat at times; was very finicky about carrots, spinach, and other vegetables. Mother "persuaded" her by "showing her the strap." She ate plentifully of what she wanted. Her toilet habits had been established. The patient was very kindly disposed toward everybody and got acquainted easily with strangers, both children and adults. She shad shown a tendency to be cruel. She would punch the other children and at the clinic she would frequently knock them down when they crossed her path. She had a very quick, violent temper and got angry when thwarted. She was extremely jealous of her younger sister because her father would tell her he loved the baby better. When scolded or humiliated she put her fingers in her mouth to keep from crying, and before going to sleep she always indulged in a period of thumb sucking. The mother had kept the child in the house most of the time on account of her marked pugnacity and the difficulty that she caused with the neighborhood children.

At the clinic she was extremely active and mischievous, teasing her mother by pulling at her dress and then running away, pulling down the curtain, and doing numerous other things for which the mother was constantly reprimanding her. She was openly rebellious toward any discipline and defied the mother when any effort was made to thwart her. Instead of crying or whining for what she wanted, she pushed and fought her way until she got it. When attempts were made by the mother to punish her she ran away, dodging and ducking into the corners and under the table, and when finally captured and punished by the mother, she showed no resentment whatever. After she was completely exhausted she went to the corner, sat down, and began sucking her right thumb and twisting her curly black hair between the fingers of her left hand, apparently perfectly happy and contented.

The psychologist stated that it was impossible to get any measurement of the child's intellectual equipment, as she was too active and unruly. She consented to look at one of the pictures presented to her, but her interest lasted only a moment. She appeared to be a bright, hyperactive child who demanded her own way at all times, expressed her ideas clearly in sentences, and played with the pencil and paper. She was interested in everything that was going on; showed marked curiosity and, when opposed, did not hesitate to scratch, bite, and kick.

The patient's father was a hard-working man earning an adequate salary and enjoying good health. The mother was also in good health and had a fair intellectual equipment, having gone through the seventh grade in school. Since coming to this country from the West Indies she had gone to trade school and learned dressmaking. She had worked as a housemaid and in a laundry. She was much interested in her children but was not particularly cooperative so far as the clinic was concerned.

*Summary.*—We were dealing with a child, not yet 3 years of age, having a normal mentality and coming from a home that presented no outstanding defects of physical surroundings or social relationships. The most prominent characteristics in the mental life of the youngster were her curiosity and tendency to investigate, and a marked hyperactivity and restlessness displayed both at home and at the clinic. Much of the pugnacity which had been attributed to the child seemed to be due to her desire for action rather than to any desire to cause pain to others. Under existing conditions the mother had felt obliged to limit the field of activities to their four-room apartment, which was quite inadequate to meet the demands of the child. It seemed that much of her mischievousness and naughtiness, so-called, could be attributed to her desire for play life and that it was not associated with any unpleasant emotional reaction. To defy and be rebellious was her method of stimulating her mother to activity. Her motive was to be chased and to be given the opportunity of romping and running. One might well expect that when the child enters a nursery school in the fall and is given an opportunity to express herself in group games and rhythmic dances accompanied by music most of her difficulties will be adjusted.

It is always important to study carefully the motives for acts rather than the acts themselves.

## DESTRUCTIVENESS

Much of the activity of the preschool child that is termed destructiveness is brought about by the attempt to satisfy curiosity. The child learns by handling, pulling, pushing, twisting, throwing, taking things apart, and exerting his own influence on his surroundings, limited as it may be. During this process of investigation at a time when the child's motor coordination is not well established, it is not surprising that he frequently miscalculates not only his strength but also the value of some of the material things with which he comes in contact. The wise parent and the intelligent child soon work out some plan which reduces damage to a minimum. Needless to say, this plan must be started early and discipline must be enforced. It must be remembered, however, that the child does not discriminate between what is valuable and what is not. For that reason the child should not be surrounded with breakable things that are expensive to replace, but should be taught to regard with proper respect the material things with which he comes in contact. There cannot be one standard for the nursery and another for the living room. If the child is taught to be careful of the linoleum on the kitchen floor he will have respect for the parlor rug. If he puts a value on his heavy china mug he will be likely to handle delicate china in the same way.

Whenever possible, the child should have some private place for himself, whether it is a room of his own or merely a corner set aside for his use. This should be a place in which he can ramble about without undue restrictions and without fear of doing something that will bring him into conflict with the adult members of the household. The continuous nagging and scolding to which many active youngsters are subjected are the cause of much emotional tension on the part of the child and continued irritation on the part of the parent. The constant fear that something is going to happen if Tom and Mary do not stop whatever they are doing, creates a bad atmosphere in which to rear a child.

Destructiveness may be a way of getting attention, the result of jealousy, a method of getting revenge, or a means of settling a grudge. Under such conditions the child is not conscious of the motive back of the conduct; and only after careful study of the child and his environment, including the personalities and experiences he encounters, is it possible to be helpful in solving the problem.

Lydia was a very attractive little girl, 10 years of age, whose medical history presented nothing worthy of note. She was in the fourth grade in school and getting on well.

She was brought to the clinic by her father, who stated that she was "viciously destructive" and "willfully stubborn." He gave the following details concerning recent happenings.

All during the winter she had persisted in going down into the cellar and turning on the cold water, permitting it to run into the steam boiler. For this she was severely scolded, threatened, and spanked, and finally her bare hands were placed in the hot furnace so that they were badly blistered and had to be bandaged for several days. Fifteen minutes after the removal of the bandages the act for which she had been punished was repeated.

Four days previous to visiting the clinic she scratched the piano with a pin. This episode was followed the next day by the mutilation of the top of the dining-room table with the cover of a tin can. For these two offenses the father scratched her arm and the palm of her right hand with a pin, leaving ugly-looking wounds which were much in evidence when the child was seen at the clinic.

Recently her father had missed several phonograph records and upon being appealed to the patient admitted taking them to school but did not return them, although her father requested her to do so. She said she had given the records to her teacher, but the father went to the school and saw both the teacher and the principal and found that the child had lied. She admitted this later. She was severely switched about the legs on the way home from school, but she maintained a sullen silence until the next day, when she told the housekeeper that she had put the records down through the cracks in the veranda. A carpenter was called and several boards were removed, but no records were found. A few days later, of her own accord, she produced the records, which had been hidden away in her room.

She wrote on the wallpaper, hammered the walls, and destroyed furniture.

She was the oldest of five children whose mother had died 3 years before the clinic visit. Her father stated, "I have had 20 housekeepers since then." The one in charge then was 63 years old; she was kindly and affectionate toward the patient, and the child was fond of her. The father was a stern, reserved, quick-tempered man who was trying hard to keep his family together, and in spite of his apparent brutality he wanted to do what was right.

At school the patient was considered bright, well-behaved, and truthful. At home she was untruthful, disobedient, destructive, selfish, jealous of material things, unaffectionate, stubborn, and resentful. Her father said, "She is willing to undergo any pain to aggravate me."

At the clinic Lydia appeared to be a happy, cheerful little girl, who frankly admitted her jealousy of her younger sister. She gleefully told about school-day experiences but suddenly became sad and tearful at the mention of her mother. She had apparently assumed the responsibility for "all the rest of the kids," as she called them. She was interested in her schoolmates. She wanted pretty clothes and liked her teachers, the housekeeper, and her father. She showed no resentment at the severe punishment she had received and offered no excuses or explanations for her misconduct. She seemed to be very friendly and approachable. One felt that a sympathetic relationship had been established which would do much to get things going right.

The father was given to understand that punishment was useless, a fact that he had appreciated for some time. He was asked to get on a more companionable basis with the children, and one Saturday he demonstrated his good intentions by bringing three of the children to the clinic en route to the movies. The father's report at this second visit was encouraging. Lydia had been "getting along fine" for a week, none of the destructive tendencies being in evidence. She had seemed happier and more cheerful, had talked more freely, and had been much overjoyed at the prospect of going to the movies.

After the picture show the child returned home. Everything seemed to be progressing well when suddenly, for no apparent reason, she gathered up several phonograph records and destroyed them. There seemed to be no particular emotion attached to this episode, it being apparently the result of an impulsive idea. She was not punished on this occasion, and everything went along smoothly for 48 hours, her father being still hopeful that another week might pass without further manifestation of her destructive tendencies. One evening he brought home a new pair of white shoes for her, a present for which she had shown a strong desire for some time. She was happy over the gift, but within an hour after her father's return she cut the upholstery on one of the best chairs in the living room with a pair of scissors. This information was reported to the clinic by the father over the telephone. He admitted that he had reached the limit of his patience and said that some plan must be made to take the child from the home.

Arrangements were made with a child-study home in Boston to take this child for an indefinite period; but although the father had demanded that such a plan be made, he let the matter drop at that point.

Nothing else was heard about the case until 6 weeks later, when the Society for the Prevention of Cruelty to Children was notified that the neighbors had been much disturbed the previous night by screams coming from the home of the patient. Upon investigation they found that the father had been whipping one of the younger boys severely. They threatened to break in, and the father explained that the boy had been damaging the furniture in much the same way as Lydia had done. The father admitted that he had a violent temper and sometimes lost control of it. It was generally agreed by those interested that the children ought to be placed out, but the father would not consent.

However, a plan was agreed upon and carried out whereby the children would be sent to Maine for the summer months. Such a plan was, of course, only temporary.

*Comment.*—This child was not under the personal observation of the author long enough to enable him to formulate any definite ideas of the underlying cause of the child's destructiveness. There were, however, several pertinent factors in the history that gave an inkling of the line of treatment that must be followed. The first and most important was the child's devotion to her mother, her inability to assimilate into her own life the situation caused by the mother's death, and her bitterness and resentment on being deprived of her mother.

In a superficial examination of the facts presented it was found that all the destructive tendencies of this patient were directed toward the house in which she lived and the furniture in it. At school, when visiting, or under any circumstances or conditions not found in her own home, she never manifested any of these destructive tendencies. It seemed that it was the association with her own home that brought out all her vicious tendencies. One also found from the history that for many years prior to the death of the mother the sole interest of both parents had been to save enough money to build a house that would be more or less of a show place in their community, a small unattractive village in the suburbs of Boston. Both parents had worked without daily recreation or vacations and had even gone without the necessities of life, until the death of the mother, in order that another dollar might be put away. It was only after the death of the mother, however, that the father finally erected the $16,000 house, which stood as a monument to his ambition and thrift. But somehow one could only feel that to the patient, consciously or perhaps unconsciously, it was but a memorial to the toil and sacrifice of the mother for whom she had always shown a very strong attachment. This may be considered merely speculative, considering the little opportunity the writer had to observe this particular case, but it was not unreasonable to expect to find an explanation for these apparently voluntary vicious acts of destructiveness in some deep-seated mental conflict with which the child was blindly struggling.

---

Martin, aged 4 years 8 months; birth and development normal. He was nursed by his mother for 3 months. From that time on he presented a difficult feeding problem. When his mother's milk gave out, he refused to take the bottle and had a great deal of nutritional disturbance during his first 2 years. He had been a restless sleeper until recently, but lately he had been going to bed at 7 p. m. and sleeping well until morning. Occasionally he had terrifying dreams, during which he had typical night terrors. There were very apt to follow some definite incident, such as being frightened as he had recently been by one of the neighbors, who told him of the bogeyman. He ate well. There was no history of enuresis or masturbation.

The general health of the patient had not been particularly satisfactory. Besides having severe nutritional disturbance during the first 2 years of his life, he had had several convulsions, the first occurring at the thirteenth month and others at intervals of about 6 months. The last one, which had occurred while he was at the hospital, was reported as being definitely epileptoid in character and lasted 30 minutes.

The patient found it difficult to get along with other children. He was unduly pugnacious; he got into many fights and was constantly teasing those with whom he came in contact. He seemed to enjoy playing with animals, but usually ended by using various methods of tormenting them. He was extremely stubborn. His mother stated that when he was told to do a thing he always did just the opposite. She felt that she could not trust him a minute. If she was in the bedroom while he was in the kitchen he would turn on the water faucet or the gas. He had knocked the parlor lamp off the table and had shown other destructive tendencies. If taken into a store he would pick up things and handle them, perhaps grabbing an apple and biting into it. Recently, while at a rest camp, he climbed into an automobile and started it. On two other occasions he had started automobiles on the street. For these reasons the mother lived in fear of what was going to happen next.

When rebuked he retaliated by using obscene and profane language. Recently, when his Sunday-school teacher, thinking he was too young to read, did not give him a Sunday-school paper, he stamped his feet, kicked her, and called her a nasty name. This habit had been growing steadily worse for the last few months. Efforts at home to discipline the child had been fruitless. The mother stated, "He is just one of them kids that is just smarty. It's his disposition to be that way, and he can't help it." She further commented that in spite of his sauciness he usually said things with a twinkle in his eye, and everybody liked him.

He had always been extremely active and destructive; lost no opportunity to get into a fight; seemed lacking in any appreciation of the rights of others; would enter any of the neighboring houses without knocking, and openly appropriated what he desired. At the nursery school he was considered a difficult child to teach, seemed unable to follow directions, and had no sense of rhythm or order. He did very poor work and would not obey—was considered a general nuisance. Of late he had been calling his teacher bad names whenever she asked him to do anything.

The family occupied a four-room apartment situated on a busy thoroughfare. The house was well furnished and homelike, well ventilated and neatly kept. Family relationships were unusually pleasant. Both the father and the mother were much interested in the children and were eager to cooperate in any way possible. The discipline had been left very largely to the mother, who looked upon the patient's behavior as something inevitable and thought that it was too much to expect results from the clinic.

*Summary.*—The patient, nearly 5 years of age, had been having convulsions at rather infrequent intervals for 4 years. It was evident from his general reactions to the problems of everyday life and his behavior in school that he was not endowed with a normal intellectual equipment or that if he had such an endowment at birth, its development had been retarded by the convulsions. In spite of the fact that the home situation was at least average and the parents were cooperative, it was perhaps useless to hope that satisfactory results would be obtained so long as treatment was carried on in the home, where the mother was inclined to take the stand that "what is to be will be." There was every reason to believe that this child would be much benefited by institutional life during the developmental period, for not only was the youngster's mental development somewhat retarded but the whole situation was complicated by the convulsive phenomena and the emotional instability. Under these conditions a very special environment, such as can be obtained only in the best institutions, was needed so that the limited abilities of the child could be developed to their fullest extent.

## DELINQUENCY

The self-regarding sentiment of most individuals is to a very large extent dependent upon the opinion that other people have of them. It is only after an individual has achieved success and established himself firmly in science, business, or a profession that he has sufficient confidence in his own achievements to ignore the opinions of others to any marked degree.

During the early years of a child's life, when imitation and suggestion play a leading part, it is particularly important that he should not absorb from those about him ideas in regard to his own qualities which might react disadvantageously on his conduct. The child who is continually led to believe that his word cannot be depended upon or that he has no regard for other people's property and other people's rights, is quite apt to accept this suggestion as representing the truth and to make no effort to avoid doing what he feels is expected of him. On the other hand, suggestions that he has certain capabilities and that a certain moral standard is expected of him may do much to stimulate his efforts in the direction of a line of conduct which will furnish in itself the satisfaction to assure its continuance. It is too much to expect that the child who is being reared in an environment where truth and honesty are held lightly will develop of his own accord standards acceptable to society. No one expresses any particular amazement over the fact that a child brought up in a German family learns to speak German or that the French child learns to speak French, but we sometime fail to appreciate the fact that conduct as well as speech is to a very large extent an imitative phenomenon.

One mother brought her child to the clinic, stating quite frankly that the child, aged 3 years, used the same swear words that her hus-

78985°—39——5

band used and that he manifested the same arrogant, defiant attitude toward her that he saw in his father. There is nothing obscure between cause and effect in this particular case. Another woman brought in her youngster, quite perturbed because the child had bought candy with a nickel which had been given her for carfare to visit the dentist. Only a week before, however, this same mother had told the child that she was going on an automobile ride and then had taken her to the dentist. One finds that a child is quite capable at a very early age of differentiating fact from fancy and that one of the first important needs in the development of honesty and integrity is conduct on the part of those with whom the child comes in daily contact which he can safely imitate.

However, the problem is not by any means one of suggestion and imitation entirely, and frequently very complicated situations arise which do not permit such a simple interpretation. A little girl was sent to the clinic by the court because of stealing. Investigation showed that the motive in this particular case was intense jealousy of her chum, whose family could afford to give her many of the little niceties which young girls crave but which the patient could not have. This feeling of jealousy had persisted over a period of years, and it was not until she was given charge of the cloakroom at school, a privilege assigned to her because of her apparent honesty, that the jealousy made itself manifest in stealing.

Delinquent behavior—that is, the type of activity which is eventually going to bring the child into conflict with society—should receive the same consideration and thorough investigation as any other symptom of maladjustment. The only approach to the problem that will bear fruitful results is interpretation of the child's difficulty in terms of his past experience, his present environmental situation, the personalities surrounding him, and his own intellectual, physical, and emotional make-up.

All children who steal cannot be treated in the same way. The child who goes into the department store and steals something which he desires although he has in his pocket a sufficient supply of money to attain the thing desired in a socially accepted way is quite a different problem from the child who steals money to buy candy for distribution among his contemporaries in the hope that he will thus be allowed to participate in their activities.

Stealing in young children often has its origin in what Dr. Healy terms "grudge formation"[5] and in sex conflicts. Such cases call for most careful, intensive study, frequently over long periods of time. They require patience and kindness on the part of the parents, and before they are satisfactorily adjusted they may tax the skill and ingenuity of the specialist.

The problem of lying also must be regarded from various angles. The lying associated with stealing is invariably of a protective nature and is quite different in its psychological implications from the problem of the child who lies in an effort to bolster up his self-esteem.

Truancy may result from varied motives, some closely tied up with the personality make-up of the child and others entirely dependent upon environmental situations. It is not a sufficient deviation from

[5] Healy, William, M. D.: The Individual Delinquent, p. 376. Little, Brown & Co., Boston, 1915.

normal conduct to be considered too serious in itself. It is only when truancy represents an effort to escape from an undesirable environment that it should cause concern, and then the environment rather than the symptom requires treatment. It is the spirit of "wanderlust" in most youngsters that prompts them to investigate whatever is strange and new. To most youngsters this means nothing more than investigating a new alley, making friends around the corner, or going to the park; with the more venturesome it leads at times to the motion-picture shows or wherever there seems to be anything exciting going on. Unfortunately most of these early truants are punished after the first offense, and the punishment in no way inhibits their desire for future adventure or satisfies the curiosity stimulated by their first experience. It is only when the moment to return home is at hand that they recall the last experience. This very often prompts them to remain away from home on account of fear. One youngster with the habit of remaining out at night with the other boys, who would leave him one by one, said he was always afraid to return home "to face the music." His mother said that he had been beaten very hard but that it did no good. Beatings do not solve these problems.

The discovery of the child's motive—that is, what he hopes to accomplish by his misconduct—is a prerequisite for any intelligent plan of treatment. The importance of this is brought out in the following cases:

Nora, aged 10; birth and developmental history quite normal. She was the third of five children. She was brought to the clinic by her mother because she told "silly lies" without any reason, stayed out at night without permission, and stole small amounts of money. The child had had measles and whooping cough, but none of the other children's diseases; had no history of injuries or operations; slept and ate well, occasionally talking in her sleep but not so as to be understood. She wet the bed at infrequent intervals. The mother said that the child was selfish and always wanted her own way. She was not affectionate and showed no attachment for her father or mother. She was extremely jealous of her younger sister, wanted everything the sister had, and resented the mother's showing any attention to the sister. She was constantly quarreling with other members of the family, and was "irritable and snappish." The mother stated that she did the punishing with a strap, as the father seldom disciplined the child. The patient was apparently afraid of her father but not of her mother. The mother said that the child got along well in school and got good marks, but subsequent investigation did not bear this out.

The following comments on the other children in this family were of interest: George, aged 15, was said to be disagreeable, troublesome, and a trial to his mother. When 8, he was arrested for breaking into the girls' high school with two other boys and destroying microscope lenses. He was put on probation, and his conduct since had been unsatisfactory. Four years later he was again arrested for breaking into and entering a grocery store, but the case was dismissed. He was always lazy at school, which he left at the age of 14, having repeatedly played truant. After leaving school he worked as an errand boy for 6 weeks at a stationery store and made $7 a week. He was looking for work at the time of the clinic visit and spent most of his time on the street. He was scornful and defiant toward his father, and refused to go to church. Joseph, aged 10, was still attending school. He had always been well behaved until 2 years before, and after that he had become irritable when crossed. He was arrested with two other boys for taking a doctor's kit from an automobile and was put on probation. The two younger children presented nothing abnormal in their physical or mental make-up worthy of note. They had no conduct disorders.

At the clinic the patient appeared to be quiet and subdued. She was rather well developed and well nourished and was fairly attractive. She manifested little interest in her surroundings. When questioned regarding her delinquencies she answered quickly but apparently without frankness, judging from the data previously obtained. She accounted for the time spent away from home as being spent with her girl friends and with the other children on the street. She said she never asked permission to go out because her mother always refused it. When she was out, she said, she was afraid to go home. She appreciated the seriousness of her present situation and her attitude toward her difficulties seemed quite normal. She admitted quite frankly that she did not like housework, but said she was willing to do it since she must. She was looking forward to learning cooking in school the next year. She admitted taking money that she found about the house, stating that the amounts varied from 10 to 45 cents and that she always denied having taken the money because she wished to avoid the punishment that always followed. She said she enjoyed most being on the street or with her friends and liked to be away from home. She read little and did not care for the movies.

The following briefly summarizes the home situation. The mother appeared to be a hard-working woman who bore the marks of her toil and hardships. She had never had good health and was obviously discouraged over the discord among the members of the family and the poorness of the tenement in which they had to live. She had always had considerable worry and anxiety over the three older children. Her husband kept her constantly upset because of his marked irritability and fits of temper, which disturbed the family most of the time. He was apparently disgusted with the lack of success they had had in raising the family, and there were many scenes between him and the oldest boy. The husband's reactions were always worse when he had been drinking. The patient seemed to be his favorite child and had considerable influence over him when he was having one of his "spells." The mother tried to adjust to this chaotic situation, but the alcoholism of her husband and the constant quarreling of the children made her very unhappy. The home situation was quite intolerable. The family occupied a five-room flat in a poor neighborhood on a noisy, crowded street. The tenement was damp and cold, and in spite of the mother's efforts to improve it it was not attractive.

During the first clinic visit little was accomplished except to get the history and an interview with the child. The mother was requested to return to the next clinic, but it was several weeks before she appeared again. The report was very discouraging. The child continued to disregard her parents' wishes, paying no attention whatever to her mother. She always avoided telling her mother where she was going and where she had been, even if her conduct had been such as to justify praise. Her school work was not satisfactory, and it was expected that she would have to repeat her grade or else take summer-school work.

On the second visit sufficient time was taken to discuss the problem in some detail with both the mother and the child. It appeared that the mother's restrictions on the girl had been rather severe. Her anxiety over the patient's whereabouts and her distrust of her ability to take care of herself made the mother feel that the only safe place for her was in the house. The family budget was such that the mother felt unable to give the youngster any allowance and she invariably refused her when she asked for money. The mother was frank in admitting that on occasions her irritability toward the other members of the household was spent on Nora, and that she rarely, if ever, had any time to devote to her except for matters of discipline. An effort was made to present to Nora some of the difficulties of the mother's position and the importance of her assuming certain responsibilities in helping out in the household and causing the mother as little anxiety as possible. It was agreed between them that the patient should have an allowance of 10 cents a week and that she would ask her mother's permission before she went out to visit other girls or to play in the street.

The mother did not return until about a month later, notwithstanding the fact that she had been urged to make weekly visits to the clinic. She said that the patient was doing better, and that she was not running away as she formerly had, but that she was still very unreliable about keeping her promises, irritable with the other children, doing poorly in school, and of little assistance in the household. The mother said it was difficult for her to get to the clinic more than once a month because her household duties made heavy demands upon her time. The whole situation was gone over again in detail, and an effort was made to have both the mother and the patient make some concessions.

The following month the mother returned to the clinic. Although she was very reluctant about admitting an improvement, she said that Nora "did not run away any more, and she did not tell silly lies" so often. She reported that Nora was still very quarrelsome and hard to get along with. Her school work was poor and her deportment mark low. At this visit, the patient got a little friendly and confidential for the first time. She said that although she did not like her teacher and hated the thought of going to school during the summer, she was very anxious to stay in the sixth grade so that she could be with her brother. The child was apparently in a very unhappy frame of mind, resenting authority and feeling that she was not having the opportunity that other children had. Her attitude seemed to be that she had to take whatever she got out of life in spite of what others thought. The mother seemed to feel absolutely hopeless. She had lost her courage to go on, was unable to see anything bright in the future of the patient, and did not hesitate to let the patient know how discouraged and unhappy she was about the outlook.

The patient did not return to the clinic for several months, and then she came alone. She stated that she was getting along well in school, that things were improving at home, and that she was getting more confidence in her mother. But the mother's report, as gathered by the social worker, was that of a harsh, pessimistic critic who saw nothing but the unfavorable side of the situation. She had just received a school report which indicated Nora's absolute failure. Her deportment, writing, and geography were poor, and the mother laid great stress on these failures. Nora said, by way of apology, that besides these poor marks she had received four marks indicating exceptionally good work—a fact that the mother admitted. When the patient was asked in her mother's presence if she was helping in the household, the mother spoke up, saying, "Believe me, she don't do much. She lies and steals money. I don't dare take her in anyone's house for fear she might take something." The mother still refused to give the child money for any purpose, in spite of the promise she had made at the clinic. The patient said that she never had a chance to go to the movies, that she got candy from other children but never had any of her own—"only what I take. The girls I play with sometimes have candy and sometimes give it to me." She thought that a little girl of her age should have 10 or 15 cents a week.

The child was given a long talk on the value of honesty, playing the game fair, and helping her mother. The mother was interviewed at length about the absolute necessity of changing her attitude toward the child. The importance of making the child believe that something was expected of her was called to the mother's attention. It was pointed out that nothing could be accomplished if she persisted in impressing the child with her delinquencies, especially if this was done in front of other people. The fact that she had unsuccessfully followed her own methods with the older children was pointed out to her with extreme frankness, and an effort was made to show her that nothing could be lost if she followed the plan outlined by the clinic.

Notwithstanding the fact that the situation seemed extremely hopeless if the child was to remain in that environment, it seemed worth while to continue the efforts in this case. Something about the patient—her honesty and frankness at the clinic as compared with her reported actions at home and her insight and appreciation of the importance of overcoming her delinquencies—gave encouragement in spite of the wretched environmental conditions in which she was living and the poor cooperation of the mother.

The latest reports from the school had been encouraging. The patient was in the seventh grade, got along much better than the year before, got a mark of "one" in effort and "two" in conduct, and had not been sent to the office for disciplinary reasons during the entire year. The patient was frank and free in her talks with the doctor and had lost much of the stubbornness which characterized her first visit to the clinic. Her mother had put her on an allowance of 10 cents a week and had recently given her 30 cents to go to a festival. There was no trouble at home about taking money, and the patient seemed to be making a fairly good adjustment. She had passed all her examinations in school and was looking for a summer job instead of having to make up school work.

Although this improvement had been in evidence for a period of only 3 months and might not continue without occasional relapses, the case was particularly interesting as an indication of what could be done in spite of wretched environmental conditions and lack of cooperation. Besides the rather infrequent visits to the clinic during which the problem had been discussed with both parents and patient, successful efforts had been made to get the girl interested in a girls' club and in taking books from the library, both of which activities gave her much-needed interests other than street life.

---

Olive, aged 6 years 4 months, third of four children—the other children being 8 years, 7 years, and 11 months old, respectively; birth and development normal except that talking was delayed until she was 26 months of age and that she had always lisped. Except for an orthopedic operation on account of a shoulder deformity, the child had always enjoyed good health. Prior to this operation she was very restless at night and frequently walked in her sleep, but since the operation her sleep had been restful and quiet. She had a good appetite and was not finicky. She was said to be domineering and quarrelsome and preferred to be alone, although she was not shy. She was extremely affectionate and sensitive and was inclined to be jealous when she saw others being petted. She got along well at home—at least her mother said the child was easy to manage. She enjoyed her play life and spent much time by herself. Her mother denied that the child had any propensity for stealing (in spite of a history to that effect obtained from outside sources) but admitted having lost money which she had left about the house. She said she could not suspect the children as she had always trusted them. The child was in the first grade. In spite of her history and the poor impression she made during the first contact because of her unattractive manner and unkempt appearance, she graded normal on the psychometric test.

The parents were separated, but the father occasionally came to the house to see the children. The mother seemed quite devoted to the children, and although the living quarters were poor—they consisted of a four-room apartment on the third floor of an extremely dilapidated building—and the home was untidy and cluttered, she attempted to do more than give them purely custodial care. She made an effort to amuse them, occasionally taking them to the motion pictures and for walks.

Olive was referred to the clinic by a settlement worker because of her persistent stealing and the conditions under which the thefts were carried out. From the settlement she had taken two hats and an umbrella. She was frequently found going through the children's clothes, rifling their pockets. She admitted these thefts only under conditions in which it was apparent that she must be caught. Even when called to account for having stolen an article, she would make attempts to take things from the person reprimanding her. It did not matter whether the articles were of particular value or whether they would naturally interest a child of her age. From the school she had taken beads, a rubber ball, a teacher's key, fruit, and numerous other articles. When confronted by one in authority with the charge of thieving, she invariably denied the thefts but always confessed later. There seemed to be no outstanding problems except the stealing and lying.

The home situation was one of filth and immorality. The father had apparently spent much of his time with other women prior to leaving home. He claimed that the mother was irresponsible in the care of the children and the household, that she used vile language, that she never had the meals ready, and that the house was always dirty. She, on the other hand, accused him of having a violent temper, saying that he frequently went into a rage and that there was nothing too mean or vile for him to say. It appeared from the history that both of them had associations of the lowest type.

Obviously little or nothing could be expected by the clinic in the way of cooperation by the parents. The only hope of helping the child lay in those with whom she came in contact outside the home. The assistance of her teacher was solicited, and her cooperation did much toward any improvement that was made. The teacher stated that the patient was a dear little girl; she seemed to be much attached to her. The child got along well with the other children in school, but it was very difficult to make her concentrate. She did not seem to have any interest in school, was poor in all her subjects, and probably would not be promoted. At school her speech defect was a great handicap. She was considered very childish for her age.

At the clinic she entered the examining room in a shy and diffident manner but did not appear frightened or resentful. At first she merely smiled at the examiner's questions. Soon, however, she became more responsive and, with a marked defect in her speech, began to repeat letters and numbers for the doctor.

She volunteered a little information about her home life—the fact that she had two brothers, that her father took her to the movies, and that she went to the beach and to school. On the first visit she was very reticent about discussing delinquencies, and the subject was soon changed to a more pleasant one. She said she liked to play ball and skip rope but did not like dolls because they break; she liked the dances at the movies and said she could dance; she told of seeing Charlie Chaplin, told the doctor what she had had for different meals during the last 24 hours, named a number of common objects in the room, and gradually became more interested in her surroundings.

A week later the patient returned to the clinic. She was much more friendly but still a little shy. She made an effort to carry on a few speech exercises, imitating the doctor. When asked with whom she played she said, "No one." When asked why, she said, "Nobody likes me." Then she discussed the subject more spontaneously, saying that she didn't see why they didn't like her—no one liked her except her father and mother and the baby. Girls didn't like her; they knocked her down. She insisted that she was the only one the other children did not like. She said she didn't like anybody but her family. There seemed to be real emotion attached to the idea that nobody liked her. She tried to hold back the tears, but it was difficult. She talked more frankly about her thefts and tried to justify herself by the fact that she did not like those from whom she took things.

At this time she was given a long talk, in which she took considerable interest, about how she might make people like her, about playing fair and square, and about how she would feel if other people took her things. She was told that a careful record was to be kept of the days on which she did not take things and that she was to bring the record to the doctor the following week. The teacher was seen, and arrangements were made to keep a chart on which a star would indicate each day that the patient's conduct had been satisfactory. This was carefully explained to the patient. She started off in a happier frame of mind than she had thus far exhibited.

Just a week later the following report was received from the school: "Olive has been getting on much better during the last week. It was not until yesterday morning that she was found peeping into the school desks in a rather suspicious way. There is no record of her having taken anything that did not belong to her at school all week." At the clinic, however, she found two pennies in the toilet, which she returned with some reluctance. She seemed quite happy while at the clinic and said she enjoyed making the visits.

The following week the report was excellent. The patient was much pleased at the interest the teacher had taken in her and was apparently making a persistent effort to get the coveted stars to bring to the clinic. At the settlement house which she visited frequently, however, she was found several times in the act of taking things that did not belong to her. Her reaction on being questioned about taking these things seemed one of remorse—she cried and seemed very much upset.

There was something very inaccessible about this child. She chattered away and answered questions very readily, but it was difficult to get close to her innermost life. The last report received from the school was excellent. "Olive has not taken anything for a long time." She came into the clinic cheerful, happy, and cleanly dressed. She had genuine pride in the fact that she had such a good report, and again it was felt that in spite of wretched environmental conditions much had been accomplished toward helping this child to overcome two very asocial reactions and to get much more happiness out of life.

---

Paul, a lad 13 years of age, was brought to the clinic by his stepmother, an unusually bright, intellectual woman, extremely fond of and interested in her stepson. For the last 5 years he had been developing certain delinquencies that had caused the family much concern. He began by taking money from the family and doing such things as mailing letters without putting on postage and short-changing when sent on errands. He would tell lies to get out of difficult situations. He would not, however, persist in the lies but would confess what he had done and then break down and cry.

About 3 weeks before coming to the clinic his stepmother lost $5. About the same time the patient came home and said that he had got a job in a store. He gave the name of the store, the man he worked for, and the streets where he had to deliver goods. He elaborated to the extent of telling what the storekeeper and the customer said to him. He said that he was treated well and was given crackers at the store. At the end of the week he brought home $5 and turned it over to his mother. Investigation revealed the fact that the lad was not employed and that the money was the same that he had stolen. Immediately after this episode, he made further attempts to take money; that is, he was found searching in places where money was usually kept.

This lad was in the eighth grade and was getting on well in school. The psychometric test showed that he had normal mental equipment. He had never worked. The father was generous to the children; he gave them a dime on Saturday with which to buy candy. Paul was interested in playing football and baseball and in skating and sledding, and got along well with other boys. He said everyone was kind to him. He admitted that he cried easily but knew no reason for doing so. He appeared to be an unusually cheerful, active boy who, in the examining room, was frank and honest. He made no effort to attribute his delinquencies to others. He said he seldom went to movies and never went with a gang.

A study of this case showed that the motive was the desire of the boy to emulate his father and play the part of a grown-up in helping to provide for the family. It was what Kirkpatrick has called "passive enjoyment rather than active effort," but the motive was obviously not a malicious one, and intelligent cooperation on the part of the parents made it quite easy to straighten out this lad's point of view. The social-service department of the clinic was very active in this case. The lad's interests were broadened, and arrangements were made for him to spend the coming summer on a farm. The last notes stated that he had been completely freed from his former delinquencies, that he had been getting on well in school, and that the family had been relieved of the worry and anxiety that were naturally associated with his former difficulties.

---

Quentin, aged 11 years, was brought to the clinic of the psychopathic hospital by his mother upon the recommendation of the principal of his school. He was under the jurisdiction of the court for entering a hotel by one of the side windows and taking $10 from a desk. He denied the theft when discovered hiding in a closet, but finally gave the money up when the policeman arrived. He had stolen many car tickets from the family. There had been a long history of delinquencies.

The patient was a keen, bright lad, with normal intellectual equipment. He discussed his trouble frankly and was anxious to overcome his "bad habits." He was kind, affectionate, generous, made friends easily, was interested in all sorts of games and sports, mixed well with other children, and never held grudges. He lacked interest in his studies and up to the time of coming to the clinic had never responded to discipline. He had been scolded, deprived of privileges, and whipped, without results. He had no fear of policemen nor of going to court.

Through the social-service department of the clinic this lad joined a boys' club, and supervision was carried on from the out-patient clinic. Results were extremely gratifying, and the last report of the lad was, "Getting on well."

It is of interest to note that although the parents attributed the lad's delinquencies to an accident which happened about 2 years before, the boy's statement was, "My mother says I do these things because I hurt my head and get crazy, but it is because I want sleds and things. My brother used to do all these things. Now he is big and he gets me to do them." Frequently parents try to attribute the delinquencies of their children to some sickness or accident, and sometimes the children themselves are prone to accept the suggestion as an excuse for doing those things which they enjoy.

---

Gordon, the older of two children, was referred by his mother to the clinic at the age of 4 years and 9 months for disobedience, masturbation, and quarreling. He was also described as stubborn and very destructive.

Birth was by Cesarean section. Developmental history was normal except that the patient had been given a bottle until he was 2 years of age, having refused to drink milk from a cup. At 4 years he had had whooping cough, followed by influenza, pneumonia, and an abscessed ear. He had been circumcised. Tonsils and adenoids were removed when he was 2 years of age. His eating habits were always a problem. He refused to eat unless fed, told a story, or offered a reward. He had enuresis until he was 4. Occasionally he bit his nails. He had masturbated since infancy, apparently without realizing it. The patient presented the picture of an undisciplined child, very stubborn and negativistic. He was prone to show off, and was very destructive of furniture and toys. He would throw objects about without any consideration of the possibility of injuring another child.

The home situation was physically good, but was undesirable from the point of view of meeting the patient's personality needs. Maternal relatives in the home dominated the situation, and the mother's attachment and dependence on them showed her own emotional immaturity. The psychological examination revealed the patient to be of normal intelligence. The case was carried in the clinic for 7 months, but service was interrupted by the mother's inability to attend because of illness. The mother lost interest and the case was closed while the boy was still unimproved. The psychiatrist considered the mother's own adjustment very poor. He observed that she seemed unable to profit by advice regarding a better technique for handling the patient's problems.

Two years later the mother referred the patient to the clinic. The same problem appeared as before, with the additional problems of lying and stealing. The previous problems were all intensified. Gordon had no idea of obedience and presented many types of habit difficulties. He was extremely jealous of his younger sister; he had begun to have nocturnal enuresis; he had developed the habit of biting his finger and toe nails; and he chewed his pajamas, blouse collars, and so forth. He took money wherever he could get it and used it for the purchase of guns. His mother threw away the guns, because of her fear that the patient would grow up like "Abe" F——, a man who had been involved in a bank-robbery case and who was well known to the patient's family.

Gordon was very inattentive and a daydreamer; in fact his mother had at times feared he was deaf. His lack of concentration made his teacher in the second grade consider him the "worst child in the class." His first-grade teacher, having had a much smaller class, had had no difficulty with him. Much of his behavior was thought to be a demand for attention.

A new psychological examination gave the patient a rating of good, average intelligence. A hearing test showed a loss of hearing in both ears, but this was not considered sufficient to account for his lack of response.

Home conditions had been somewhat improved, as relatives no longer lived with the family; but the mother was still very dependent on the relatives. She also rebuffed the patient and favored his sister. She had not wanted a boy. The father worked long hours, saw the children seldom, and thought that the problem was the mother.

The problem of stealing was treated by arranging for an allowance to the boy from the parents to take the place of former gifts from the grandfather. Attempts to give the mother a more objective point of view and a knowledge of mental-hygiene principles were not very successful because of her own emotional immaturity. In spite of this, however, the patient's behavior showed some improvement. Arrangements were made for "attitude therapy" for the mother. It was also recommended that the father attempt to give the patient more of his time.

---

Mildred was 6 years and 8 months of age when first seen at the habit clinic. She had been referred by a school teacher because of lying, stealing, truancy, and swearing. She also had temper tantrums.

Mildred was born of an illegitimate union, and nothing was known of her parents. She had been adopted shortly after birth by Irish parents of a low intellectual, economic, and social level. At the time of the clinic visit the adoptive mother was over 60 years old and the father about 44. The reason for the adoption was the mother's desire to compensate for her inability to have children of her own, since she was past the child-bearing age at the time of her marriage. Besides the patient and the adoptive parents, a maternal aunt was in the home.

The patient's early development was normal and she was in good health. She had had no diseases, operations, or accidents. She had good eating habits but was a restless sleeper. She had the habit of hiding in bed such stolen articles as scissors, nails, and pencils. She had been masturbating since she was 2 years old.

This child lied about everything. She had stolen candy from the five-and-ten-cent store, and she frequently took things from about the house and hid them. She had started to swear at about the time that she was referred to the clinic.

Her temper tantrums dated back to the age of 17 months. They were resorted to when she could not have her own way. When having such a tantrum, she would scream, kick, pick up anything handy, and threaten her mother with it.

She usually played with younger children, and whenever she become angry with them she would hit them with the first weapon she could find. On several occasions she had hit a neighbor's child on the head with a hammer.

She was hyperactive, stubborn, willful, and quite unaffectionate. She completely dominated her parents, who no longer made any effort to discipline her.

It seemed unlikely that the patient would improve in this environment, as she had complete control of the situation and her parents were too ineffectual and ignorant to profit much from attempts at reeducation. Mildred was accordingly placed for observation in the study home of a child-placing agency with the possibility of long-time placement in a foster home. The clinic, however, was unable to convince the parents of the advisability of such a placement, and the patient returned home.

Intensive therapy was then carried on by the social-service department. For several weeks the patient showed improved behavior and the mother appeared to make an earnest effort to help carry out the clinic's recommendations. The maternal aunt refused to cooperate, however, and the home situation became worse when the patient realized that she was the cause of friction between her mother and her aunt. The case was closed after 7 months, as it seemed useless for the clinic to try further treatment until the home situation should be improved by the aunt's departure from the household or by a change in her attitude.

Truancy, which is a common problem among urban children, may be motivated either by the desire to escape from an unhappy situation or by curiosity about the unknown and longing for something new. As with much undesirable behavior, however, once a pattern is established it seems to become self-perpetuating; and although the original motive may be forgotten, the habit has become so strong that no new motive is necessary.

Sam was a colored boy, 6 years and 10 months of age when first seen at the clinic. There was nothing unusual in his birth or developmental history.

The patient went to bed, when he was at home, at about 9 o'clock and slept until 8. Often he did not come home until after midnight. He sometimes had nocturnal enuresis. His appetite was excellent and he would eat anything. He was quarrelsome, hyperactive, and stubborn. He could not be trusted and he tried to be very independent. He ran away whenever he had a chance and often did not come back until late at night. His family picked him up in police stations and on the streets. According to his mother he had "business ability." He sold newspapers, ran errands, and shined shoes. He either gave the money to his mother or bought food with it. The patient was curious and liked to look at books, but he had a reading disability. He was very imaginative and invented stories. Once he made up a story from the illustrations in a book he was supposedly reading aloud.

This patient had an intelligence quotient of 99.

The family occupied a six-room apartment on the first floor of a tenement house. The apartment had a bathroom and three bedrooms. The furnishings were adequate. Sam slept in a room with two brothers, sharing a bed with one of them.

The problem as presented by the father and mother was that of truancy and difficult behavior. Sam had been a truant off and on ever since he had left kindergarten. He would wander away with the other neighborhood children. The family moved away from the neighborhood and the first Sunday in their new home Sam wandered back to the old district. He might go as far as 5 miles in his wanderings, sometimes riding on the back of a streetcar.

A week before his first visit to the clinic he had left home about 2 p. m. and had been found by the police at 3 a. m. after an 8-hour search. He picked up a dime to a dollar a day from his various activities, such as dancing, singing, or getting papers and selling them. He would often bring home rolls which he had bought. At other times he would bring home money. He was in and out of restaurants, eating until he no longer had an appetite for meals at home. Sometimes larger children took his money from him.

The patient, when interviewed about his truancy, stated, "I sell papers; I work in a barn; I mind the horses and keep people from taking them away; I work in a show—pick up papers so I can get in for nothing. Sometimes I clean automobiles; for a dollar I do the wheels and the windows and clean the seats and everything."

It was suggested that the patient be placed out in the country in order to determine the importance of environment in his conduct. He was placed in a suburb by a child-placing agency and he got along very well. His problems have been minimized and there is no evidence of truancy at present.

## RETREAT AS A METHOD OF MEETING FAILURE

Unlike children who develop a resentful, rebellious attitude toward restraint are those who respond by retreat. These children do not battle in an endeavor to break down the barriers but are inclined to retreat in the face of obstacles, to become submissive rather than rebellious. The mental characteristic known as plasticity seems to play an unduly important part in their make-up. They offer no resistance to factors in the environment which play upon them. These children as a rule are timid, shy, and cautious. They find little satisfaction in the activities of their more venturesome companions. Thus, while one child is thrilled by the experience of playing truant from home or school, another finds his satisfaction in the overprotective atmosphere provided by an oversolicitous mother. One lad finds life crowded with so many interesting and exciting episodes that he spends but little time thinking what it is all about. To another child life is dull, barren, and boresome. He runs away from it, and only in his daydreaming does he get enough satisfaction to justify his existence. These children are self-centered, critical, jealous; they have limited interests and few friends. They get but little satisfaction from the ordinary, everyday activities of life. They turn their headlights in upon themselves rather than out upon the world. They are inclined to be extremely dependent on one or two people but are quite withdrawn from the world at large. Many of these children in early life are looked upon as being resourceful, capable of entertaining themselves and providing their own amusements. This in itself is of value if it is not just part of the activity of an asocial child.

These children invariably suffer from a sense of inferiority. They do not enjoy any feeling of security about life, and in comparing themselves with other children they are vaguely conscious of their own inadequacies so that they seek to avoid competition when failure seems inevitable. The importance of preventing the child from developing what is commonly known as an inferiority complex is apparent to all who are concerned about his happiness and efficiency. The child is so dependent upon the opinions of others, especially those from whom he seeks approbation, that adults cannot be too careful about helping him to build up his self-esteem. A father who thoughtlessly tries to stimulate his boy to greater effort by constant teasing may be quite unaware that this humiliates the child and does something to his pride that will not easily be eradicated.

When the standards set for the child, whether in conduct or in school work, are so high that failure is the rule rather than the exception, the child is losing the one great motivating force to further effort—success. Children who are unfavorably compared with others in the home or neighborhood develop a sense of inferiority very easily, especially when the comparison is unfair because of their inherent deficiencies in mental equipment or physical strength. Habits like enuresis and masturbation, when managed unwisely by the parents, may also cause the children to feel that they are different, leading them eventually to build their lives around their liabilities instead of around their assets.

Of course, mental and physical handicaps necessarily impose certain limitations upon a child, but even when these are present every effort should be made to see that the child has an opportunity to develop to the fullest extent of his capacity. The child who is conscious of doing this will not feel inferior.

When the child, no matter what the reason, develops this feeling of inferiority, many things may happen. As has been shown, some children bolster up their self-esteem by aggressive measures such as stealing, truancy, and defiance toward authority. Others assume the protective attitude of always being right while everybody else is wrong. But the group we are concerned with at the moment succumb to their feelings and take the passive course which appears to them to be easier. Shyness is a mode of behavior that serves as a retreat for individuals of all ages, but the emotional experience leading to this behavior is often obscure. In the following case shyness was associated with stammering and both conditions seemed to bear a definite causal relation to an unhappy home situation to which the child had been unable to make a satisfactory adjustment.

Adele, a Negro girl, 4 years and 9 months old, was referred to the clinic because of shyness.

Birth and development were normal. She had had chickenpox, measles, whooping cough, mumps, and sore throats. Her habits were regular.

Adele was a shy, quiet, unassertive child who did not appear to be interested in her environment. She asked few questions, being content to sit back and watch what was going on. When speaking, her voice was scarcely above a whisper. Although quite able to take care of her own wants, she was never very active or noisy and spoke only when necessary. Her shyness had been apparent at so early an age that her mother thought it must have been inherited. At times the child stammered considerably, according to the mother, although the school and the clinic saw no indications of this. In kindergarten the patient did good work, but she talked little and never made advances to the other children of her own accord. Aside from kindergarten she had little or no contacts, for the mother treated her as a "hothouse flower" and considered her too delicate to play outdoors except in very pleasant weather.

When tested at the clinic the child showed normal intelligence; her intelligence quotient was 105. As usual, she was shy and bashful.

There was considerable friction at home. The father was cruel and abusive to his wife and was interested in other women. He paid no attention to the children. The mother had no social outlets. There were, moreover, religious differences between the parents. All this resulted in many bitter quarrels in the presence of the children.

Careful study of this case showed that after one of the parents' quarrels the child's stammering increased noticeably and her withdrawal became more apparent. The mother was urged to allow the child to play outdoors without too much supervision from herself and to encourage the child's social contacts. Arrangements were made to have the mother and the children attend a camp. The harm of overprotection and the results of marital difficulties as they related to the child's problem were discussed. The mother tried to cooperate with the clinic as far as she could, and the child developed more independence.

In the following case shyness was associated with general timidity.

Pauline was referred to the clinic at the age of 5 years and 9 months because of her extreme shyness. She was also described as oversensitive and timid and given to crying easily.

This child's birth had been difficult (breech presentation) but her development was normal. She had been in good health until her fourth year and then within 1 year she had measles, whooping cough, and mastoiditis. She recovered from all these infections. She wore arch supports to correct flat feet.

but suffered from no other defects. Her eating, sleeping, and toilet habits were normal.

Her mother described her as being very shy and as having a tendency to be unduly anxious and worried over minor matters. When she was with other people she was likely to hang her head and seem embarrassed, especially in large groups and in school.

These traits were demonstrated at the clinic. In the clinic playroom the child stayed close to her mother and was very reluctant to join the other children. She was overconscientious about the order of the toys, chairs, and other equipment in the room.

The parents were intelligent and the home atmosphere was harmonious in spite of financial strain. There were two other children, who seemed entirely normal. A sister of the patient had died during the preceding winter and this experience had a serious effect on her. She was sensitive to her mother's grief over this loss and would try to comfort her. At the same time she was apparently having reactions of her own to this experience as well as to the family financial difficulties. Her mother observed that she seemed to be "walking in a trance."

In the psychological examination this child proved to be of good intelligence, having an intelligence quotient of 113.

In the absence of either physical or mental handicap, treatment was directed toward increased socialization of the child and a change in the family methods of discipline. The mother cooperated well with the clinic. She not only allowed the child to play more freely with other children, but she restrained herself in the use of peremptory commands and in her constant emphasis on cleanliness and manners. In the more relaxed atmosphere the child soon lost some of her tenseness and no longer found it necessary to hide behind a wall of shyness.

The death of some member of the family is often the source of behavior difficulty in a child—not that death in itself is a cause of behavior problems but that members of the family are often unwise in their explanation of it or in the display of their own emotions and attitudes.

The following case is interesting in its presentation of an unusually complex method used by a 4-year-old child to escape the mental anguish associated with the death of his grandmother. It also indicates that even at this early age the child meets his problem quite differently in relation to different individuals. The symptoms in this case were such as to cause real anxiety, for the child's regression from reality into a world of fantasy seemed complete at times. However, responses of this type to difficult life situations are not particularly uncommon in children. Although every effort should be made to so organize the child's mental outlook on life that he may become more objective and deal more efficiently with reality, the implications of such symptoms during the preschool years are quite different and of less significance in relation to actual mental disease than would be the case in a preadolescent child.

A mother brought a lad of 4 years to the clinic because of persistent masturbation and stubbornness. An analysis of the case revealed a complicated situation. The family history disclosed tuberculosis on both sides of the family. The general background was poor and unstable. The maternal relatives and the patient's immediate family were dependent upon public aid.

The home atmosphere was far from serene. The father was in poor health and took only a passive part in family life. The mother was erratic and inconsistent in her discipline and showed definite favoritism toward the boy's younger sister and an antagonistic attitude toward the boy. The home was shared by an aunt and an uncle, the latter adding to the difficulties by calling the boy a "sissy" and constantly teasing him in this way.

Further study of the case showed that the boy had been much attached to his grandmother, with whom he had spent much time. At the time of her death he had stayed with the family upstairs and had cried bitterly for her, saying, "My grandma's gone." He was told by his mother that grandma had gone to New York. Two months later, however, he told his mother that his grandmother was dead, that she "went down a big hole." He continued to talk incessantly of his grandmother. Whenever he had a pencil he would write letters to her, often saying that he heard his "grandma calling him"; and when punished, he would say, "I'll go to grandma." He called for her in his sleep. His mother at times found him gazing at his grandmother's picture and holding imaginary conversations with her. When his mother interrupted him he would be very angry with her, saying he hated her, telling her to get out and stay out, and even trying to strike her.

The mother claimed that his attitude had changed completely since the grandmother's death. Whereas, formerly, she had had no fault to find with him, he now cried for the least little thing, had become bold, and was unkind and disagreeable to her.

From the account given by the mother one felt that the child presented certain symptoms quite malignant from a mental point of view and that he was in need of careful study and supervision.

The boy was normal physically but had many personality defects in his make-up. He was very jealous of his little sister and selfish with her, probably because his mother openly favored her. He held a bitter, antagonistic feeling toward his mother and said that he hated her. She interpreted everything he did as being "fresh and bold" and expressed herself as too disgusted with him ever to bother to praise him. His uncle's teasing made him feel inferior, and he resented being called "sissy." He preferred to play with dolls and games about the house, and it was not surprising to find that he had always been kept close to his family and was not allowed to play with other children. He was afraid of the dark and cried out in the night that pigeons were biting him. His mother admitted that she had at times frightened him in order to make him obey. He wet his clothes and had temper tantrums.

In the treatment of this case there were several factors to be dealt with. The most important was the mother, who had to be reeducated in her attitude toward the patient and in her methods of discipline. The father had to be made to realize his responsibilities and the child had to be educated to meet his problems in a more satisfactory manner.

The treatment consisted of frequent visits to the clinic and long talks with the doctor. The mother's attitude was changed; masturbation was stopped by means of diversion and the substitution of other interests; the child was desensitized to the dark through education and through his love of approbation; enuresis was stopped by the institution of routine measures; the boy was allowed to play outdoors with other children; and he was no longer teased or called "sissy." Within a few months the child made a perfectly satisfactory adjustment to his home and to his play activities. Subsequent investigation showed that he continued to make a very good adjustment to life.

*Comment.*—The foregoing case is not particularly different from other cases cited, except for the reaction of the patient to the death of his grandmother. With his playmates he met the situation in a fairly satisfactory way. He would talk about making trips with them to New York to see his grandmother, apparently refusing to think of her as being gone in the sense that she would never return, and undoubtedly lessening the sting by handling the situation as a child might be expected to do. With his mother he apparently faced the question openly and frankly, and his antagonism toward her indicates that he felt her to be responsible in some way for the grandmother's death. He stated that the grandmother was "in a hole in the ground." This was his conception of death, the child having none of the conceptions of the hereafter which those of his age usually entertain and which help them to face such sorrowful situations during their early years. When alone, however, he withdrew more completely from the realities surrounding the situation and carried on imaginary conversations. If these symptoms had been presented in a child 10 or 15 years older, they would have appeared to be rather definite psychotic symptoms, but in children it is extremely difficult to separate the products of daydreams and unfilled wishes from symptoms that have graver significance.

There is no cause for alarm if children have playmates of an imaginary character or if they hold conversations with their dolls or other toys. Not infrequently their own personalities split up temporarily so that they are dealing apparently with two or three distinct individuals at the same time, asking and answering questions, praising one and punishing the other. It is these more imaginative children who make up the dreamers of later life, some of them achieving success because of these dreams, other falling by the wayside, unable to cope with their more materialistic brothers.

There is cause for concern only when these definite retreats are used by the child to meet some definite problem which has made unusual demands upon his powers of adjustment. Here it indicates, perhaps, a type of reaction which later in life may be developed and utilized to the disadvantage of himself and all others concerned.

Isolated fears are often found to be due to threats thoughtlessly made by parents or other people who are concerned with the problem of breaking some undesirable habit acquired by a child. This may be seen in the case of Gladys.

Gladys was 3 years and 1 month old when she was first brought to the clinic by her mother because of fears.

Birth was 3 weeks premature but normal. Her development was normal and her health history, except for pneumonia in infancy and several severe colds, was good. She was still wetting the bed at night and was receiving considerable attention during mealtime and bedtime. She slept well except after an attack of fear, during which she would stand up in bed and cry for her mother. She often had "muscular spasms," which came during the night, waking her out of her sleep. At such times she would scream violently, clutch at her mother convulsively, and become limp after a few minutes. The physician who examined her reported that these were not convulsions.

Being the only girl and considerably younger than her two brothers, Gladys was always the recipient of much attention from the family. She was, moreover, a much-wanted child, her parents having longed to have a girl for some time preceding her birth. An atmosphere was built up in which "everybody always shushed for Gladys." She became self-confident, happy, friendly, and affectionate, with no fear of people.

Her chief fear seemed to be of the wind. As a small child she had been in the habit of getting up in bed during the night and her mother had tried to stop this by threatening that the wind would blow over her and she would get sick if she did not stay under the covers. She began to think of the wind as a terrifying monster leaning over her, and she would become especially frightened when she heard the autumn wind blowing through the trees. Thunderstorms were terrifying to her. She was very much afraid of the vacuum cleaner and always stayed on a chair when her mother used it.

During one of her "muscular spasms" the patient began looking around in her bedroom as if fearing some horrible specter. She gave her parents the impression that her acute fear was due to the imagined approach of some dreadful monster whom she referred to as "pain."

This child had at one time had the habit of pulling her hair out and chewing it to such an extent that she actually had bald spots on her head. To break her of this habit, a friend of her mother told her that "some awful thing" would come and grab her hand away from her head. Although at that time she stopped pulling her hair, she began to have a continuous fear of this monster.

Another group of cases in which fear plays a very important part during the early part of the individual's life and is often carried into late adolescence and sometimes never completely eradicated, includes those cases in which some form of sex activity has played a part. Frequently sex problems are created in this way by the parents. One little girl who was battling the problem of masturbation happened to live near one of the State hospitals for the insane, and it was firmly impressed upon her that if she continued the habit she would eventually end there. She was taken around the institution in order that the threat might be more firmly imprinted upon her mind. The child was told that everybody would soon know what she was doing—that they could tell by her expression and by the way she acted. Other children are threatened with operations under the same conditions. It is not unusual to find parents mutilating the fingers of young children, either by burning them or by pricking them, because of this habit.

It is hardly necessary to say how acutely sensitized the young, immature mind becomes to the habit of sex when such drastic measures are taken by interested but injudicious parents. Many of the inadequacies of adult personalities undoubtedly had their origin in feelings of inferiority that were stimulated during childhood. Apparently everything is done to make these children feel that they are different, and it is not surprising that they become shy, timid, and self-centered. Finding themselves in association with others who are quite intolerable to them, they seek solitude and build up in fantasy a dream world in which they can reside unmolested.

The situation of the child who flees from reality and finds consolation for his feelings of inferiority in a world of fantasy is well illustrated by the following case:

Harry had not quite reached 10 years of age when he was first seen at the clinic. He was described by his grandmother as being a lonesome, friendless child. She stated that her earliest recollection of the boy was that of hearing him tell her about an imaginary "friend boy" and that up to the time of his coming to the clinic his chief companions were various insects and imaginary children. He did not get on well with other children in school and was regarded as queer. He was very fond of old people and very sympathetic with them, being "very much upset," for example, over seeing an old lady crying in church. He was very responsive to music, singing church litanies to himself and improvising songs about fairies.

In spite of the fact that this lad had a good intellectual equipment, with an intelligence quotient of 121, his adjustment to school had been rather poor.

The boy was very restless during his sleep, talking as if he were fighting with someone, shouting, and tossing about, and occasionally laughing. His general health was good. He lived with his paternal grandparents, who had adopted him and his sister at the time of the death of their parents. The home, although small (a three-room apartment) was comfortable but obviously lacking in space for play. The problem presented was mainly one of withdrawal, daydreaming, and running away from life as it actually exists. The boy had an unusually acute imagination, was very keen in his observations, and could occupy himself with his fantasies for hours at a time. He would carry on imaginary conversations with a grasshopper, philosophize over the different cloud formations and what they might mean, and discuss with himself the observations that he had made upon the different kinds of trees and other living things. He appeared to be on intimate terms with fairies and he symbolized them by taking a couple of match sticks wrapped in silver paper and describing them as the fairy king and queen to whom he would sing. According to his grandmother these imaginary figures became so real to him that he would leave them with great reluctance, saying he was afraid to go away lest they be unhappy. He also had imaginary children as playmates.

During his psychological examination at the clinic he talked to himself a great deal, seemed to be thinking aloud, often about things that were irrelevant to the examination. His manner to the examiner was, however, responsive and friendly.

After helping his grandparents to build up a more objective sort of existence for this child by getting him promoted to the fourth grade where he belonged and by helping him make contacts with children in a "play group" who were more congenial than those of his immediate neighborhood, the clinic was able to close the case at the end of 11 months with the report that the child was making a satisfactory adjustment.

78985°—39——6

## PROBLEMS ASSOCIATED WITH THE DEVELOPMENT OF THE CHILD'S SEX LIFE

Parents who at some time have received help from the clinic in the handling of a specific problem often come to regard the clinic as an educational center to which they may turn for advice and suggestions on various subjects connected with child training. They may wish guidance in choosing toys and play equipment or suggestions for children's books, or advice regarding a child's speech development, or help in considering a summer camp. No less frequently, however, they want help in handling some aspect of their child's sex education.

The question how reproduction occurs is one that every child with average curiosity will ask sooner or later unless some experience has made him unduly self-conscious and prematurely reticent. By the time a child is four, he has probably asked about the origin of babies many times. The answer given by the parents depends largely on their own sex adjustment and their attitude toward the subject. The clinic can be of great help, however, in giving parents an opportunity to think out and talk over some of the concepts which they wish to give the child.

The whole task of sex education can be made easier for parents if they are encouraged to keep these two thoughts in mind: First, that they must be absolutely honest as far as they go at any one time so that they will not be obliged to retract some of their statements later; and second, that they are telling the child about the normal, natural process of reproduction and not about sexual intercourse. The young child has no curiosity about adult emotional relationships or the actual process of conception. He is, however, vitally concerned and intensely curious about his origin, and the facts are so simple and understandable if presented frankly and unemotionally that the child can be completely satisfied. If parents will answer the question of the preschool child about reproduction without making him feel that he has introduced an unclean subject which only naughty children speak of, something will have been accomplished. It is a real achievement if the parent can make the child feel that he has brought up one of the most interesting topics in the world and if he can show the child, so far as his age and intelligence will permit, why it is interesting.

The knowledge of reproduction is in itself not so important as the attitude and emotional response which such an approach will foster in the child. In this connection the clinic can be of great help in giving parents an opportunity to rehearse—at least in their own minds—what their own attitude and emotional response will be. It is not enough for the clinic workers to tell a timid and inhibited parent that he must state the facts truthfully, for in that case the clinic worker is actually being as evasive as many parents. The workers should be as frank as they advise parents to be. For many parents the experience of hearing another person speak of the sex organs by name, simply and correctly, is of the greatest benefit in helping them to overcome self-consciousness in approaching the subject.

Clinic groups that find it impossible or impractical to give this type of help to individual parents may accomplish similar results by arranging to have part of a parents' conference or one of a series of lectures for parents devoted to this subject. The clinic may provide the speaker or leader from its own staff, or may sponsor presentation by an outside person.

Reproduction is a topic to be neither featured nor ignored. Not all problems will be eliminated even when reproduction and sex are wisely presented to children, but the problems will be easier to manage, and parents will be in a far better position to help if they have been accepted by the child as guides and counselors. It is fortunate, indeed, that some of the taboos regarding sex are being lifted and that older children are no longer entirely dependent upon the parent and the home for honest information regarding these vital matters. The preschool child, however, must still depend on parents and parents must therefore assume the responsibility of seeing that the child embarks upon life with a wholesome outlook and an intelligent understanding of the process of reproduction.

In addition to helping parents in the matter of sex education, the clinic offers help in handling the various habits and attitudes arising in connection with the child's sex development. Common among these is the habit of masturbation.

Mothers of problem children frequently say that the habit of masturbation began at such an early date in the life of the child that it is impossible to tell when it did start. One child said that he had "handled himself" ever since birth. Such statements bear witness to the fact that the child may become aware at an early age that he can arouse pleasurable sensations by manipulating the genitals and other erogenous zones. This awareness is usually brought about by some external stimulation such as may be caused when the child is given a bath, when uncleanliness gives rise to various irritations, when the child makes a rather minute investigation of his own body, and all too frequently when older children become curious about sex and make investigation of smaller children. In certain cases sexual precocity has been deliberately stimulated by irresponsible nursemaids.

It is not desired to convey the impression that masturbation begins so early in the great majority of children. When it does begin in these immature years it invariably lasts a short time. It may recur between the ages of 10 and 14. In fact it is so common during this period that a transitory period of masturbation about the age of puberty is generally considered quite normal.

The masturbatory act is usually carried on by irritating the external genitals with the hand, but children occasionally use sticks, pencils, and other small objects for this purpose. The act is often complicated by other manipulations which apparently add to the pleasure. Thumb sucking, rectal irritation, and rubbing the navel are most common, and any one of these acts may be performed alone to the satisfaction of the child.

Visits to the toilet are frequently events of great interest to children, and it is not unusual to find that masturbation occurs only at these times. Not only their own visits to the toilet but those of the adult members of the household are of interest. One little girl was brought to the clinic on account of her interest in seeing people nude. She was accustomed to secrete herself behind the bed or in the closet or to peep through the keyhole and put many other ingenious schemes into operation to see any of the adult members of the family nude.

Other children are unduly sensitive about being in the presence of any member of the family while disrobing, and at a very early age they are what we commonly term "prudish" regarding the problem of sex.

Most of these youngsters, from a therapeutic point of view, fall into two groups: (1) Those who cling very tenaciously to these pleasures and in fact to all the pleasures of their lives, and (2) those who give them up with little reluctance. Members of the latter group need little or nothing more than to have their energizing forces sublimated along some more desirable path, and stress should be laid on the development of some new interest rather than on the undesirable habit. The treatment must be outlined to cover not a few days or a week but a period of several weeks. The parents' fears and anxieties over the outcome of the habit must be allayed so that they can carry out the treatment without undue emotion. All that is usually required in such cases is to attract the child's attention with a picture or a game when he is in the act of performing the undesirable habit. Other methods that require ingenuity may be used, such as directing the child's attention to some situation, even though it is only of passing interest, if it is sufficiently unique to hold his attention for the moment. The habit, of itself, gradually subsides. This habit in young children is not so serious as in older children with whom masturbation occurs only in seclusion, for in the early years the asocial quality of the act is not yet appreciated. Parents may be assured that no undue anxiety regarding these cases is justified if the child is directed with intelligence.

The cases that present the most difficult problem for treatment are those of children who turn to masturbation only when they are in unhappy or despondent moods. They find in this habit a source of comfort, and a comfort which is always at hand. As they grow older they may continue to indulge in the habit much as children turn to thumb sucking, especially as a means of inducing sleep. They may not experience any particular sex urge at the time, but they are bothered by a general, indescribable feeling of unrest, both physical and mental, which they find can be subdued if a sufficiently strong sex feeling can be stimulated.

The most practical method of treatment is as follows:

(1) Careful physical examination to determine whether there are any definite sources of irritation.

(2) Absolute cleanliness.

(3) Knowledge of those with whom the child is making intimate contacts.

(4) Knowing the child well enough to be able to understand his moods fairly well and appreciating the fact that masturbation is frequently sought as a retreat from unhappiness.

(5) Allaying the fears and anxieties of the parents and helping them to realize that dangers to the physical and mental well-being of the child are more apt to come from injudicious treatment than from the habit itself.

In any attempt to dispense with an undesirable habit something must be substituted for what is being taken away. Not only must approval replace disapproval, pleasure replace pain, and reward replace punishment, but some very definite and tangible method of sublimating energy must be presented to the child and presented in such a way that it can be utilized.

Considerable experience has shown that mechanical appliances which are used for restraining children are of little value unless the child is at an age when he can fully appreciate why the restraint is being used and can develop a state of mind in which he is quite willing to cooperate instead of resenting the treatment. If restraint is used forcibly the situation resolves itself into an open battle between the child and the parents in which both are doomed to lose; for invariably the child clings to the undesirable habit in spite of these drastic measures.

The following case is presented in considerable detail because it brings out several important points regarding the early development of sex interest in children and because it is further complicated by convulsions of an epileptoid character, which was the symptom that brought the patient under observation.

Frances, a 9-year-old girl, was brought to the clinic by a social worker for two definite reasons: (1) Because of convulsions which resembled epilepsy and (2) because of her precocious sex interest and sex delinquencies, which had begun when she was between 5 and 6 years of age. The episode that brought the child to the attention of the referring agency was that the child's teacher found an obscene picture in her possession.

Physical findings were negative, except for a positive tuberculin test and the "spells" which resembled petit-mal attacks. The gynecological examination that was made on account of the social history indicated a certain amount of irritation of the genital organs. The child was well developed and well nourished.

The child's intelligence quotient was found to be 111. Mental findings graded the child 1 year above her chronological age, which gave her an intelligence quotient of 111 on the Stanford scale. All the tests given were responded to at about the same level except that for rote memory, which was particularly good, and that for practical judgment, which was below her mental age. She was much interested and entered eagerly into the spirit of the tests. She was in the third grade at school and was capable of doing work above the average. The teacher considered the child very bright but stated that at times she appeared extremely absent-minded.

The parents reported that the child had "immoral habits," that she never sought girl friends but was always in the company of boys, and that she had immoral relations with them.

No information was obtained regarding the grandparents of the patient, but her father appeared to be a fine, self-respecting man, who was making every effort to do all he could for the welfare of his family. The child's mother had died 4 years previous to the time of the clinic visit. She had been epileptic and hypersexual to a marked degree. She died at a psychopathic hospital in a toxic psychosis. The child's father had married a second time and the stepmother seemed to be kindly and affectionate toward the child and interested in her welfare. In matters of discipline concerning the younger children, she received but little support and encouragement from the three older married sisters in the family.

The child had been living at home with her father, stepmother, and brother John, aged 13. The latter was said to be a quiet boy but it was learned that he indulged in petty stealing and had been arrested twice. There were three older married sisters who continually interested themselves in the father's household, much against the wishes of their stepmother and probably to the disadvantage of the home. The father stated that none of his children seemed normal. He had always had difficulty in bringing them up. They were delinquent, misbehaved, and had bad reputations. On the whole there seemed to be nothing obvious in the immediate household to account for the delinquent tendencies of the children.

For the last 3 years Frances had interested herself in boys, although according to her own story she did not exclude girls as companions in her erotic indulgences. From the history it appeared that the patient had been more of an influence on the environment than the environment had been upon her. The father stated that since the child was 3 years of age she had shown an abnormal interest in sexual things and had been quite aware of her own sex feelings and how to stimulate them. When returning from the moving pictures she appeared to remember nothing but the sensual aspect of the picture. On several occasions the patient had been found in the cellar of an unoccupied house, with three or four boys of her own age. She told her father what had happened and showed no sense of shame in speaking of the active part she played in these episodes.

In the doctor's office she answered all questions frankly and showed herself an extremely precocious individual with an intimate knowledge of sex affairs which could have had its basis only in personal experience. She made no effort to minimize her part in these events and voluntarily expressed a desire to overcome these hypersexual tendencies. She discussed the entire situation without embarrassment, went into the minutest details, and discussed her innermost thoughts and dreams in an interesting and enlightening way. She appreciated the effort that she must make in order to overcome the cravings and desires responsible for her past difficulties. She was also anxious to develop other interests to substitute for her erotic daydreams. At no time did she blame others for her trouble, and she stated that she was extremely anxious to overcome her undesirable habits in order to make it easier for her stepmother, to whom she was apparently very much attached.

This case presented two definite problems for solution: (1) The convulsive tendency and (2) the precocious sex interest and sex delinquencies. Physical findings in the case were essentially negative. Mental findings indicated that the child had more than ordinary intelligence. Her teacher considered her bright. The delinquent behavior might have been considered accidental in origin and as being continued because of hypersexual cravings. Home conditions were not ideal, yet they were not sufficiently difficult to account entirely for the strain of delinquency found in this family. Associations were neither better nor worse than those found in many districts. Nothing in the mental make-up of the child or in the environmental conditions stood out distinctly as the exciting factor of her difficulties.

The effect of such a series of experiences upon the development of character and personality in the child is open to conjecture. The reason for the particular experiences at such an immature age in this individual case may well be considered as environmental or accidental. The effect of such an experience depends upon circumstances and conditions that are beyond the control of the child, and the solution is quite as dependent upon accident as was the origin of the primary experience.

The fact that this child was of rather high-grade mental equipment and somewhat precocious in her interests other than her sex interests was indeed fortunate, for the experience could be very well assimilated and digested by the child, minimized by the parents, and perhaps turned to some good purpose. On the other hand, the habit might be repressed so completely as to lose its own identity entirely, only to appear in some quite pathological condition or some definite asocial act—as apparently occurred with this patient in her hysterical episodes. Again, the experience might be rather imperfectly repressed; and continually and persistently forcing its way into consciousness, might produce disintegration of the personality such as is manifested in many of the psychoneuroses of the neurasthenic and anxiety types.

From a physiological point of view it is not difficult to conceive of such early sex experiences as sensitizing the individual to subsequent emotional experiences of a sexual nature and producing a hypersexual individual whose sexual outlet may be prostitution, homosexuality, or other perversions. Notwithstanding the fact that this tremendous physiological sexual drive may exist, it is not unlikely that such an experience would produce a psychological repugnance to sex, the two forces combating each other and resulting in conflicts that torment and incapacitate.

While the child is passing through these experiences she needs all the help and understanding that she can get from those having the case in charge. To wait 20 years and then begin philosophizing about the effect of such early sexual experience and its relation to the nervous breakdown of an adult is perhaps easier than to get a clear, concise picture of just what is taking place when the child is passing through the experiences. But there is no comparison in real value between gaining information while the forces are operating and guessing later what actually happened, how the mental mechanism worked, and what effects the experience had on the development of the individual.

## PERSONALITY CHANGES FOLLOWING ILLNESS AND INJURY

Parents are frequently inclined to blame an illness, an operation, or an accident for some change in the behavior of the child, when a careful examination and thorough investigation of all the facts surrounding the problem would indicate that the illness or accident has been to blame only in so altering the relationship of the child to his environment as to allow these personality problems to develop.

It is only natural that parents are deeply concerned when a child is ill, especially if the condition is at all serious. Their anxiety over the welfare of the child is often out of all proportion to what the situation really warrants. Whether the child has been cared for at home or in a hospital, the period of illness and convalescence is one during which the entire household revolves around the child. The other children are instructed to give in at all times to the ailing member. His every want is anticipated, and his demands, however numerous and varied, are satisfied at the earliest possible moment. He is in a position to commandeer everything in his environment and, needless to say, it is not an unattractive situation in which he finds himself.

For the first time, so far as he can remember, he is the center of attraction and attention. He never before appreciated just how important he really was. Before this illness he had had to give and take with the rest of the family. He had his responsibilities and he was expected to "carry on" like the other children in the family. He took his shares of punishment and accepted it, but now everything has changed to his advantage. It is therefore not surprising that the child who finds himself in this situation should get an exaggerated idea of his own importance and that after he has enjoyed these indulgences on the part of the oversolicitous parents he should cling rather tenaciously to his new position, being reluctant to give up the symptoms which created it.

A typical example is that of James, whose mother said, "James is very restless, cries easily, twitches his arms and body muscles, is very irritable, flies into tempers, and cannot sleep nights." This change appeared after his return from a hospital where he had been treated following an accident. He became very surly, always looked ugly, seldom smiled, and appeared unhappy and discontented. He had become so different since the accident that the boys started to call him "Empty-head." The problem confronting the mother was whether she should follow the advice of her lawyer and sue for damages. Fortunately, however, her primary interest was in the recovery of the lad. Inquiry revealed that since the accident the routine of the household had revolved around the patient. Every whim was gratified regarding his food; other children were notified that they must accede to his every wish; all the toys were his to accept or to reject; and the lad found himself in the limelight.

After a careful physical and neurological examination had been made, it was planned to change the regime of the household. The mother was to revert to the old plan of making the child give and take and battle for what he could get with the rest of the children. In just 1 month his mother reported that he was happy and contented and played with the other boys, had lost his surliness, was getting along well in school, and showed no evidence of the personality change which was so apparent when he first came under observation.

Many of these problems might have been avoided had the parents appreciated just what all this attention might mean to the child. The most important part of most illnesses is the convalescing period. At this time the parents must use the best judgment to avoid not only prolonging the illness but creating attitudes on the part of the child toward the illness which cause trouble later. Quarrelsomeness, jealousy, selfishness, disobedience, sullenness, tempers, and many other undesirable personality traits may have their origin during the convalescent period.

Although many of these personality changes have a definite psychological basis, it has been recognized within the last 10 years that many cases of marked personality change are the result of encephalitis. These changes may manifest themselves in a deep apathy or a marked hyperactivity characterized by irritability, destructiveness, and not infrequently by violent temper. Occasionally delusions and hallucinatory experiences are also associated with them. Such changes are usually preceded by a fairly typical history of encephalitis, which should ordinarily not be confused with other diseases. There are, however, a number of cases in which the attack was so mild that the diagnosis of encephalitis was not made but which were nevertheless followed by marked change in personality.

This point should be kept in mind in making a diagnosis and planning treatment. Obviously the ordinary clinic measures carried out on a psychological level or any reconstruction of the environment do not materially alter the conduct of these children. The treatment to a very large extent is one of reeducation under adequate supervision.

Another situation that may arise with reference to personality changes and their relation to accidents is brought about when parents take the opportunity of blaming illness and accidents for undesirable behavior. Thus, the mother of an 8-year-old child gave a history of the child's lying, stealing, being cruel, and other asocial conduct as beginning after a coasting accident which took place about a year before the time of her coming to the clinic. A subsequent social investigation revealed, however, that this child had been a serious problem at home, at school, and on the street for several years; that he was well known to the police and the truant officers; and that although the accident itself and the attention which the child received may have exaggerated the situation, it could in no way be regarded as the cause.

Undoubtedly certain peculiar personality traits are developed by children who suffer from such chronic diseases as diabetes and cardiac conditions which have limited their activities and prevented them from participating in a normal way with children of their own age and by children who have been the victims of illnesses like infantile paralysis which leave physical handicaps. Usually, however, those children who are handicapped by infantile paralysis in early life are remarkably free from personality changes. This may be due to the fact that the limitations imposed by the illness are present at such an early age that the child learns to live with the difficulty from the very beginning. Furthermore, the handicap is of such a nature that his contemporaries make certain allowances for it. The cardiac and diabetic children, however, have no such obvious defect. Children with heart conditions become overwhelmed by their inability to compete with other children after they have recovered from the disability and so may develop a feeling of inferiority. But the diabetic child is more likely to become critical, irritable, resentful, and defiant unless wisely managed from the beginning of his illness. These personality traits are not characteristic of the respective illnesses, but they are observed with sufficient frequency to be worthy of comment.

It should always be remembered that every family has its own history and its own associations which color its attitude in a new situation. Prolonged and exaggerated solicitude over a child who is ill with measles may seem quite out of proportion to the cause until one learns that an older child lost his hearing following an attack of measles. It is important to get a complete history in order to interpret these situations correctly and arrive at a practical therapeutic approach.

The following case, discussed in some detail, is of interest in this connection.

Randolph was referred to the clinic at the age of 3 years because of a personality change first noticed on his return from the hospital, where he had been confined with diphtheria. He was quarrelsome and had frequent temper tantrums, during which he threw himself on the floor and kicked and screamed for long periods. At night he refused to go to bed unless accompanied by his mother, and occasionally he had night terrors. In addition, he was capricious about food and had developed the habit of soiling himself daily.

This boy's birth and early development were uneventful except for a mild attack of scurvy when he was a year old, and the attack of diphtheria already mentioned.

The father had suffered a nervous break-down a year before. Although he was occasionally irritable he was, on the whole, a generous and considerate father and an excellent provider. The mother was well meaning, but highly neurotic and unstable and she had many superstitious interpretations of the simplest incidents. An older boy had died of diphtheria and she had not fully recovered from her sorrow, a fact which had considerable bearing on her present condition. Besides a younger brother there was in the household the maternal grandmother, who interfered greatly with the discipline. According to the mother the grandmother "would turn the house upside down to please the children, as she hated to hear them cry."

Prior to the boy's illness his mother had noticed nothing peculiar in his behavior, but following his return she had observed a decided change. He was sullen, irritable, seclusive, and unreasonable. He expected more than his share of attention and went into a tantrum when it was not forthcoming. He went to the window every night before retiring and, looking upward, bade good night to God and his older brother—a practice which his mother considered uncanny and unexplainable. He had not been permitted to play with the other children in the neighborhood because of his peculiarities and because none of them were his age. The mother complained that it was impossible to have the child remain in the bedroom alone before going to sleep—he begged her to remain with him to make sure there were no wolves outside the door. He entertained this constant fear of having wolves enter the room.

On his first visit to the clinic the boy refused to leave his mother or to permit her to enter the examining room without him. When she left he flung himself upon the floor and remained there in a rigid state until her return. She then picked him up and allowed him to bury his head in her bosom, simulating a nursing child. He later began to pout and talk in a babylike fashion but refused to converse with the examiner.

The intellectual equipment of this boy was about average. He had an intelligence quotient of 98.

This is a case which superficially would impress one as having all the essentials of an early mental aberration, were one to base one's conclusions entirely on the mother's interpretations and findings without further analysis of the situation. Indications which the mother accepted as being highly ominous were really nothing more than would be expected in a child of this particular make-up living in such an environment and influenced moreover by a factor which will be mentioned shortly.

The mother, grief-stricken over the death of her older son (who had died while the patient was convalescing), attempted to compensate for her loss by indulging the patient to an unlimited degree. Everything began to center around him. He was the one attraction in the house and all the members of the household exhibited their joy at his recovery. The child saw himself in this prominent and not unpleasant position and it was not long before he took full advantage of it by making numerous demands which the family readily granted.

At one time the family had employed a maid who had nightly threatened the child with a wolf story before he went to bed. She used this story in an attempt to hurry him to bed and always warned him to remain in the room lest he be captured by the wolf. This bit of information revealed the origin of his fear of wolves.

Later it had been the grandmother's privilege to prepare the patient for bed. She would undress him, hear his prayers, and, before putting him to bed, take him to the window and have him bid good night to his deceased brother, who, she explained, was watching over him with God. When the development of this particular practice was explained to the mother she no longer looked upon it as being a mysterious procedure but realized that it was simply what his grandmother had taught him.

Much of the success of the treatment in this case rested on the mother's acceptance of modern methods of dealing with the child's problem and the destruction of many of the superstitions which had previously handicapped her. After a short psychotherapeutic talk she was found to be most cooperative and willing to carry out the treatment in detail.

A chart was given to the mother to help her solve the feeding problem, and measures were taken to desensitize the child to fear of wolves. He no longer was to assume the role of invalid but was to take his place in the household on an equal footing with his younger brother.

The child made three visits to the clinic. On his last visit his mother reported that he went to bed unaccompanied, that he no longer talked about wolves, and that he had earned his complete quota of stars on the chart. His marked aversion for milk had been overcome and he drank it unprotestingly with every meal. The family was leaving for a summer resort where it was hoped he would be given a wider opportunity for contacts with children of his own age.

## CONVULSIONS, TICS, MANNERISMS

When one considers that more than half of all individuals suffering from chronic convulsive disorders in adult life, the so-called epileptics, had their first convulsion prior to the fourth year of life, the importance of convulsions in children becomes apparent. This does not mean that the isolated convulsion which sometimes ushers in an acute infectious disease in children need be taken too seriously or cause parents undue anxiety. Any child, however, who has a series of convulsions or is prone to react to infections, falls, and emotional stresses and strains by having a convulsion is in need of the best medical attention.

A study was made of a group of children under 4 years of age who had been patients in hospitals and had suffered from convulsions associated with acute infections, spasmophilia, gastrointestinal upsets, rickets, and whooping cough. These cases were carefully followed up to discover their subsequent history. A surprisingly large number of these children eventually died of convulsions and many of those who were still living continued to have convulsions or were mentally deficient. The implication of this study is that convulsions in children should no longer be looked upon as a mere incident in their medical history nor as something that happens to every child, like an increase in temperature or a gastrointestinal upset. The convulsion itself must rather be considered as a certain criterion of the inherent instability of the nervous system. Some children are so inherently stable that the convulsions associated with actual irritation of the nervous system (such as is seen in encephalitis) may subside and leave no ill effects. This indicates that there is no well-defined limit to the amount of brain irritation that may occur without leaving ill effects. It appears that some nervous systems are capable of withstanding a rather severe disturbance such as would naturally be produced by an acute inflammatory condition of the brain. Others will succumb to a mild infection or a slight trauma, leaving behind an increased instability which responds more or less periodically to the minor vicissitudes of life and manifests itself in convulsions.

From the standpoint of preventive medicine it does not matter whether these early convulsions are of psychogenic or of biochemical origin. There seems to be little doubt in the minds of those most interested in the subject of epilepsy that each convulsion paves the way for the succeeding one, and that the path becomes deeper and the line of demarcation sharper and more easily traversed by the excess of liberated nervous energy. For this reason it is tremendously important for the future welfare of the child that a careful investigation be made, by both clinical examination and laboratory tests, to determine the exciting factor in the production of these infantile convulsions.

It is important for the pediatrician and the psychiatrist to work hand in hand. The former usually sees the child over a short period of time, but it is an extremely important time when the undesirable forces, whether they are psychogenic or chemical, are operating. The latter, on the other hand, sees the child over a longer period of time, but invariably at a period somewhat removed from that in which the exciting factors actually operate. Until a better working knowledge is obtained of the baffling phenomenon called epilepsy, it is especially important for the psychiatrist and the pediatrician to cooperate and to have a clear knowledge of each other's technique. In almost every case of a convulsive disorder it is necessary to look for both a predisposing and an exciting factor.

There is no group of cases today more worthy of the attention of those best qualified in the practice of medicine than those of early infantile convulsions. It has been said that "the child, for the first 5 years of life, is an organism so tender, so easily broken, so easily damaged, that it needs all the care that first-class intelligence can give it."

Susan, a poorly nourished and underdeveloped girl, 6 years of age, was brought to the clinic by her mother for a series of problems of which fainting spells were the most important.

There was no history of epilepsy or mental or nervous diseases in the family. The child's birth and early development had been normal; she had had the ordinary diseases of childhood. There was no history of convulsions, but the mother stated that the child, since she was 8 months of age, had had spells during which she had momentarily lost consciousness. These fainting spells, so called by the mother, usually took place when the child found herself in any difficult situation. When threatened with punishment she would fall to the floor in an apparent faint. She would hold her breath and get blue in the face. The mother would then pick her up, fondle her and put her on the bed, and the episode would be over. At other times these "fainting spells" would follow one of her temper tantrums. She would lie on the floor, kick, and yell, holding her breath for varying periods and apparently losing consciousness. She might, however, have one of the temper tantrums without the fainting spell.

The mother stated that the child was very affectionate but domineering. She always wanted "to be the boss," whether at home or at play, and usually got her own way. She was extremely stubborn and when refused she responded in the manner already described. She was said to be friendly and generous. She was jealous to the extent that she demanded at least as much attention as was given to the other children in the family. The mother repeatedly stated, "The child must have her own way. The only way to manage her is to give in to her."

*Comment.*—The foregoing history, in association with the negative physical examination, stamped these "fainting spells" as belonging to a psychogenic group of reactions. It seemed quite obvious that the child was utilizing this method to gain her own way. It is always difficult in a case of this kind to divorce the physiological aspects from the purely psychological. For example, the effect on the oxygenation of the blood of holding the breath might in itself produce unconsciousness. This case was stamped as being psychogenic by the fact that the treatment, which dealt entirely with teaching the mother how to deal with the child during one of these "fainting spells" or temper tantrums, completely relieved the symptoms. At the time of the last visit the child had not had a spell for over 2 years, although she occasionally met an unpleasant situation with the cruder method of tantrums.

---

The case of Theodore may also be mentioned. The child, aged 2 years and 5 months, was brought to the clinic on account of severe temper tantrums, which only recently had terminated in convulsions. When one considered the complete disintegration of the mental life of this patient as indicated by violent temper, insomnia associated with night terrors, enuresis, pugnacity, extreme jealousy, selfishness, destructiveness, and masturbation, it was not very difficult to explain the convulsions as one of the numerous manifestations of an inherently unstable nervous system. This manifestation at times might follow the sexual excitement of masturbaton or the extreme emotion attached to a temper tantrum, and at other times it might be the manifestation of more definitely physiological causes, such as would be associated with excessive fatigue, lack of sleep, or marked indiscretions in diet. The treatment had to be directed not toward the convulsions but rather toward rehabilitating the individual as a whole.

---

Billy, aged 4 years, was brought to the clinic because he was extremely stubborn and difficult to manage and was seemingly quite insensitive to the praise or blame of those in his environment.

In this case the first convulsion occurred at the age of 13 months and was associated with an acute infection of the influenza type. Since that time the child had had nine convulsions, occurring at intervals approximately 6 months apart. These convulsions had invariably been associated with some acute illness. One spell was associated with an acute febrile condition which lasted several days. One occurred after circumcision. Several others were in association with definite gastrointestinal upsets at the hospital. The convulsions in this case never occurred with any emotional experience, but always at such times and under such conditions that it was difficult to determine the exciting cause.

Another important factor in this case was the fact that the child was retarded mentally. When the convulsions begin at such an early age mental retardation is common. Mental deficiency of this type should not be looked upon as congenital or due to defective germ plasm. It must be assumed that the child whose nervous system is so unstable that he reacts to an acute infection with a convulsion is somewhat handicapped from the start, but that does not by any means indicate that he would have been mentally deficient if he had not had the convulsions. Many of the physical abnormalities seen in children, such as monoplegias and hemiplegias, are not congenital but appear during the first 2 years of life, following convulsion. This is a practical as well as an interesting point to be kept in mind when considering the general subject of heredity.

The treatment in such a case, so far as the convulsions are concerned, is obviously not one of psychotherapy. A special regime should be instituted in which the amount of physical and mental stress should be definitely limited. Diet is of paramount importance and one should avoid all the more indigestible articles of food and the methods of preparing food which render it less digestible. Tea, coffee, and other stimulating as well as irritating articles of diet should be eliminated. Constipation is invariably found in these cases and should be guarded against. It is best combated by a carefully selected diet, which should include much fruit, green vegetables, and bread made of whole wheat. After such a case has been carefully studied to eliminate every possible physical cause, and the proper regime has been instituted, it may also be necessary to use some drug. The treatment of such cases should always be directed by a physician.

There are many and varied physical manifestations indicating disturbance of the nervous system in children, and from the beginning all such symptoms should be considered as having a physical basis and should be referred to a physician. Chorea is one of the most common examples of what an infection may do to the nervous system, especially in a child who is inherently unstable. Chorea is usually associated with rheumatism, and the symptoms are undoubtedly due to a mild form of meningitis. Motor unrest and mental irritability invariably precede the characteristic, involuntary movements which involve the arms, legs, and frequently facial muscles. These movements may become very violent at times and the child will throw himself about in a manner that may do him bodily harm. Although it is now generally recognized that chorea is due to an infection, fatigue and excitement markedly exaggerate the symptoms.

Habit spasms sometimes present a picture that is closely allied to chorea, but the muscular involvement is less extensive, usually affecting only one group of muscles of either the upper or the lower extremity.

The spasm may take the form of blinking the eyes, wrinkling the forehead, and making a pulling movement of the facial muscles, especially the nose, which result in peculiar grimaces. Spasms of spitting, coughing, and peculiar types of breathing are also observed frequently. When these involuntary movements have been present over a period of months or years, they frequently resist treatment and an absolute cure is not always possible. This accounts for the fact that many adults are still afflicted with habit spasms that were acquired during early life. There is undoubtedly a predisposition on the part of some children which permits the ordinary stresses and strains of everyday life to throw the coordinating mechanisms of the brain out of adjustment. The first evidence of this instability may be precipitated by fright, grief, intense anger, or physical fatigue. These habit spasms are not infrequently seen in children when there is a history of prolonged mental exertion, as for example, the child who is subjected to a school program plus outside activities such as music and dancing lessons that make up an intellectual and physical load beyond his ability to carry. These symptoms are but the first evidence that the child is working too hard.

One must keep in mind, however, that in dealing with these problems it is not the symptoms but the child who needs treatment, and every effort should be made to determine the emotional stresses to which he is being subjected. Such an investigation leads in various directions. The discipline in the home may be too rigid; an ambitious parent may be pushing the child too hard; the child may be suffering from extreme anxiety in his personal relationships with his teacher or over failure in his work. Often teasing and bullying by his contemporaries supply the answer to the problem. Besides these more obvious situations, fears and anxieties of which the child is not aware may be operating below the level of consciousness. The symptoms are of such a nature that parents are sometimes worried and irritated and are prone to put considerable pressure on the child to make a greater effort to overcome what they consider an unattractive habit. They do not realize that the more conscious the child becomes of his difficulty the more likely it is to be exaggerated, so that nagging, scolding, and punishment are not only useless but harmful. Under a physician's direction the child should be removed from the irritations of his environment. He should have complete rest, and general routine measures for building up physical health, such as proper food, sleep, and elimination should be put in force. After the acute symptoms have subsided, it may be necessary to make important changes in the child's daily routine.

The early manifestations of these involuntary muscle spasms are often detected in a clinic when the child is brought in for some other reason. It is during the early and incipient stages of these emotional upsets that valuable preventive work can be done. These problems in themselves are not serious medical problems, but certain attitudes that develop around the problem have important implications. The child may become very self-centered, shy, and diffident, showing marked feelings of inferiority which lead him to refrain from entering into activities with other children and prevent him from developing a normal, healthy outlook upon life. Early recognition and treatment are therefore imperative.

## THE CRIPPLED CHILD

The White House Conference on Child Health and Protection in 1930 called attention to the fact that "there are more than 10,000,000 children in the United States who are 'handicapped'—in the sense in which the term is here used—i. e., children who are blind and partially seeing, deaf and hard of hearing, crippled, who are mentally deficient or disordered, who are suffering from tuberculosis, cardiac or parasitic diseases."[6] This is a very conservative statement, yet it indicates the magnitude of the problem and is a challenge to those responsible for rehabilitating, so far as possible, the physically and mentally handicapped child. The problem is further complicated when consideration is given to the interdependence of the physical, intellectual, and emotional aspects of life and the extent to which the individual's personality, his general outlook on life, and his capacity for happiness and efficiency may be materially and permanently affected by the wisdom with which handicaps are treated in early life.

The effect of physical disease, injuries, and accidents on the personality of the individual has already been discussed (pp. 82–85). The chronically ill and the permanently physically handicapped have some general problems that are not unlike those found in persons suffering from acute conditions, though it must always be taken into consideration that a particular handicap may exert a specific effect upon the personality make-up of a particular individual. The fact that one's mood or feeling of well-being is affected by the condition of the bodily organs—that is, the functioning of the liver, the gastrointestinal tract, the thyroid gland, and so forth—is so well understood that it needs no further discussion. It is not so commonly understood, however, that emotional responses toward life, such as worry, grief, or anger, affect the functioning of the bodily organs; that high blood pressure, indigestion, diarrhea, pains, or hyperacidity may be the result of a love affair, a disastrous speculation, or the loss of a job; and that cause and effect can be demonstrated, whether from the point of view that feeling tone is affected by physical ailments or vice versa. The whole problem may become very much involved, but for practical purposes it is important to keep in mind that the patient's mental attitude toward his illness or his physical handicap is of paramount importance—so important, in fact, that this attitude in itself may account for so-called personality changes and for much of the resulting incapacity.

During the last 2 decades the attitude toward the crippled child has gradually changed. Society, families, and individuals have been in the past rather prone to view these unfortunate individuals sympathetically yet pessimistically, accepting them as responsibilities for home and institutional care who were entitled to kindly consideration

[6] White House Conference, 1930: Addresses and Abstracts of Committee Reports, p. 292. Century Co., New York, 1931.

and adequate custodial supervision when facilities were available. With the development of improved surgical techniques, deformities and resulting handicaps have been greatly reduced. This has meant that certain children who were suffering from a form of physical handicap previously considered permanent have had complete correction of that deformity. Other children whose deformities could not be corrected have had normal function restored through treatment so that the deformity is no longer a handicap. With better insight into the incapacitating aspects of the mental attitude toward the handicapped, efforts have been made to consider the individual as a whole and to find some life occupation in which his deformity would be minimized and his assets given the fullest opportunity for expression. This attitude on the part of society toward the crippled child has opened many new channels through which the handicapped individual has been able to find adequate outlets for his potential physical achievements and his emotional and intellectual satisfactions. Parents, having been awakened to this new social optimism in regard to the handicapped child, have felt less sensitive about these unfortunate members of the family and as a group are seeking all available assistance as soon as they recognize the problem. Under such conditions we have a right to anticipate earlier recognition of the child's needs, better medical care, help and guidance in the selection of a vocation, improved mental attitudes on the part of the handicapped child, and in general an increase in his happiness and efficiency.

The most important therapeutic contribution that can be given to the crippled child is the assurance that there is a place for him in life, that he has a contribution to make to justify his existence, and that effort on his part is worth while. Only in this way can the will to attain the maximum degree of independence be established within the child. When this is accomplished the handicapped individual no longer indulges in introspection and self-pity but turns his attention to the outside world, where he can now find guidance and direction in preparing himself for a life of usefulness. It must be kept in mind that the attitudes which the crippled child assumes toward his handicap will invariably be but a reflection of attitudes shown by those with whom he comes in contact during his early years. The parent who is constantly reminding the child that he cannot do this or that because of his limitations or the dangers involved will contribute little toward helping him build up the attitude of confidence which is essential if he is to utilize his assets to the fullest extent. On the other hand, if the child is reared in an environment where his physical limitations are relegated to the background, where he is being constantly presented with opportunities and tasks that are well within his ability, and where his attention is focused toward intellectual interests, he soon learns that there are many ways and many opportunities by which he may compensate for his particular handicap. Every handicapped child should be not only permitted but encouraged to do everything he can possibly do for himself, and the assistance that he receives should be limited only to those tasks which are definitely beyond his ability. Only in this way will he attain that sense of normality and independence which is essential

78985°—39——7

to his ultimate success. The child who has acquired a healthy attitude toward his handicap and a sense of independence will embark upon the task of fitting himself for life with confidence and courage.

The next important step perhaps is that of selecting a vocation. Here again guidance and training are important, and the problem of determining the work which is best suited to his particular abilities and in which his handicap will be least in evidence needs careful consideration. The wise counselor will realize that the work should be selected with the idea of giving the individual not only the opportunity of doing his particular task efficiently but also the maximum amount of emotional satisfaction.

Especially careful consideration should be given to the type of vocation selected for the handicapped child. One naturally selects a field of training that offers opportunity for subsequent employment. Insofar as it is humanly possible, this particular group of individuals must be safeguarded from failure. They are invariably sensitive and are inclined to compare themselves, to their own disadvantage, with those unimpaired by handicaps; and they are prone to think in terms of what they might have achieved were it not for their handicap. It is, therefore, important that they attain success regardless of what the job may be. This is essential if confidence is to be acquired and if they are to become self-sustaining in the field of industry. It is obviously more difficult for the handicapped to throw aside training in one activity and start over in something new. No effort is too great nor time too precious to spend in helping the handicapped child to overcome those difficulties and surmount those obstacles which obstruct the path to a happy, useful, productive life. Every handicapped child must be considered as an individual needing special consideration. These children should not be looked upon as cases to be dealt with in any routine, mechanical way, as one might deal with a piece of defective machinery. They are human beings struggling to make a place for themselves in an environment in which they will meet keen competition, under conditions which, to say the least, call for all the help that science and human consideration have to offer.

One need not look far afield to find shining examples of the victory which modern surgery, wise counseling, and vocational guidance, associated with confidence and courage, have won for the handicapped child. Many of these individuals have reached peaks in their achievements, not in spite of their handicaps but because of them. Many of these young people have been stimulated to greater effort, have acquired a finer sense of values, have been aroused to loftier ambitions, and have been generally stimulated in the right direction by virtue of their handicap.

It is impossible to lay down specific rules and give definite information on how to direct the activities of any individual handicapped child. Keen appreciation of the desired objectives and of the fact that the case involves a human being and not just a deformity will do much to help the handicapped child develop to his highest degree of usefulness from a physical and an economic point of view. It will also create in him attitudes toward himself and the world that will give him assurance of his own worth, a feeling of independence, and a sense of security about life in general.

## MENTAL DEFICIENCY

Although the problem of mental deficiency is not one of primary concern to the habit clinic, it is an important problem of childhood and one that is directly related to behavior problems. Imbeciles and idiots are obviously cases for institutional care, but high-grade defectives must often be cared for in the community. The social maladjustments of the latter group are due not to the mental defect as such but rather to the accompanying mental instability. Since the advent of so-called intelligence or psychometric tests, the large number of mental defectives in the population has become more apparent, and it is realized that but a limited number can possibly be cared for in institutions. As a group they are, moreover, neither bad nor vicious, and they may serve a very useful purpose in the industrial world.

Mental tests are of real value in determining within reasonable limits the intellectual load which any child is capable of carrying. The results of such tests should receive serious consideration, however, only when the tests have been both given and interpreted by one who is expertly trained.

In testing the preschool child there are several points to keep in mind:

(1) Considerable time is required to establish friendly relationships with the child.

(2) In addition to having the child in a cooperative state of mind, it is frequently essential to get the intelligent cooperation of the mother. The child who embarks upon a psychological examination after having just overheard his mother say, "He is stubborn and won't do a thing unless I am right with him," has been given every incentive to do nothing whether the mother is present or not.

(3) It is absolutely essential to have a clinical psychologist who has sufficient imagination and flexibility and has had sufficient experience to elicit the child's maximum efforts and to evaluate the results. He must keep in mind that these children have not had the standardized training of the school. Children of preschool age who come to the clinic are often shy and reticent, afraid of new surroundings, indifferent, or inattentive. They may come from homes where little training or stimulation has been offered them. There may be language difficulties. Giving mental tests by any rule of thumb is therefore even less practical with the preschool child than it is with older children. If they are so applied, a shy, diffident, unstable child of superior intelligence may appear backward or even defective.

(4) In spite of the advances that have been made in tests to measure the intelligence of preschool children, there are still relatively few that are standardized. Nonlanguage tests are practically essential, and in checking test results a certain amount of leeway must be given the examiner, thus allowing for the child's interests and

activities at home and for his fund of general information. If it appears worth while to make a psychological examination of a child, as full a sample as possible should be made of all his abilities and disabilities.

The advantages of these examinations may be summed up briefly as follows:

(1) Unfortunate and deficient home training is shown by these examinations at an age when those trends of mental development which are stunted can be stimulated. In many cases this implies the possibility of preventing special disabilities and intensifying special abilities. The child who shows underdevelopment in ideational or verbal fields can be given special story-telling advantages—can be read to more. The child with inferior manual ability can be given more and better opportunities for manual work.

(2) Children who have unusual precocity of a specialized type (for music, color, and so forth) or of a general sort may have this precocity appreciated and developed.

(3) Children examined before starting public-school work can be put into special classes to see how much of the retardation is real and how much apparent, thus avoiding the undesirable sequelae of early school failure, the clogging of normal primary grades, and the stunting of a precocious mentality.

(4) It is essential for successful therapy with neurotic children that their intelligence be known. Obviously the feeble-minded and the precocious cannot be given the same treatment.

A careful psychological examination should be considered an important and essential part of every attempt to understand a child and his particular problem. It is important to keep in mind that the clinic has not only an obligation to the defective child but also a responsibility to the family in which that child lives. It is invariably necessary to point out to parents that the home and the lives of the normal people in that home cannot be built around the feeble-minded child. Parents of mentally defective children are not inclined to accept the diagnosis regardless of how thoroughly the case has been studied; or if they accept the diagnosis they are prone to seek every available source of help. This state of mind often leads to constant pursuit of a cure for something that is incurable. The emotionally overwrought parents feel that there must be an operation, a drug, or some bit of medical magic that will create or restore what never existed. This tragic and pathetic situation, however, is not alleviated by offering false hope. All too frequently parents devote their time and practically all their available money to building the home around the abnormal child. This deprives the normal children in the home of the opportunities to which they are entitled and at the same time creates in them jealousy, resentment, and other undesirable personality traits which prevent happy family relationships.

It is the duty of the clinic to see that physically and mentally healthy children with potentialities for worth-while achievements are not neglected because of the undue sentimentality of the parents for the mentally defective child. Whatever can be done for the defective child must be done by adequate methods of education and training. Direction as to how this training may be best obtained can be given by the clinic or other sources that are available in the community.

Extensive surgical and medical procedures are rarely called for after the child has had a careful physical examination and the necessary laboratory tests. In order to help these distraught parents to meet their problem in an intellectual rather than an emotional way and to safeguard the interests of the home, the clinic must present the problem to them with absolute frankness, regardless of how difficult such frankness may be.

The following case, although not belonging to the preschool group, is an example of what may happen to the mentally defective child who is also the victim of unintelligent parents and a sordid, immoral, poverty-stricken environment.

A girl 13 years of age was seen in jail while being held for trial because she had pushed a little boy 4 years old into the water, causing his death. The family background in this case was particularly bad; poverty, ignorance, and vice each played a part. For a long time the girl had been recognized as a menace to the community, and efforts had been made by the Society for the Prevention of Cruelty to Children to have her cared for in an institution. The mother, however, resented any interference from outside, and the case was allowed to drift along, one unhappy incident following another until this final tragedy, which demanded the attention of the law.

It was said that 2 years before, while bathing, this girl had held a youngster's head under water until the youngster was nearly drowned. A year before she had voluntarily had sexual relations with a man. At frequent intervals less serious incidents had been brought to the attention of the family and various social organizations.

In the psychological examination she graded at a mental age of 9½ years. Her emotional reaction during the examination, however, was a fair criterion of her irresponsibility.

When first visited in the jail she was very much concerned over the fact that she was being detained and could not go to the beach with her aunt. She showed little or no concern about the death of her playmate or about what would eventually happen to her. She did, however, manifest some anxiety over what the deceased lad's older sister would do to her, as the sister had threatened her before she had been sent to jail.

At the time of the next visit she was very much upset because she was not allowed to have the papers in order to read about herself and what had happened. It was almost impossible to hold her attention on any subject. She would constantly revert to the fact that "she wanted to read about herself and see what it said" and "the other prisoners who had the papers wouldn't permit her to see them." The lack of normal emotional response and the absence of concern regarding the youngster whose death she had caused are characteristic of many of the higher grade mentally deficient individuals, and it is this insensitiveness to praise and blame and lack of ability to learn from previous experience which make them a menace to society and require some type of institutional training for an indefinite period. Many of these individuals, however, eventually become stabilized through institutional care and are able to make satisfactory adjustments in the community in later life.

This case was disposed of by commitment to an institution.

## CONCLUSION

The material as presented indicates two things: First, that there is still much to be learned about the art of training children and that we are still in search of more adequate ways of overcoming undesirable habits and straightening out twisted personalities; and second, that there is an orderly, systematic, scientific approach to these problems which will produce increasingly satisfactory results as our knowledge advances.

Habits of eating, sleeping, and elimination are of fundamental importance in the development of the child's early life, and it is around these normal functions that many more serious difficulties occur in later life.

It has been pointed out that there are inherent differences in the way children are constituted mentally as well as physically. Therefore, it is not reasonable to expect all children to meet the same type of life situation in exactly the same way. In fact, it has been shown and demonstrated by case material that their responses may be very diverse. One child fights while another flees; one basks in the warmth of attention and affection while another is made self-conscious and uncomfortable by the same experience; Johnny worries over any minor deviation from the family moral code while Tommy rejoices in his success in outwitting his parents, his teacher, or the policeman. The point is that each child is in need of personal study and investigation, and no general scheme for handling problems of behavior is likely to be of any great value.

The attitudes of parents which may result from their own inadequate training and unhappy experiences in life have been shown to be among the most detrimental influences to the child during the formative years, and much that is of value in clinical and educational efforts results from helping parents with their own personal problems as they are reflected in their attitudes toward the children. One must continually remind those dealing with parents that it is not sufficient to point out the faults in their attitudes and techniques. They must also be made to understand why they persist in carrying out these attitudes in spite of the fact that they have been confronted with failure over a period of years. The point is that parents are quite unconscious of the fact that they are reacting on an emotional rather than on an intellectual level.

It is, therefore, important that the existing emotional attitude toward the child should not be exaggerated by the parents' visit to the clinic. It requires nice judgment to impress the parents with the necessity of giving serious consideration to the mental health of the child in order to avoid difficult problems later on while at the same time giving them understanding and confidence to replace worry and anxiety.

The responsibility for the mental health of the child must rest in the hands of parents, teachers, nurses, and the family physician. The same cooperative spirit in the management of the child's behavior as is evident in dealing with physical health and education will contribute much to the future happiness and efficiency of a large army of children who would otherwise embark upon life handicapped by habits, attitudes, and personality traits which result in delinquency, peculiar social behavior, antagonistic attitudes toward parents and society, and in an introspective, analytical approach to life where self is always so much in the foreground that it prevents the individual from getting the proper perspective of his environment as a whole. These distortions in outlook, when they are not caused by mental disease, are invariably the product of what the child has acquired from his early training and experience. Insofar as possible, it is the duty and responsibility of parents to see that the early career of the child is so guided and planned that he will avoid the shoals upon which many are wrecked.

# CHILDREN AND YOUTH
Social Problems and Social Policy

**An Arno Press Collection**

Abt, Henry Edward. **The Care, Cure and Education of the Crippled Child.** 1924

Addams, Jane. **My Friend, Julia Lathrop.** 1935

American Academy of Pediatrics. **Child Health Services and Pediatric Education:** Report of the Committee for the Study of Child Health Services. 1949

American Association for the Study and Prevention of Infant Mortality. **Transactions of the First Annual Meeting of the American Association for the Study and Prevention of Infant Mortality.** 1910

Baker, S. Josephine. **Fighting For Life.** 1939

Bell, Howard M. **Youth Tell Their Story:** A Study of the Conditions and Attitudes of Young People in Maryland Between the Ages of 16 and 24. 1938

Bossard, James H. S. and Eleanor S. Boll, editors. **Adolescents in Wartime.** 1944

Bossard, James H. S., editor. **Children in a Depression Decade.** 1940

Brunner, Edmund DeS. **Working With Rural Youth.** 1942

**Care of Dependent Children in the Late Nineteenth and Early Twentieth Centuries.** Introduction by Robert H. Bremner. 1974

**Care of Handicapped Children.** Introduction by Robert H. Bremner. 1974

[Chenery, William L. and Ella A. Merritt, editors]. **Standards of Child Welfare:** A Report of the Children's Bureau Conferences, May and June, 1919. 1919

**The Child Labor Bulletin, 1912, 1913.** 1974

**Children In Confinement.** Introduction by Robert M. Mennel. 1974

**Children's Bureau Studies.** Introduction by William M. Schmidt. 1974

Clopper, Edward N. **Child Labor in City Streets.** 1912

David, Paul T. **Barriers To Youth Employment.** 1942

Deutsch, Albert. **Our Rejected Children.** 1950

Drucker, Saul and Maurice Beck Hexter. **Children Astray.** 1923

Duffus, R[obert] L[uther] and L. Emmett Holt, Jr. **L. Emmett Holt:** Pioneer of a Children's Century. 1940

Fuller, Raymond G. **Child Labor and the Constitution.** 1923

Holland, Kenneth and Frank Ernest Hill. **Youth in the CCC.** 1942

Jacoby, George Paul. **Catholic Child Care in Nineteenth Century New York:** With a Correlated Summary of Public and Protestant Child Welfare. 1941

Johnson, Palmer O. and Oswald L. Harvey. **The National Youth Administration.** 1938

**The Juvenile Court.** Introduction by Robert M. Mennel. 1974

Klein, Earl E. **Work Accidents to Minors in Illinois.** 1938

Lane, Francis E. **American Charities and the Child of the Immigrant:** A Study of Typical Child Caring Institutions in New York and Massachusetts Between the Years 1845 and 1880. 1932

**The Legal Rights of Children.** Introduction by Sanford N. Katz. 1974

Letchworth, William P[ryor]. **Homes of Homeless Children:** A Report on Orphan Asylums and Other Institutions for the Care of Children. [1903]

Lorwin, Lewis. **Youth Work Programs:** Problems and Policies. 1941

Lundberg, Emma O[ctavia] and Katharine F. Lenroot. **Illegitimacy As A Child-Welfare Problem, Parts 1 and 2.** 1920/1921

New York State Commission on Relief for Widowed Mothers. **Report of the New York State Commission on Relief for Widowed Mothers.** 1914

Otey, Elizabeth Lewis. **The Beginnings of Child Labor Legislation in Certain States;** A Comparative Study. 1910

Phillips, Wilbur C. **Adventuring For Democracy.** 1940

Polier, Justine Wise. **Everyone's Children, Nobody's Child:** A Judge Looks At Underprivileged Children in the United States. 1941

**Proceedings of the Annual Meeting of the National Child Labor Committee, 1905, 1906.** 1974

Rainey, Homer P. **How Fare American Youth?** 1940

Reeder, Rudolph R. **How Two Hundred Children Live and Learn.** 1910

**Security and Services For Children.** 1974

Sinai, Nathan and Odin W. Anderson. **EMIC (Emergency Maternity and Infant Care):** A Study of Administrative Experience. 1948

Slingerland, W. H. **Child-Placing in Families:** A Manual For Students and Social Workers. 1919

[Solenberger], Edith Reeves. **Care and Education of Crippled Children in the United States.** 1914

Spencer, Anna Garlin and Charles Wesley Birtwell, editors. **The Care of Dependent, Neglected and Wayward Children:** Being a Report of the Second Section of the International Congress of Charities, Correction and Philanthropy, Chicago, June, 1893. 1894

Theis, Sophie Van Senden. **How Foster Children Turn Out.** 1924

Thurston, Henry W. **The Dependent Child:** A Story of Changing Aims and Methods in the Care of Dependent Children. 1930

U.S. Advisory Committee on Education. **Report of the Committee, February, 1938.** 1938

**The United States Children's Bureau, 1912-1972.** 1974

White House Conference on Child Health and Protection. **Dependent and Neglected Children:** Report of the Committee on Socially Handicapped — Dependency and Neglect. 1933

White House Conference on Child Health and Protection. **Organization for the Care of Handicapped Children, National, State, Local.** 1932

White House Conference on Children in a Democracy. **Final Report of the White House Conference on Children in A Democracy.** [1942]

Wilson, Otto. **Fifty Years' Work With Girls, 1883-1933:** A Story of the Florence Crittenton Homes. 1933

Wrenn, C. Gilbert and D. L. Harley. **Time On Their Hands:** A Report on Leisure, Recreation, and Young People. 1941